"Ever since the centuries of burning women ~~as witches~~ they taught women how to govern our ~~lives, our~~ reproduction—the medical world hasn't included all of humanity. *Doing Harm* shows what is left to be done and directs both women and men toward healing."

    —Gloria Steinem

"Maya Dusenbery's exhaustively researched book is equal parts infuriating and energizing. No woman will see the medical establishment, and perhaps even more profound, her own body, the same way after reading it. In a just world, it would be required reading in medical schools from this day forward."

    —Courtney E. Martin, author of *Perfect Girls, Starving Daughters*

"Maya Dusenbery brings new life to one of the most urgent yet under-discussed feminist issues of our time. Anyone who cares about women's health needs to read this book."

    —Jessica Valenti, author of *Sex Object*

"Maya Dusenbery shines a harsh light on the sex bias that pervades every level of medicine, from physician training to research to patient care. It is outrageous that such malignant neglect exists more than two decades after the federal government acknowledged the gaps in knowledge about women's health. *Doing Harm* challenges a new generation of women and practitioners to fight for medical equity."

    —Leslie Laurence, coauthor of *Outrageous Practices*

"We like to think of medicine as an objective and incorruptible science. In this groundbreaking book, Maya Dusenbery shows how the same forces that hold women back in society more broadly—sexist condescension, white male dominance, treatment of women as secondary and men as the default—also lead to sub-par medical care and inadequate attention to health issues that impact women. Every doctor, scientist, health care provider and researcher should read this book. And so should every woman: you'll come away armed with information that will allow you to advocate for yourself in the doctor's office, and it could save your life."

    —Jill Filipovic, author of *The H-Spot*

"*Doing Harm* is a thoroughly researched and much-needed exposé, weaving together different stories that illuminate an unfortunately repetitive theme: The recognition of the lag in women's health care is long overdue, and it's time to relieve the burden placed solely on women to fight not just for reproductive care, but for a more holistic approach to women's health care."

—*Pacific Standard*

"Dusenbery peels back the sick layers of America's paternal healthcare system. She plays both patient and journalist, seamlessly combining history, research, and interviews into an easily digestible must read. 5/5."

—*Bust* magazine

"Dusenbery digs deeper into the issue, exploring the way gender bias in medicine often leaves women struggling for proper care."

—Tonic (VICE)

"Filled with sharp analysis of the current state of women's medicine, historical context for women's health care and health care activism, and moving stories from patients who have been subject to the kind of harm these gender biases can cause, Dusenbery presents a well-balanced, thoughtful, and impassioned argument for change in health care for American women."

—*Harper's Bazaar*

"Through interviews with patients, doctors, and experts, as well as a deep cultural analysis, Dusenbery presents a horrifying picture of what it means to be a woman who's dismissed by her doctors."

—Bitch Media

"Dusenbery's book, based on two years of research into a host of conditions, exposes the systemic causes of these disparities and provides critically relevant information for the public—and for those in medicine, psychology, and the research sciences."

—Greater Good Science Center

"In *Doing Harm*, Dusenbery explores how biases and sexism in medicine lead to harmful outcomes for women."

—*Popular Science*

"Dusenbery says these experiences fit into a larger pattern of gender bias in medicine. Her new book, *Doing Harm*, makes the case that women's symptoms are often dismissed and misdiagnosed."
—NPR, *Fresh Air*

"Her new book is all about how women receive sub-par medical care because the medical community knows comparatively less about their bodies and diseases and too often doesn't trust women's reports of their own symptoms."
—WNYC, *The Brian Lehrer Show*

"Maya Dusenbery explores how medicine often leaves women on the periphery of real medical advancement. She explores the horrific reality of how medical practitioners and academic researchers completely dismiss women."
—*Marie Claire*

"Dusenbery writes about women's pain and illnesses being overlooked because of their menstrual cramps, menopause, even entering motherhood."
—*Dame* magazine

"In her book, Dusenbery traces how women are overlooked in every corner of illness, from autoimmune diseases to chronic pain (which disproportionately affects women and includes everything from irritable bowel syndrome to migraines to arthritis)."
—The Cut

"Maya Dusenbery's book, *Doing Harm*, explains how women's health issues have historically been dismissed—and what we can do about it now."
—Broadly

"*Doing Harm* is a fearless account of the incompetence of our culture when it comes to treating women properly. Dusenbery writes about the institutional systems that are against women—from philosophy to pharmacy to popular culture—in an accessible, engaging, and organized narrative."
—*The Rumpus*

"Maya Dusenbery has added immensely to the literature on women's health."
—*NY Journal of Books*

DOING

HARM

The Truth About How Bad Medicine and
Lazy Science Leave Women
Dismissed, Misdiagnosed, and Sick

MAYA DUSENBERY

HarperOne
An Imprint of HarperCollinsPublishers

HarperOne

HarperCollins books may be purchased for educational, business, or sales promotional use. For information, please email the Special Markets Department at SPsales @harpercollins.com.

FIRST HARPERCOLLINS PAPERBACK EDITION PUBLISHED IN 2019

Designed by Paul Barrett

Library of Congress Cataloging-in-Publication Data is available upon request.

ISBN 978-0-06-247083-6

23 24 25 26 27 LBC 10 9 8 7 6

For Martha and Lisa

CONTENTS

INTRODUCTION

A FEW YEARS AGO, I was diagnosed with rheumatoid arthritis. Illness, like love or grief or any other important aspect of human experience, is difficult to talk about without falling into clichés. One of the truest, in my opinion, is that your health is something you take for granted until you lose it. As someone who was healthy for twenty-seven years before becoming ill, I had come to expect that I could count on my body. It had always provided a comfortable, resilient home, one that, as a lifelong athlete, I felt a great deal of control over. Before, it was often a source of pleasure, and when it was in pain, it was a pain I chose willingly to make it stronger and faster. Most of the time, though, I forgot my body entirely. It was the loss of this luxury that I felt most acutely when my immune system started attacking my joints. Suddenly, I was always aware of my body; no matter what I was doing, some part of my attention was pulled to the constant aching in my knuckles and knees, and I deeply resented the intrusion.

When you get diagnosed with an autoimmune disease, especially if you're a woman of a certain age, it's a lot like when you buy a new car and promptly start seeing the same make and model everywhere. It's estimated that as many as 50 million Americans suffer from autoimmune diseases, a class of diseases of which rheumatoid arthritis (RA) is just one, and rates are on the rise. Yet as I learned more about this epidemic, there seemed to be little awareness of it, both in the public and within the American medical system.

Certainly, medicine seemed frustratingly short on answers. It couldn't tell me why my immune cells had suddenly turned against my own joints. It could offer only intense drugs that suppressed my entire immune system, caused my hair to fall out, and required regular monitoring of my liver. Most perplexingly, despite how common autoimmune diseases are, the medical system appeared to be remarkably bad at recognizing them. While I had been diagnosed with RA relatively quickly, I learned that many others weren't nearly so lucky. According to a survey by the American Autoimmune Related Diseases Association (AARDA), it takes nearly four years and four doctors, on average, before a patient with an autoimmune disease is properly diagnosed. Nearly half report that before they were diagnosed, they were dismissed as "chronic complainers" who were overly concerned with their health.

As a feminist writer, I was inclined to think that this state of affairs might have something to do with the fact that women make up more than three-quarters of those with autoimmune diseases, while they constitute less than a third of practicing doctors in a medical system that has, until recently, been even more overwhelmingly male dominated. As someone who'd written about reproductive rights for several years, I was hardly a stranger to thinking about women's health. But while I was well versed in the overt ways the politics of contraception and abortion affect access to reproductive health care, I didn't feel like I had a comprehensive understanding of how a more insidious gender bias—born of centuries in which biomedical knowledge was produced by men—has left its impact on the care that sick women receive today.

I realized that my relationship to the medical system, like my relationship to my own body, had been very much influenced by my status as a fairly healthy person. Just as I'd had the luxury of not thinking very much about my body until it broke, I'd also given little thought to how well the medical system was equipped to care for me if it did. I'd always known, of course, that there were thousands of ways a body could break, but such theoretical possibilities don't matter much to an invincible twentysomething. Likewise, I knew, intellectually, that doctors and scientists are just fallible human beings, affected by the biases we all are, and that biomedical knowledge is incomplete. But as long as I didn't personally have much need of medicine, it was easy to not think about its limitations.

But once I started to think about them, I quickly realized that auto-immune disease isn't the only women's health problem that is comparatively neglected. Indeed, it felt like every disease that experts described as an overlooked, and often growing, "epidemic" disproportionately affects women. Women make up about two-thirds of people with Alzheimer's disease, which experts now consider the third leading cause of death (after heart disease and cancer), though it receives only a fraction of the research dollars. They're at least twice as likely to have chronic pain conditions that affect 100 million American adults but that are woefully undertreated and under-researched. Then there are conditions like fibromyalgia, chronic fatigue syndrome, chronic Lyme disease, and multiple chemical sensitivities that are 70 to 80 percent female dominated and so poorly understood they have yet to be fully accepted as real diseases by the whole of the profession.

Meanwhile, I was somewhat surprised to realize that, apart from our reproductive health concerns, medicine pays little attention to potential differences between men and women, instead taking a one-size-fits-all approach to clinical research and practice. (Ironic, given that medicine, historically, had often declared women to be fundamentally different from—and inferior to—men.) For decades, that one size was specifically a seventy-kilogram white man; women of childbearing age were largely excluded from clinical research, particularly drug studies, altogether. While their numbers have increased since the early nineties, when federal law began requiring women and racial minorities to be included in research funded by the National Institutes of Health (NIH), we are still feeling the legacy of years of foundational research conducted on men, with the assumption that it could be extrapolated to women. And despite a wealth of evidence that has emerged over the past couple of decades showing that that was not a safe assumption—that there are, in fact, plentiful differences between men and women in everything from drug responses to risk factors for various diseases—researchers still don't routinely analyze and report such differences.

I also didn't have to look very far to find that it wasn't just women with autoimmune diseases who found that their symptoms initially weren't taken seriously by health care providers. Just a quick survey of my own network revealed that women with a wide range of problems were similarly dismissed. For a month, multiple health care providers insisted that one friend's stabbing chest pain was likely just anxiety before they realized it was pericarditis, an inflammation of the lining around the heart that causes symptoms similar to those of a heart attack. Two ob-gyns attributed the abdominal pain and incontinence of another's ureaplasma infection to stress. When another friend complained of dizziness, wooziness, ringing in her ears, and floaters in her eyes, an infectious disease specialist suggested that she see a therapist; it turned out she had West Nile virus. The list went on.

Anecdotes like these abound on the Internet too. Often, women's symptoms are brushed off as the result of depression, anxiety, or the all-purpose favorite: stress. Sometimes, they are attributed to women's normal physiological states and cycles: to menstrual cramps, menopause, or even being a new mom. Sometimes, other aspects of their identity seem to take center stage: fat women report that any ailment is blamed on their weight; trans women find that all their symptoms are attributed to hormone therapy; black women are stereotyped as addicts looking for prescription drugs, their reports of pain doubted entirely. Whatever the particular attribution, there is often the same current of distrust: the sense that women are not very accurate judges of when something is really, truly wrong in their bodies.

There is research to back up these anecdotes, though not as much as you might imagine, only because, I came to learn, there's little research on diagnostic errors in general, which are described by experts as an enormous blind spot within the profession. But where it exists, it paints a fairly consistent picture: women are often not taken as seriously as their male counterparts when they enter the medical system. Women wait sixty-five minutes to men's forty-nine before getting treatment for abdominal pain in the emergency room. Young women are seven times more likely to be sent home from the hospital in the middle of having a heart attack. Women face long delays, often years long, to get diagnosed even with diseases that are quite common in women. And they experience longer diagnostic delays in comparison to men for nearly everything, from brain tumors to rare genetic disorders.

THE RISE OF THE AMERICAN MEDICAL PROFESSION

For much of Western history, caring for the sick and dying has been women's work. Women were respected healers in ancient times, but their standing declined in Europe during the Middle Ages and early modern period as university-trained male physicians gradually turned medicine into an elite occupation among the wealthy. Since medicine is so closely aligned with the sciences these days, it's easy to assume that the medical profession naturally followed from the scientific knowledge it claims as its foundation. As Barbara Ehrenreich and Deirdre English write in *For Her Own Good: Two Centuries of the Experts' Advice to Women*, the rise of modern scientific medicine "has often been told as an allegory of science versus superstition: on one side, the clear-headed, masculine spirit of science; on the other side, a dark morass of female superstition, old wives' tales, rumors preserved as fact." But in fact, the cart came before the horse: medicine became a male-dominated profession long before it came to be rooted in science.

In the United States, this takeover happened relatively late. European physicians didn't come to America, so women remained the primary healers in the colonial era and beyond. Female "root and herb" doctors often combined the passed-down medical lore of their cultures in the old world— Europe and Africa—with knowledge of local medicinal plants learned from Native American tribes. In women's hands, healing was not a profession but a "neighborly service." By the late eighteenth century, though, a new class of professionals, "regular" doctors, were seeking to turn healing into a commodity that could be bought and sold. This was a difficult task, especially at a time when even the university-educated physicians in Europe had little knowledge that lay healers lacked; they had studied ancient philosophy, but their imaginative medical theories weren't based on any scientific study or even much interaction with patients.

The regular doctors dealt with this dilemma by offering treatments that had the most extreme impact on the patient possible; though they rarely helped, their dramatic (side) effects justified the doctors' fees. Bloodletting (sometimes by leeches) to the point of fainting, purging (through vomiting, laxatives, and enemas), and poisons (like arsenic and calomel) were offered as cure-alls. To say that the herbal remedies and received wisdom based on centuries of observation that female lay healers offered were superior to the methods of the regular doctors (which became known as "heroic medicine") is an understatement. One eighteenth-century commenter described heroic medicine's bleeding and purging as "one of those great discoveries which are made from time to time for the depopulation of the earth."

In the early nineteenth century, the regular doctors made their first attempt at establishing themselves as a profession with a monopoly on healing, convincing seventeen states to pass laws restricting the practice of medicine to those with a medical license. But this move sparked a mass backlash in the form of the Popular Health Movement. Women, small farmers, shopkeepers, artisans, and factory workers united against this power grab by doctors who had no claim to superior expertise and whose methods many considered barbaric. By 1830, every state with licensing laws had loosened or repealed them. Initially, this populist movement opposed the whole idea of a medical profession, instead calling for the democratization of health knowledge, but eventually it birthed a number of organized "irregular" medical sects (eclectics, botanists, homeopaths, hydropaths) that began establishing their own medical schools.

Women were a key part of the Popular Health Movement and were active in the irregular sects. By the middle of the nineteenth century, they were increasingly pushing to become regular doctors too. When men's schools refused to let them in, they opened their own. In 1847, Elizabeth Blackwell became the first woman admitted to a regular medical school in the United States. By 1900, the number of female physicians had climbed to more than 7,000—or 5 percent of all the doctors in the country—and there were nineteen women's medical colleges and nine women's hospitals.

These pioneering women doctors often argued for their inclusion in the profession on the grounds that it was improper for male doctors to treat female patients, a fairly compelling argument during a time when there were rigid norms of modesty for upper-class ladies and little public trust in the emerging medical profession. The male doctors' intense resistance to women entering the field speaks to just how threatened they were by the prospect of competition from female doctors. As one irregular woman doctor pointed out in 1861, whenever female doctors "made their appearance, a general uprising of the people to welcome them, and the most vigorous attempt of the regular masculine dignitaries of the 'profession' to quell the 'insurrection' [were] the result." A professor at one women's college told medical students in 1855, "They will raise the cry, 'She is out of her proper sphere' because they are afraid they will be pushed out of places they are not fit to fill; 'A woman can't practice medicine,' because they are afraid she can."

As the twentieth century approached, medicine in Europe was becoming more rooted in science thanks to advances in biology, pathology, and anatomy. But in the United States, there were still few standards to become a doctor. The most elite of the American regular doctors, who aspired to turn the profession into the gentlemanly occupation it was in Europe, sought to eliminate the "low-class" competition from an increasingly crowded field. The American Medical Association (AMA), which had formed as the professional group for the regulars, asked the Carnegie Foundation to conduct a review of the state of the country's medical schools. In 1910, the resulting Flexner Report concluded that the nation had too many doctors and too many were poorly trained. It recommended sweeping reforms of medical education: stricter acceptance standards, more years of study, training in the basic sciences, and laboratories in every school. In the aftermath of the report, as foundation money flowed to the minority that the report declared to be on the right track, about half of the country's medical schools closed or merged.

One of the "unintended" consequences of the Flexner Report was the near-total exclusion of women and people of color from medicine for the next several decades. The report had concluded that there wasn't a need for many women doctors since there lacked "any strong demand for women physicians or any strong ungratified desire on the part of women to enter the profession"—a bald-faced lie on both counts. Meanwhile, the report claimed that the country needed only enough African American doctors to serve black communities. By 1915, the portion of medical school graduates who were women had declined to an all-time low of 2.9 percent. Most of the women's and black medical schools had closed. By 1930, only one women's school remained. The new requirement that all applicants have two years of college education ensured that a medical education was accessible only to the upper classes. Meanwhile, state medical licensing laws were

changed so that only graduates of the regular, scientific schools could pass
them, and most states made practicing medicine without a license a crime.

The regular doctors had finally gained a legal monopoly over the practice of medicine, and in the process created a profession that was overwhelmingly white, male, and wealthy.

THE MORE THINGS CHANGE . . .

For the next half century, thanks to overt discrimination, the percentage
of doctors who were women never climbed into the double digits. In 1970,
when less than 10 percent of medical school students were women, a survey of admissions officers found that nineteen of twenty-five American
medical schools admitted that they gave preference to male applicants unless the female applicant was head and shoulders superior. A class-action
gender-discrimination lawsuit was soon filed against every medical school
in the nation. In 1972, the landmark legislation Title IX of the Education
Amendments prohibited discrimination on the basis of sex in educational
programs that receive federal funding, and by the midseventies, the number of female medical students had nearly tripled.

Since the mid-aughts, women have made up just under half of all medical students. For the last several years, about a third of practicing physicians have been women, and their ranks are destined to grow as older,
male-majority generations of physicians retire.

As women have entered the profession, they have tended to disproportionately go into the primary care specialties. The proportion of practicing
ob-gyns who are women increased dramatically from 12 percent in 1980 to
just over half today. Currently, 60 percent of pediatricians are women. And
the trend will just continue: In recent years, women have made up about
85 percent of ob-gyn residents and 75 percent of pediatric residents. They
also make up a smaller majority of those going into family medicine and
psychiatry.

Because of this trend, it may be easy for the average patient to underestimate just how male dominated much of medicine remains. For many
healthy women, the kinds of physicians you're most likely to see routinely,

for your own health care or your family's, are precisely those specialties that are the most gender balanced, or even majority women. But they are, in fact, the *only* specialties where women are well represented. There remain large segments of medicine where women are vastly outnumbered: women make up about a quarter of emergency medicine physicians, neurologists, and anesthesiologists; less than 20 percent of general surgeons; 12 percent of cardiologists; 7 percent of urologists; and less than 5 percent of orthopedic surgeons.

Another reality that's largely hidden from patients is the stark gender inequalities within the hierarchy of academic medicine. Women now make up 38 percent of full-time medical school faculty. However, they remain concentrated in the lower ranks; the higher up on the leadership ladder you go, the fewer women there are. In 2014, only 21 percent of full professors, 15 percent of department chairs, and 16 percent of deans at American medical schools were women. According to a 2015 analysis of data on over 90,000 physicians, men were nearly two and a half times more likely than women to be full professors, even after accounting for factors that affect promotion, like differences in age, experience, and specialty, and measures of research productivity. The people making the key decisions about where funding and resources go, what gets taught to the next generation of doctors, and who is hired and promoted are still overwhelmingly white men.

Women continue to lag behind men when it comes to getting their biomedical research funded and published. Only about 30 percent of researchers receiving NIH funding are women. A 2016 study published in *The BMJ* found that growth in the number of biomedical studies authored by women has stalled in recent years. According to their tally of thousands of articles published in six of the most prestigious medical journals, the proportion of studies that list a woman as the first author has increased from 27 percent to 37 percent since 1994. But this progress has plateaued, and at some journals actually declined, since 2009. Interestingly, the journals that had women editors in chief had higher rates of female first authorship. But of course, there is a gender gap among editors too: women make up just 17.5 percent of all editorial-board members of sixty major medical journals.

Women doctors also earn less than their male counterparts. According to a 2016 study published in *JAMA: The Journal of the American Medical Association* of roughly 10,000 physician faculty members at twenty-four medical schools, the women earned over $50,000 less per year, on average, than their male colleagues. This gender pay gap is often blamed on the fact that the primary care specialties that women often go into tend to be lower paying. But even after adjusting for specialty and several other factors that affect pay—including age and experience—there was still a difference of almost $20,000 that wasn't explained. In fact, some studies suggest that the gap has actually been increasing in recent years.

Surveys of women in medicine attest to the persistent discrimination they face. A 2000 study of over 3,000 full-time faculty at twenty-four American medical schools found that 47 percent of the youngest female faculty and 70 percent of the oldest female faculty had experienced gender-based discrimination. About half the women had experienced some form of sexual harassment. In 2016, a *JAMA* study of over a thousand successful midcareer clinician-researchers suggested that little has changed. Though these women had received their medical education during a time when women made up nearly half of all medical students, their experiences were disturbingly similar to those of their pioneering foremothers: 70 percent of the women perceived gender bias, and two-thirds said they had experienced it firsthand. A third reported that they'd been sexually harassed.

We should all care about the sexism that women continue to face within medicine for its own sake, of course. Working women in every profession deserve equal pay for equal work, freedom from sexual harassment and discrimination, and supportive workplaces that allow them to reach their full potential. We would also do well to support gender equality within medicine simply because women tend to be better doctors—to all patients. A 2013 Canadian study of 870 doctors treating patients for diabetes found that the women outperformed the men on every standard of quality care. Women doctors spend about 10 percent more time with their patients than their male counterparts do. They tend to be more "patient-centered," expressing more empathy and concern, and better eliciting information about their patients' symptoms, lives, and emotions.

But this book is, ultimately, about how gender bias affects the care patients receive. And while the underrepresentation of women in the medical profession has been a major source of the gender bias in the medical system, simply getting more women into the profession will not automatically fix it. Women doctors do tend to bring new perspectives. As researchers, they are more likely than men to conduct research on women's health or gender disparities. But, at this point, the gender bias in medicine runs much deeper than the gender of its practitioners. It is largely unconscious and systemic, and women doctors are not immune to it.

A SYSTEMIC PROBLEM: THE KNOWLEDGE GAP AND THE TRUST GAP

What I've come to see is that a historically male-dominated medical system has created two interlocking problems that affect the quality of care women receive.

First, there is a knowledge gap: the average doctor does not know as much about women's bodies and the health problems that afflict them. It starts at the most basic level of biomedical research, where investigators overwhelmingly use male cells and animals in preclinical studies. And it continues throughout the clinical research process, where women remain underrepresented, analysis by gender is rare, and women's differing hormonal states and cycles are usually ignored entirely. Meanwhile, conditions that disproportionately affect women have often not been deemed worthy of research funding and time. As Dr. Janine Austin Clayton, associate director for women's health research at the NIH, put it in a 2014 *New York Times* article, "We literally know less about every aspect of female biology compared to male biology."

Second, there is a trust gap: women's accounts of their symptoms are too often not believed. For centuries, Western medicine tended to throw many of women's inexplicable symptoms into the catchall diagnostic category of hysteria. The explanation offered for this mystery female malady shifted over the centuries, but at the end of the nineteenth century, hysteria came to be seen as a psychological problem. Ever since, a medical profession that increasingly understands the underlying cause of many diseases—and can objectively confirm patients' reported symptoms with blood tests and high-tech scans—has tended to attribute to "the mind" any that it can't see and explain. The terminology has morphed—from hysteria to somatization and conversion disorders to "medically unexplained symptoms"—but the idea has remained remarkably unchanged. And the idea that women are especially prone to such psychogenic symptoms has endured too. In other words, a stereotype that women's symptoms are likely to be "all in their heads" has been hard baked into medical knowledge itself.

These two problems—the knowledge gap and the trust gap—are mutually reinforcing to such a degree that they've become stubbornly difficult to correct. Are women's complaints so often dismissed because doctors simply don't know enough about women's bodies, their symptoms, and the diseases that disproportionately affect them? Or are women's complaints so often dismissed because doctors hold an unconscious stereotype that women are unreliable reporters of their symptoms? Is it a lack of knowledge or a lack of trust? It seems to be both. The knowledge gap and the trust gap are so tightly interwoven at this point that they could be thought of as two sides of the same coin: Women's symptoms are not taken seriously because medicine doesn't know as much about their bodies and health problems. And medicine doesn't know as much about their bodies and health problems because it doesn't take their symptoms seriously.

This book, then, is not about a few sexist bad apples within the medical profession. It is about how bias is embedded into the system. It is about how all health care providers, like all of us, have unconscious biases by virtue of living in a culture that holds certain stereotypes about women. And it is about how even the very best doctors know relatively less about women's health compared to men's, not because of any individual failure on their part but because they are not taught as much about women's health, often because, quite simply, less is known.

This book is about both sex and gender bias within medicine. *Sex* refers to differences in biological traits, like chromosomes, hormones, and reproductive organs. *Gender,* on the other hand, refers to the social expectations and experiences associated with identifying as a man or woman in a particular culture. Gender identity and sex often, but don't always, match: Cisgender (cis) people identify with the same gender as their sex;

transgender (trans) people identify with the other one. Though sex and gender are often talked about as binaries, in reality, nature is a lot more diverse than the two categories we try to impose on it. A not-insignificant proportion of people are intersex, born with some biological traits we associate with one sex and some that we associate with the other. Some people are gender nonconforming and do not identify strongly as either gender.

When I discuss differences between men and women—whether in relative risks of certain diseases or in how they're treated by health care providers—I generally mean cis people simply because our knowledge of such differences has been derived largely from research on them. But it should be noted that the problems explored in this book don't solely affect cis women. All women—cis or trans—are affected by the trust gap. And the knowledge gap affects anyone, regardless of their gender, whose sex is assigned female.

In fact, since relatively few diseases target *solely* women, the bias within medicine affects everyone. Plenty of cis men have been hurt by the dearth of knowledge about conditions that disproportionately affect women. And putting comparatively less effort into understanding the bodies of one half of the population, and the ailments that happen to especially affect them, has left gaps in our scientific knowledge that have deprived us all.

BARRIERS TO ACCESS

This book focuses on how gender bias affects medical knowledge and the care women receive when they enter the medical system, but it is worth spending some time considering the obstacles that many women have to overcome to access the medical system at all.

The Affordable Care Act provided some key benefits to women especially, which, as of this writing, they still have. Before it went into effect, approximately 20 percent of women ages eighteen to sixty-four were uninsured. By 2015, that figure had dropped to about 11 percent. Health care reform also corrected some long-standing unjust practices of the insurance industry. Insurers are now required to cover basic preventive care that's critical to women's health, like contraception, annual well-woman visits, testing for sexually transmitted infections, breastfeeding support and supplies, and domestic violence screenings, without any co-pays or deductibles. They're no longer allowed to charge women higher premiums than men for the same coverage simply because they're women, a practice known as "gender rating" common in the pre-Obamacare days. They can't deny women coverage for "preexisting conditions," like having had a Cesarean section, being pregnant, or experiencing domestic violence. And they can no longer refuse to offer maternity-care coverage, as the vast majority of plans on the individual market previously did.

Still, 11.2 million women, many of them low-income women of color, particularly immigrant and Latina women, remain uninsured in the United States. Since they make up the majority of poor uninsured adults, women have been especially impacted by the refusal of nineteen states, mostly Republican-controlled states in the South, to expand Medicaid eligibility. Meanwhile, regardless of insurance status, women have more trouble affording health care than do men. According to a 2013 nationally representative survey conducted by the Kaiser Family Foundation, 26 percent of women reported that they have had to delay or forgo medical care in the past year because of the cost, compared to 20 percent of men. Cost is a problem especially for uninsured women, of course, but even insured women often can't afford to see a doctor: 35 percent of women with Medicaid and 16 percent of women with private insurance also said they delayed or skipped care out of cost concerns.

Furthermore, it's not only financial barriers that affect women's access to the medical system. A quarter of women, regardless of income, reported that a reason they went without health care was that they simply didn't have time to go to the doctor. For low-income women especially, not being able to take time off from work, a lack of transportation, and problems finding childcare are also common barriers. Women make up a majority of workers in low-wage and part-time jobs that often don't provide sick days. Until we have federally mandated sick days, medical leave, and affordable childcare for all, too many women will remain unable to get the medical care they need. It doesn't matter whether you have insurance and can afford your co-pays, if you don't have the kind of job flexibility that allows you to go to an appointment, let alone two or three.

A lack of access to the medical system, of course, can often supersede any of the problems women patients face within it. If you can't afford to see a doctor at all, whether that doctor would take your symptoms seriously is a moot point. And all the biomedical knowledge in the world is meaningless if the people who need it most can't benefit from it. On the other hand, for many women, their tenuous connection to the medical system just compounds the problems discussed in this book. With limited access comes higher stakes. Millions of women in this country literally cannot afford for the medical system to be this bad at caring for them. They don't have the co-pays or sick days to go to specialist after specialist in search of the proper diagnosis. When they are dismissed once or maybe twice, it may not be the start of a long diagnostic delay; it may be the end of the line.

Indeed, for many of the conditions discussed in this book, less privileged women simply go undiagnosed and untreated altogether. The result is that about a fifth of low-income women say their health is poor or fair and even more report that they have a disability or chronic disease that limits their activity, rates that are more than twice that of higher-income women. Yet, at the same time, an equal proportion of poor and affluent women say they receive ongoing medical attention for a medical condition. In other words, lower income women are sicker, but many of them are not receiving the care they need.

REPRODUCTIVE HEALTH CARE

I won't be discussing routine reproductive health care in this book—that is, contraception, abortion, and care during pregnancy and childbirth. That's ultimately because I'm interested in exploring how gender bias affects the health care women receive when they are sick. That's a question that I think has sometimes been overshadowed because even the healthiest among us rely on the medical system to control, manage, and monitor our perfectly normal reproductive functions. "Women's health" is so routinely conflated with "reproductive health" that it's easy to forget that the latter is just one aspect of the former. Women's health is impacted by many conditions besides those that affect the uterus, ovaries, and fallopian tubes.

That isn't to say that women's health activism's focus on reproductive health issues is unjustified. Most American women rely on contraception, usually a form that requires a doctor's visit, during the thirty-plus years they're fertile. As many as one-quarter will at some point get an abortion, and 80 percent will eventually have a child. The fact that women have become largely dependent on a male-dominated medical system for the ability to prevent, end, and safely bring to term a pregnancy—a freedom that's so fundamental to women's equality—has led to some tensions, to say the least. Undoubtedly, women have benefited in many ways from this medicalization of their reproductive lives; it's given us more effective birth control, safer abortions, and lifesaving interventions in complicated pregnancies. On the flip side, women have had to constantly fight on a variety of fronts to maintain control: to simultaneously push for greater access, resist overmedicalization, and defend their autonomy in making reproductive decisions.

That fight has often become primarily a political, legal, and cultural one. Indeed, the biggest problem with abortion care in the United States is that it's treated as if it's not medical care at all. Thanks to state lawmakers, the provision of the procedure is often dictated by politically motivated regulations, not evidence-based standards of quality patient care. Doctors in some states are required to lie to patients about risks of the procedure that simply do not exist. In others, they're required to prescribe a medical abortion according to an outdated protocol that is less effective and causes more side effects. They're forced to perform medically unnecessary ultrasounds on patients who do not want them. In states with mandatory-waiting-period laws, they have to delay providing a time-sensitive procedure that gets more expensive and more risky the further along in the pregnancy, for no medical reason whatsoever. This book is about how gender bias has shaped medical knowledge; when it comes to abortion, politicians have required medical knowledge to simply be ignored.

Still, while not the source of this politicization, the medical system deserves some blame for failing to forcefully stand up to it. While medical groups like the AMA have certainly objected to lawmakers masquerading as ob-gyns, mainstream medicine can hardly claim to be a staunch defender of abortion's important place within women's health care. In a country in which about a million abortions are performed each year, a 2005 survey of ob-gyn programs found that over half didn't offer any clinical exposure to the procedure and about a fifth provided no formal education on it at all. While 97 percent of practicing ob-gyns have had a patient seeking an abortion, just 14 percent perform them. Abortion care is usually physically relegated to stand-alone specialty clinics. The doctors who do offer the procedure often face stigma from their colleagues and are left largely on their own to fight against political interference in the doctor-patient relationship, which should provoke mass outcry from the entire profession.

One of the unfortunate consequences of having to constantly safeguard reproductive health care from threats originating outside of the medical system is that problems within it tend to get overshadowed. For example, in recent years, women's health advocates have found themselves in the ridiculous position of having to defend Obamacare's requirement that insurers cover contraception—which is used by 99 percent of sexually active women at some point—without a co-pay. Were we not stuck having such 1960s-era debates over our right to birth control, we might spend more time demanding *better* birth control. More than half a century after the pill was invented, the range of birth control options remains remarkably limited, dominated by varying types of hormonal contraceptives that can cause significant side effects. A medical system that took women's symptoms more seriously surely would have figured out some more appealing contraceptive options by now.

Many of the problems with reproductive health care come to a head in American women's experience of childbirth. The United States is the only country in the developed world where the maternal mortality rate is on the rise, more than doubling in the last twenty-five years. At least half of maternal deaths in this country are preventable, and there are stark racial disparities: black women are nearly four times as likely as white women to die in childbirth. Experts believe a number of factors contribute to this shameful record. First, while medical interventions have certainly helped make high-risk births safer, unnecessary interventions in normal births are putting women at increased risk of complications. In the last two decades, the C-section rate has climbed by almost 60 percent to more than three times the rate recommended by the World Health Organization, and they are too often performed not out of medical need but for the convenience and profit of the doctor. Meanwhile, a planned pregnancy is generally a safer pregnancy. But with 4.5 million women lacking access to affordable family-planning services, nearly half of pregnancies in this country are unintended.

Finally, a healthy woman tends to have a healthier pregnancy, and American women's high rates of chronic, often unmanaged conditions also contribute to our poor maternal health. That fact should serve as a reminder that while I'm leaving routine reproductive health care out of this book, there's no such option in real life. While reproductive health is not synonymous with women's health, neither is it separable from it.

A WAKE-UP CALL

Paula Doress-Worters, one of the original members of the Boston Women's Health Book Collective, has recalled the workshop that would eventually result in the classic women's health manual *Our Bodies, Ourselves*: "Everyone had a 'doctor story'—that is, a tale about male physicians who were sexist, paternalistic, judgmental, or simply unable to provide the information women needed." In many ways, the medical system—as well as our society at large—has been radically transformed since then. In the late sixties, over 90 percent of physicians were men, and women couldn't get their own credit cards.

But women still have "doctor stories"—and they have not changed quite as much as we might like to think. There was the friend who, as a black teenager fully informed about her birth control options, told her gynecologist that she would stick to condoms; he passive-aggressively prescribed prenatal vitamins, saying it was obvious she'd be pregnant soon. Or the Latina woman with breast cancer I heard from, who wanted a mastectomy but whose doctor objected, saying, "But you aren't married." Or the queer woman whose orthopedist asked if the swelling in her dislocated finger had gone down enough for "Mr. Right to put a ring on it." Or the mom of a child with physical and intellectual disabilities who noticed that the only item listed in her daughter's chart under "Developmental Concerns" was "Mother works outside the home."

These kind of overt microaggressions may be less common these days, or at least easier to brush off in an era when women have more power. But it is the more subtle stories that are more pervasive—and more dangerous, because the gender bias they reflect is harder to pin down if you see each story only in isolation. The doctor who didn't listen—but perhaps that's just how he is with everyone? The time your symptoms weren't taken seriously—but, in retrospect, maybe you could have done more to advocate for yourself? The many misdiagnoses of "stress" that you can't really imagine a male patient receiving—but then again, how can you know that for sure? I hope that this book helps women who've felt dismissed and unheard in these ways see that their experiences aren't just the result of bad luck or their own failings, but instead that they reflect deeper, systemic problems in the medical system.

And I hope it will be a wake-up call especially for my fellow millennial women. I'm too young to remember the 1990 congressional hearings that drew widespread media attention to the underrepresentation of women in clinical research. My own doctors were mostly women when I was growing up. By the time I started college, roughly equal numbers of women and men were attending medical school. And like many women of my generation with a certain amount of privilege, I've always expected be taken seriously. The feminist revival of the last decade or so seems to be what happens when a generation of women who take for granted their equality realizes that our society—its institutions, policies, and norms—has not changed nearly as much as our expectations have. Before I began researching this book, I had no idea just how far behind the medical system lagged. It's high time that millennial feminism turned its attention to the gender bias remaining in medicine at large and tackled this unfinished revolution.

Now is an especially urgent time to do so. Many women in the United States are sick, and they're getting sicker. Since the turn of the twentieth century, women have lived longer than men, on average. But the gap has been narrowing since the eighties, when men's life expectancy began increasing at a faster clip than women's, largely thanks to a decline in deaths from cardiovascular disease. And the additional 4.8 years of life expectancy that women currently have do not come with better health. Women report poorer health, both physical and mental, and are hospitalized more than men throughout adulthood. In their later years of life too, women are worse off than men. When it comes to "active" life expectancy—the number of years living free from significant limitations that prevent you from doing everyday tasks—men have overtaken women over the past three decades. Women still live longer, but men live *better* longer.

This difference—women's lower mortality but higher morbidity—has been known as the "gender paradox." Tellingly, from the seventies through the nineties, some researchers questioned whether women were really as sick as they claimed, suggesting instead that women are actually healthier than men (after all, they aren't as likely to die!) and only rate their health as worse because they're less stoic. Today, it is well accepted that the paradox has a different, straightforward explanation: women have higher rates of debilitating but not life-threatening chronic diseases. Women are not any more likely to report poor health than men with the same medical condition; they're just more likely to have one. More than half of all American women have at least one chronic health condition, and women are more likely than men to have multiple chronic problems. What's more, prevalence rates of many of the conditions that disproportionately affect women—from autoimmune disease to Alzheimer's—are increasing.

These days, my RA is in remission, and I try my best to not take my health for granted. I remind myself occasionally what a gift it is to again be able to forget about my body, and how amazing it is that, when all goes well, immune cells attack only pathogens automatically, without thought or effort. Too often, it doesn't go well. And though bodies will always break, doctors will always make mistakes, and science isn't about to know everything there is to know about the mysteries of the human body anytime soon, our gender should not be a factor in the mistakes made and the knowledge left unknown. Above all, we should be able to expect that in medicine's ongoing quest to understand and ameliorate human suffering, women's experiences are taken seriously and that our voices are heard.

PART 1

OVERLOOKED AND DISMISSED:

A SYSTEMIC PROBLEM

CHAPTER 1
THE KNOWLEDGE GAP

WOMEN'S HEALTH ACTIVISM HAS shaped American medicine through-out its history. In the 1830s and 1840s, as the Popular Health Movement resisted the regular doctors' attempt at gaining a professional monopoly, women formed "Ladies' Physiological Societies" to learn about their bodies and trade home remedies. In the early twentieth century, women reformers agitated for public health campaigns to combat infant and maternal mortality and fought for the legalization of birth control. The women's health activists of the 1960s and 1970s successfully transformed many aspects of medicine: they won the legal right to abortion, established women's health clinics, and secured important patient rights from a condescending medical system that often withheld information about the risks of drugs and procedures. And through self-help groups and popular manuals like *Our Bodies, Ourselves*, they sought, like their nineteenth-century predecessors, to give women the knowledge to better take care of their health.

It wasn't until the late eighties, when women finally made up a critical mass of those within the medical community, that they were in a position to successfully call attention to one of the most insidious ways gender bias was embedded in medicine: the medical knowledge that had been accumulating over the course of the twentieth century, and especially in the previous few decades as biomedical research exploded in the United States, was disproportionately benefiting men. Science simply knew less about women's bodies and the diseases that befell them—and, worse still, the medical community was not attuned to this failure and seeking to correct it. In 1990, a coalition of women's health advocates, biomedical researchers, and lawmakers came up with a strategy to put this knowledge gap on the public's radar—and we've been playing catch-up to close it ever since.

In 1985, a Public Health Service task force had released a report, spearheaded by Ruth Kirschstein, the first and only woman serving as an institute director at the NIH at the time, warning that "the historical lack of research focus on women's health concerns has compromised the quality of health information available to women as well as the health care they receive." In response, the NIH had announced a new policy that "urged" researchers who received federal research grants to include women in their clinical studies unless there was a good reason not to. But women within the NIH—who at the time occupied less than a third of senior policy and research positions—knew the policy hadn't changed matters much.

So in the late eighties, a group of women scientists, working both within and outside of the NIH, formed the Society for the Advancement of Women's Health Research—now called the Society for Women's Health Research (SWHR)—and teamed up with allies in Congress to expose the problem. They decided to demand an audit of the NIH's efforts by the independent oversight arm of the federal government, the General Accounting Office, now called the U.S. Government Accountability Office (GAO). In 1990, the GAO released its findings: As expected, it turned out that the NIH had done little to implement its policy on women's inclusion at all. The application guidelines for researchers didn't mention it, and in fact, many NIH staff weren't even aware the policy had been adopted. Of the NIH-funded studies reviewed by the GAO, one-fifth didn't mention the gender of the study subjects, and a third claimed the study would include women but didn't specify how many. The NIH couldn't actually say with any certainty how many women were included in the research it funded, with billions of taxpayer dollars, to further the nation's health.

Just as the members of Congress and advocates had planned, the GAO report garnered widespread public attention. In hearings flooded with reporters, the cochairs of the Congressional Caucus for Women's Issues lambasted NIH leaders, and the medical research community as a whole, for compromising women's health. "American women have been put at risk by medical practices that fail to include women in research studies," said Rep. Patricia Schroeder. "NIH's attitude has been to consider over half the population as some sort of special case," Rep. Olympia Snowe charged.

Given the NIH's lack of record keeping, it was impossible to say exactly how underrepresented women were, but the public learned that women had been left out of many of the largest, most important clinical studies conducted in the last couple of decades. The Baltimore Longitudinal Study of Aging, which began in 1958 and purported to explore "normal human aging," didn't enroll any women for the first twenty years it ran. The Physicians' Health Study, which had recently concluded that taking a daily aspirin may reduce the risk of heart disease? Conducted in 22,071 men and zero women. The 1982 Multiple Risk Factor Intervention Trial—known, aptly enough, as MRFIT—which looked at whether dietary change and exercise could help prevent heart disease: just 13,000 men.

The default to studying men at times veered into absurdity: in the early sixties, observing that women tended to have lower rates of heart disease until their estrogen levels dropped after menopause, researchers conducted the first trial to look at whether supplementation with the hormone was an effective preventive treatment. The study enrolled 8,341 men and no women. (Although doctors began prescribing estrogens to postmenopausal women in droves—by the midseventies, a third would be taking them—it wasn't until 1991 that the first clinical study of hormone therapy was conducted in women.) An NIH-supported pilot study from Rockefeller University that looked at how obesity affected breast and uterine cancer didn't enroll a single woman. While men can develop breast cancer—and a small number of them do each year—as Rep. Snowe noted drily at the congressional hearings, "Somehow, I find it hard to believe that the male-dominated medical community would tolerate a study of prostate cancer that used only women as research subjects."

In 1992, a couple of years after taking the NIH to task, the Congressional Caucus for Women's Issues asked the GAO to review the state of affairs at the Food and Drug Administration (FDA). While the NIH is the largest public funder of biomedical research, most studies of drug treatments are funded by the private pharmaceutical companies that develop them and are reviewed by the FDA as part of the drug-approval process. Since 1977, the agency had had in place a policy forbidding women of "childbearing potential" from participating in early-phase drug trials. While women were allowed to be included in later studies—after basic safety and dosage had been established—the GAO report found that women were underrepresented in 60 percent of recent clinical drug trials. And while 1988 FDA guidelines urged drug companies to analyze their data by gender when women were included, nearly half the studies reviewed by the GAO failed to do so. Furthermore, despite the fact that millions of American women were on the pill, a mere 12 percent of the recently approved drugs had been studied for potentially dangerous interactions with oral contraceptives.

Advocates had always intended the GAO report on the NIH's poorly implemented policy to serve as a spotlight that could be shined on other ways women's health was being shortchanged in the biomedical community. They charged not only that health conditions that affected both men and women equally or were more prevalent among men had been studied primarily in men, with no attention to the possibility that there might be sex/gender differences, but also that conditions that predominantly affected women had been a low priority on the research agenda altogether.

Among the conditions that predominantly affected women was, of course, all of reproductive health. In the wake of the GAO report, other medical-professional organizations, including the Institute of Medicine (IOM) and the American College of Obstetricians and Gynecologists, joined the growing chorus claiming that funding for research on women's reproductive health was inadequate. The political controversy around abortion was part of the problem, but such research was also marginalized because, with no obstetrics and gynecology program, there was no clear home for it within the NIH. In fact, there were only three gynecologists on staff at the NIH, compared to thirty-nine veterinarians.

And it wasn't just reproductive health—which is what "women's health" tended to get reduced to—that was getting short shrift. One of the advocates' important claims was that, to the extent that medicine paid attention to women's unique needs at all, it had been myopically focused on the parts of women's bodies that most obviously differed from men's. "The medical community has viewed women's health with a bikini approach, focusing essentially on the breast and reproductive system," Dr. Nanette Wenger, a leading expert on women's heart disease, wrote. "The rest of the woman was virtually ignored in considerations of women's health." This kind of "bikini medicine" overlooked the fact that women had the same top three causes of death—heart disease, stroke, and cancer of all kinds—as men did, and also suffered disproportionately from many nonreproductive health conditions that had been long neglected.

Indeed, in the late eighties, a Public Health Service task force had crunched the numbers and found that only 13.5 percent of the NIH's most recent budget had gone toward research on conditions "that are unique to or more prevalent or serious in women, have distinct causes or manifest themselves differently in women, or have different outcomes or interventions." This was an extensive list that included reproductive health concerns but also extended to an array of other not-at-all-uncommon conditions that are more common in women, including breast and gynecological cancers, Alzheimer's disease, depression, osteoporosis, and autoimmune diseases. And many of the conditions that will be discussed in this book weren't yet receiving any federal research funding at all.

In the immediate aftermath of the GAO report, the NIH formed the Office of Research on Women's Health (ORWH), and the new office summed up the state of affairs in its first research agenda in 1991, noting a "pervasive sense in the research community that many of the health issues of women are of secondary importance, especially those that occur solely in women and those that occur in men and women but have already been studied chiefly in men."

It went on to say, concerning the three leading killers of all Americans, "The startling realization is that most of the biomedical knowledge about the causes, expression, and treatment of these diseases derives from studies of men and is applied to women with the supposition that there are no differences."

WHY WERE WOMEN NEGLECTED?

Perhaps the most generous explanation for women's exclusion from clinical studies is that they had gotten caught up in the protectionist spirit of the era. In the seventies, there'd been a growing recognition—long overdue—of the risks of medical research. And, in part, women had been excluded from clinical research, especially drug studies, for their own good—or at least for the good of their hypothetical fetuses.

This paternalistic concern was quite new, however. Women had not been spared from the rampant, unregulated, and largely uncontrolled experimentation that constituted heroic medicine in the eighteenth and nineteenth centuries. The well-off women who could afford regular doctors' fees were subjected to bloodletting, purging, all manner of drugs, and, as is discussed more in the next chapter, a smorgasbord of useless or dangerous procedures performed on their reproductive organs. And, as Ehrenreich and English point out, "Though middle-class women suffered most from the doctors' actual practice, it was poor and black women who had suffered through the brutal period of experimentation." In the nineteenth century, for example, Dr. J. Marion Sims, known as the "father of modern gynecology," developed a groundbreaking cure for fistulas by practicing the surgery on enslaved women, whom he purchased specifically for that purpose, and later on poor Irish immigrants.

In the twentieth century, medicine slowly but surely became more rooted in science. The post–World War II period saw the rise of modern clinical research—with its gold standard of the double-blind, randomized, controlled trial—and a huge influx of federal funding turned the United States into a world leader in biomedical research. But this expansion preceded any consensus that the patients involved in clinical research shouldn't be treated as unwitting guinea pigs. At least through the sixties, it remained socially disadvantaged and/or institutionalized groups—like the poor, prisoners, soldiers, and the mentally ill—who were most likely to be used in medical studies. Finally, a few shameful examples of vulnerable Americans experimented on without their consent—most infamously, the Tuskegee experiment, in which poor black men were left untreated for syphilis—made headlines. In the aftermath, in the late seventies, the United States finally put in place some enforceable ethical standards for research involving human subjects.

Meanwhile, two high-profile disasters had underscored the risks experimental drugs could pose to pregnant patients and their fetuses. In the late fifties, thalidomide was used in dozens of countries as an over-the-counter sedative and antinausea remedy in early pregnancy. Though it was never given FDA approval, some women in the United States nonetheless received it. By the early sixties, it was determined that the drug was to blame for severe limb deformities in over 10,000 children. Then, in the late sixties, many of the daughters of patients who'd taken the synthetic estrogen diethylstilbestrol (DES) while pregnant started developing a rare vaginal cancer. The drug had been widely prescribed to prevent miscarriage, despite large studies suggesting it was ineffective. At a few respected American academic medical institutions, doctors had informed their pregnant patients only that DES was a "vitamin" that would help them grow "bigger and better babies."

The public outcry over these cases helped spur some much-needed federal drug regulation. Since 1938 drug manufacturers had been required to show the FDA that their medication was safe before marketing it, but the agency's regulatory power was fairly minimal. In the aftermath of the thalidomide tragedy, however, Congress passed the Kefauver-Harris Amendment, which significantly beefed up the drug-approval process, essentially putting in place most of the regulations we take for granted today. Companies seeking FDA approval for their drugs were now required to demonstrate not just safety but also efficacy in well-controlled studies, they had to secure the fully informed consent of their study subjects, the drug's advertising had to be up-front about its side effects and potential risks, and the FDA would track reports of any adverse reactions once the drug hit the market.

Along with these welcome reforms to clinical research and drug regulation, however, were some that crossed the line from overdue protection to sexist paternalism. The new federal guidelines on the ethical treatment of clinical subjects identified groups that may be in need of special safeguards because they "are likely to be vulnerable to coercion or undue influence"—a list that included pregnant women alongside children, prisoners, mentally disabled people, and the economically disadvantaged. While the ethical inclusion of pregnant women in research is certainly complicated, as two women's health advocates mused in the nineties, "one wonders what aspect of pregnancy renders women particularly vulnerable to 'coercion' or 'undue influence.'"

Meanwhile, the 1977 FDA policy didn't stop at excluding patients who were actually pregnant. It expressly prohibited women of "childbearing potential" from participating in early-phase drug studies, except in the cases of life-threatening diseases. Critics pointed out that this treated every menstruating woman as if she were potentially pregnant—a "walking womb"—an infantilizing position that implied women couldn't be trusted to know their risk of unintended pregnancy, take steps to prevent it, and make their own decision should they accidentally become pregnant during the trial. Even lesbian women, single women, women using contraception, and women whose partners had had a vasectomy weren't allowed. In a stark double standard, the policy evinced little concern at all that men of reproductive age could be exposed to drugs that harm the genetic material they contribute to their future offspring. And while the FDA ban was limited to only early-phase studies, it ended up having a broader chilling effect, making drug researchers hesitant to enroll women during their fertile years at all.

Women's health advocates had certainly been part of the chorus of voices calling for better drug regulation and respect for research subjects' informed consent. Policies that completely stripped women of their agency to weigh the risks of participating in studies—of treatments that would potentially benefit themselves—because of theoretical harm to their hypothetical fetuses were quite a different matter. Not only was such a stance patronizing to individual patients, it also didn't help ensure women as a whole got safe treatments. Indeed, the irony is that while the thalidomide and DES debacles are usually credited with spurring the FDA's 1977 ban and the broader hesitancy about including women of childbearing age in research, neither would actually have been prevented by banning pregnant patients from clinical research, let alone all potentially pregnant women. The problem was that these drugs had been inadequately studied before being released to the public and evidence of their risks ignored. Studying them exclusively in men and then marketing them to women would hardly have been a solution.

While the pendulum swing toward protectionism helps account for women's underrepresentation in drug trials, what about the rest of biomedical research? It doesn't explain why women weren't included in the MRFIT study on risk factors for heart disease, even though heart disease was the leading cause of death in women too. Nor why, despite making up two-thirds of the elderly population, they weren't represented in the study on "normal human aging." (Actually, we have an explanation for that one: according to the researchers, they enrolled only men because there wasn't a women's bathroom at the research site.)

The research community tended to offer two contradictory defenses for their exclusion of women. Sometimes, they claimed that, apart from their reproductive systems, men and women were so alike that any findings derived from studying the former would be perfectly valid for the latter as well. Women's health advocates countered that such a claim was simply an assumption, one that should be investigated. Since little medical research had actually looked to see if there were sex/gender differences, no one could say for sure that there were any differences, but no one could say for sure that there *weren't* either. Besides, this argument was more a post hoc attempt at validating the results from all-male studies, as opposed to an explanation for them. After all, if there really were no significant differences between the sexes, then there were also no grounds for excluding women. It also raised the obvious question: If researchers were so confident that it was fine to extrapolate findings on one sex to the other, why didn't it ever seem to go the opposite way?

This excuse looked especially suspect since the biomedical community also offered the exact opposite argument. Instead of claiming that the sexes were so similar that women could be properly represented by men in a study, researchers claimed women were so different from men that including women would destroy the homogeneity of the study population and "confuse" the results. A mixed-sex study would require a larger subject population in order to get statistically significant results for both men and women, making it more expensive. Furthermore, they argued, women's various hormonal cycles and states make them a more biologically heterogeneous bunch than men; not only are women different from men, they're too different from each other. With hormone levels that vary depending on where they are in their menstrual cycle, whether they are on hormonal contraception or hormone replacement therapy, whether they are pregnant, postpartum, or postmenopausal, women introduce too much "noise" that would make it harder to get "clean" findings. In short, studying only one sex was cheaper and easier, and men were the chosen ones because women's bodies were thought to be too complicated.

Of course, that suggested that the research community's blind spot about potential sex/gender differences was somewhat willful and more than a little self-serving. It would have been one thing to plead pure ignorance, insisting that it simply hadn't occurred to anyone that knowledge gained from studying men might not apply to women. Instead, the very justification offered for not including women in studies underscored exactly why they needed to be included: it might actually matter. As medical journalists Leslie Laurence and Beth Weinhouse wrote in their 1994 book on gender bias in medicine, *Outrageous Practices*, "It defies logic for researchers to acknowledge gender difference by claiming women's hormones can affect study results—for instance, by affecting drug metabolism—but then to ignore those differences, study only men, and extrapolate the results to women."

As for why conditions that disproportionately affected women seemed to have sunk to the bottom of the research agenda, the reason was perhaps more straightforward but no less challenging to fix. Advocates pointed out that most of the people proposing the studies, granting the funding, and publishing the results were men, who inevitably brought their own perspectives and concerns to their work. "I don't think it was malicious or intentional," Dr. Florence Haseltine, at the time one of the handful of ob-gyns at the NIH, told Laurence and Weinhouse. "You want doctors to study what they're interested in, so you have male doctors in their fifties studying other male doctors in their fifties for heart attacks." More precisely, when it comes to medical research, what you're "interested in" tends to be what feels most urgent to you. As Rep. Schroeder put it in 1990, "You fund what you fear. When you have a male-dominated group of researchers, they are more worried about prostate cancer than breast cancer."

"ADD WOMEN AND STIR": INCLUSION IS NOT ENOUGH

In the early nineties, some swift and important steps were taken to close this knowledge gap. The NIH immediately formed the ORWH to help monitor enforcement of their policy—which now mandated, rather than merely recommended, women's inclusion as research subjects—and coordinate research on women's health issues across the agency. Shortly after that, Dr. Bernadine Healy became the first woman to head the NIH and announced the launch of the Women's Health Initiative, a massive, long-term study into the effects of diet, hormone replacement therapy, and vitamin D supplementation on cardiovascular disease, cancer, and osteoporosis among older women. As if trying to make up for lost time in one fell swoop, it was the largest study ever funded by the NIH, enrolling more than 161,000 women. "Basically, we're trying to get the type of data that we already have on men," Healy explained. "We can't go forward on women's health research without it."

Meanwhile, Congress pushed to get these reforms codified into law. In 1993, President Bill Clinton signed the NIH Revitalization Act, which mandated that NIH-funded studies include enough women, as well as racial minorities, that a "valid analysis" of any difference could be determined. It also made the ORWH a permanent part of the NIH and earmarked funding for research on breast and ovarian cancer, osteoporosis, contraception, and infertility. The same year, in the wake of its own GAO report, the FDA dropped the 1977 policy excluding women of childbearing age, admitting that it now seemed "rigid and paternalistic" and "may have led to a more general lack of participation of women in drug development studies, and thus to a paucity of information about the effects of drugs in women."

Yet a quarter century later, there's still work to do. In 2015, Carolyn M. Mazure, director of the women's health research center at Yale School of Medicine, and her colleague reviewed how much progress had been made over the past two decades to "fully represent women in clinical trials and ensure the study of sex and gender in biomedical research." They concluded that despite some important steps, "progress has been painfully slow—stalling for long periods or sometimes reversing direction—and, consequently, not nearly enough progress has been made."

In part, that's because for all the steps taken in the early nineties, a few steps were not taken. During the hearings on the GAO report in 1990, indignant members of Congress railed against the fact that the default subject at every level of biomedical research was male, including preclinical studies using animals, tissue, and cells. Yet the NIH Revitalization Act ultimately mandated the inclusion of women only in studies with human subjects, and only Phase 3 research (the final trials conducted in thousands of patients after earlier, smaller studies have suggested a new treatment is safe and promising) had to include enough women to analyze the results by gender. It was only in 2014 that the NIH announced a policy to address the overwhelming male bias in preclinical research.

Meanwhile, the FDA didn't do much to ensure women's inclusion in drug trials apart from dropping the policy that actively excluded them. While the agency encouraged the pharmaceutical industry to consider how the effects of their drugs might be influenced by the menstrual cycle or interactions with hormone therapy and oral contraceptives, it still didn't actually require drug companies to enroll women or analyze their results by gender. In 1998, the rule was strengthened slightly, calling for pharmaceutical companies to provide efficacy and safety data for different subgroups (by age, race, and gender) in their applications to the FDA if they had collected it, but it still didn't mandate that they collect that data to begin with. In 2000, the agency issued a new regulation reserving the right to halt research on drugs for life-threatening diseases if either men or women were excluded.

Then there was the matter of enforcement. In a 2000 review of how well the NIH had implemented their inclusion policy, the GAO concluded that while women were better represented in NIH-funded studies, the studies still weren't always designed to make it possible to analyze the results by gender, and when such analysis was done, it often wasn't published. The next year, the GAO gave a similar evaluation to the FDA: Women were now adequately included in studies of recently approved drugs overall, but they made up less than a quarter of those in smaller, early-phase studies. More than one-third of applications still weren't following the rule to present any subgroup data that had been collected. Even when differences were identified, often neither the drug sponsors nor the FDA reviewers were acting on that information. Underscoring the ongoing problems with drug studies: of the FDA-approved drugs that had been pulled from the market between 1997 and 2001 because they were found to have "unacceptable health risks," eight out of ten were more dangerous to women than to men.

More recently, in a 2015 report requested by Congress, the GAO concluded that since the NIH keeps track of only the aggregate number of men and women in all the studies it funds, it's still hard to say if women are being well represented in every arena. All told, women now make up a majority of patients enrolled in federally funded research. But, the GAO report warned, a couple of large all-female studies, like the Women's Health Initiative, can mask the fact that there may still be specific areas where women remain underrepresented: "By not examining more detailed data on enrollment—such as data aggregated by research area or specific to various diseases and conditions—NIH cannot know whether it is adequately including women across all of the research it supports."

Indeed, outside analyses of published NIH-funded studies tend to paint a slightly less than equal picture. A review of federally funded randomized controlled trials published in nine prominent medical journals in 2004 found that, on average, women made up 37 percent of the trial subjects. When the researchers redid the analysis for studies published in 2009—same journals, same methodology—there had been no improvement: 37 percent.

And of course, the NIH, while the largest, is not the only funder in town. There's no federal law that says research funded by private industry or foundations has to include women. Consequently, while women are rarely completely left out of studies these days, they remain underrepresented in many. A 2013 review, for example, found that in 304 studies on cancer treatment and prevention conducted between 2001 and 2010, nearly 60 percent of subjects were men and over 80 percent were white. "Women and racial/ethnic minorities," the authors concluded, "remain severely underrepresented in cancer clinical trials, thus limiting the generalizability of cancer clinical research."

But perhaps the biggest problem is that actually analyzing study results to determine whether they differ by gender has not yet become the norm. After all, the point of requiring women to be represented in clinical research is not to include them just for the hell of it but to increase scientific knowledge by finding out whether there are or, just as importantly, are not any differences between men and women.

The NIH can't do much more than "strongly encourage" researchers to actually follow through on doing a gender analysis, much less get them to include these findings in their published studies. When the policy was first announced in the early nineties, some researchers admitted they'd try to wiggle out of it. "When an NIH staff member brought this up in a meeting, white male scientists got up and said it was outrageous," one women's health researcher recalled in the midnineties. "Several people even got up to the microphone and said they would lie, would say they're going to analyze gender but then not do it."

Whether or not they're deliberately being misleading, more often than not, researchers still don't do a gender analysis. In the review of federally funded trials mentioned above, 75 percent of the studies did not report any outcomes by gender, and 64 percent did not provide any analysis by racial or ethnic groups. In 2010, a review of 150 recent studies of treatments for depression found that only half the studies analyzed the results by gender. Of over 700 ongoing studies, nearly 90 percent of the researchers said they planned to include women, but less than 1 percent said they planned to analyze their results by gender. A 2011 review of 750 studies focused on emergency medicine between 2006 and 2009 found that while the majority reported gender as a variable, less than one-fifth examined health outcomes by gender.

Advocates often describe what's happened as the "add women and stir" approach. There was a sense in the nineties that just getting women enrolled in studies would "take care of the problem," explains Dr. Jan Werbinski, executive director of the Sex and Gender Women's Health Collaborative. "But it's been twenty-five years and we now have a lot of research that includes women but women are still invisible. Researchers said, 'Okay, we included women,' but they weren't required to report their research by sex, so women's side effects and responses to medications and diseases were still invisible."

Unsurprisingly, given the less strict rules set by the FDA compared to the NIH, drug studies are especially likely to fall short. "It's still a struggle to get the pharma companies to analyze; inclusion is one thing, analysis is something else. And that's not there yet," Phyllis Greenberger, the former president of the SWHR, says. In 2012, Congress asked the FDA to review how well it was doing at collecting safety and effectiveness data by demographic subgroups, including gender/sex, race/ethnicity, and age. While most of the seventy-two applications they reviewed included that data, the agency acknowledged that women—and racial minorities and the elderly—were often not included in sufficient numbers to make statistically significant analyses possible. "You just have to include what you have," Susan Wood, the former director of the FDA's Office of Women's Health, explains. And that's not always enough to actually detect differences.

The FDA concluded that there was room for improvement and, in 2014, released a twenty-seven-point action plan to increase inclusion of underrepresented groups and improve the quality of the analyses. It's also working to make the information more publicly accessible. To that end, it launched the Drug Trials Snapshots initiative, which puts the subgroup data included in drug applications, previously available only to those willing to wade through the voluminous review packages on the FDA's website, on a user-friendly website so that doctors and patients could see whether efficacy and side effects varied by sex, race, or age. Though advocates applauded the move, they noted that the database includes only late-stage studies and covers only new drugs going forward, not the many drugs already on the market. Plus, a website isn't exactly the most direct way to get the information out to the public. "Eventually we would like it on the label, where the patient can see it," says Wood.

There's one obvious way to make sex/gender analysis a standard of good scientific research: make it a requirement for publication in a peer-reviewed journal. Once the NIH Revitalization Act became law, the ORWH spent years encouraging medical and science journals to change their submission guidelines to do so. "We found great resistance for many years for some reason from journals," Dr. Vivian Pinn, the former director of the ORWH, says. "We tackled this over and over, and there were some leading journals that were very resistant for what they called 'scientific reasons.'" They offered various justifications: they didn't want to take space to publish negative results if no differences had been found; if the study wasn't federally funded and hadn't been designed in such a way that those analyses would be statistically sound, they couldn't very well tell researchers to redo their whole study.

Finally, in just the last several years, journals have started to come around. In 2010, the SWHR did an informal survey of eleven popular science and medical journals and found that only two—*Journal of the National Cancer Institute* and *Circulation*—included anything about reporting sex/gender differences in their guidelines for authors. The same year, in a progress report on women's health research, the IOM recommended that the International Committee of Medical Journal Editors and other journal editors "should adopt a guideline that all papers reporting the outcomes of clinical trials report on men and women separately unless a trial is of a sex-specific condition." Today, according to Stanford University's Gendered Innovations project, thirty-two peer-reviewed journals worldwide have editorial policies requiring that researchers include information on results by gender/sex when they submit articles for publication. Still, Pinn says, the years of foot-dragging have meant that even as the NIH's inclusion policy spurred new knowledge, "not as much was getting in the literature as it might have."

PREGNANT PATIENTS: "THERAPEUTIC ORPHANS"

There's one group of women that has been entirely left out of the progress toward greater inclusion of women in clinical research: pregnant patients. In 1994, the IOM recommended that pregnant women should be "presumed eligible for participation in clinical studies" and be "treated as competent adults capable of making their own decisions." Federal guidelines, however, continue to take the opposite position: while pregnant women may be included in studies under limited conditions, by default, they are not. The FDA, meanwhile, does not require the drugs it approves to be tested in pregnant women, and most are not.

With no incentive to enroll them and widespread fears of liability for harm to the fetus, the research community has left pregnant patients to be "therapeutic orphans," all but entirely left out of biomedical studies. In a 2013 analysis, 95 percent of industry-sponsored clinical drug trials excluded pregnant people, and only 1 percent were designed specifically to study them. Only eight medications are currently approved by the FDA for use during pregnancy. And all of them are used for conditions related to the pregnancy itself, like alleviating nausea or inducing labor; any drug used to treat other diseases during pregnancy is prescribed "off-label"—without the prior testing needed for FDA sign-off. "Pregnant women," a 2011 report by the ORWH declared, "may be the most underrepresented group in the entire clinical research process."

Of course, pregnant people are no less in need of safe, effective medical treatments than anyone else. Each year, over 400,000 women in the United States battle significant illnesses while pregnant. And many women have chronic conditions, from hypertension to autoimmune diseases to depression, that they must manage with medications. As bioethicist Françoise Baylis wrote in a 2010 *Nature* article, "Pregnant women get sick, and sick women get pregnant." Indeed, 90 percent of women take some medication during pregnancy, and about 70 percent take a prescription drug, according to the Centers for Disease Control and Prevention (CDC). The average woman receives 1.3 prescriptions per obstetric visit, and nearly two-thirds of women use four to five medications during pregnancy and labor.

But with little actual research to go on, doctors are simply guessing at how drugs will affect a pregnant body, and their best predictions can be disastrously off. The Second Wave Initiative, a coalition of women's health researchers that formed in 2009 to advocate for pregnant patients' inclusion in research, describes pregnancy as a "wild card." The profound changes it causes to just about every system of the body—from extreme fluctuations in hormone levels to a 30 to 40 percent increase in blood volume to alterations in metabolism and cardiovascular function—can "surprisingly and substantially" affect the way drugs are processed and act. Just as the average woman can't be considered only a slightly smaller version of the average man, "a pregnant woman is not just a woman with a bigger belly," and knowledge about the effective dose and risks can't simply be extrapolated from studies on nonpregnant patients.

The result is a medically and ethically unacceptable situation: pregnant patients and their health care providers are left between a rock and a hard place. As the Second Wave Initiative explains in a call to action, "In the absence of information about the safety and efficacy of medications, pregnant women and their providers are left with two unsavory options—take a drug, with unknown safety and efficacy; or fail to treat the conditions, thus leaving the woman and fetus vulnerable to the consequences of the underlying medical problems."

One of the results, of course, is that pregnant women may end up taking drugs that harm their fetuses—the very risk that has justified excluding them from research in the first place. A 2011 analysis found that less than 10 percent of the prescription medications approved by the FDA between 1980 and 2010 had sufficient data to determine the risk to the fetus. In 2004, one of the largest studies of drug use during pregnancy concluded that "approximately one half of all pregnant women are prescribed drugs for which there is no evidence of safety during pregnancy in humans or for which there is evidence of fetal risk in animals or humans." All pregnant patients in effect become guinea pigs: "We learn on the backs of [pregnant] women while pretending we don't experiment on pregnant women," Ruth Faden, a member of the Second Wave Initiative and director of the Johns Hopkins Berman Institute of Bioethics, explained in a 2016 ProPublica article. And we learn slowly. For drugs approved between 1980 and 2000, it took an average of twenty-seven years for enough data to accumulate to be able to determine the risks.

But the opposite consequence can be equally dangerous, and perhaps more common. Worries about risks to the fetus may result in pregnant women going untreated, or undertreated, for dangerous medical conditions. In the absence of good data, doctors—and women themselves—may be so fearful of theoretical risks to the fetus that they err on the side of avoiding all treatment, without properly appreciating the risks of *not* treating a condition. As the Second Wave Initiative explains, "If research is important to tell us when medications are unsafe, it is also important to reassure us when drugs are safe." After all, fetal and maternal health are intimately linked; generally, anything that hurts the pregnant person is not going to be good for the fetus either. And all medical treatment involves accepting risks; the question is whether the benefits outweigh the costs. While that calculus may be more complicated during pregnancy, where the magnitude of the risks to the pregnant person and fetus may, in some cases, differ, it's ultimately no different.

But in the absence of much hard data to help guide decision making about these trade-offs, experts say there's a tendency for doctors to focus on the potential dangers of treatment to the fetus over the benefits of treatment to both. For example, women with depression are often urged to go off their antidepressants during pregnancy if at all possible, which leads to higher rates of relapse compared to those who continue taking their medication. But untreated depression during pregnancy is also risky for fetuses: it is linked to premature birth, low birth weight, fetal growth restriction, and postnatal complications. Likewise, women with asthma are often undertreated during pregnancy, increasing their own risk of hypertension, preeclampsia, and uterine hemorrhage, while also placing the fetus at a higher risk of fetal growth restriction, premature birth, and low birth weight. In fact, experts say, even when there is good evidence that treatment won't harm the fetus, pregnant women sometimes receive inadequate care out of a totally unfounded, and ultimately counterproductive, overabundance of caution.

There have been some recent efforts to finally bring pregnant patients into the fold. The FDA has drafted guidelines for the industry on how to ethically determine the biochemical and physiological effects of drugs on the pregnant body, and has urged companies to set up pregnancy registries to track adverse effects once drugs hit the market, though it hasn't made the collection of this data mandatory. In 2014, the CDC launched an initiative to improve the quality of data and information on medication use during pregnancy.

But for now, their exclusion from research leaves all individual pregnant patients in the same spot all women of childbearing age were in back in the nineties: in an uncontrolled experiment nearly every time they take a medication. This is not a solution to ethical challenges of including pregnant people in research. As the Second Wave Initiative concludes in their article, "The alternative to responsible research in pregnancy is relegating pregnant women to second-class medical citizens—something, it turns out, that is not good for pregnant women nor the fetuses they carry."

AN EMERGING SCIENCE: SEX/GENDER-SPECIFIC MEDICINE

In 2005, sixteen years after the Physicians' Health Study (which enrolled 22,071 people, 100 percent of whom were men) found that low-dose aspirin lowered the risk of heart attack in men over fifty, women finally got an answer about whether these results applied to them. A study of nearly 40,000 women concluded that aspirin had no effect on heart-disease risk for those under sixty-five but did help those over sixty-five, in addition to reducing the risk of stroke, a benefit not found in the men.

The aspirin example served as a vindication of the concerns raised by women's health advocates in the early nineties. Back then, while there were certainly hints that studying men and extrapolating the findings to women wasn't always valid, since there hadn't been very much attention paid to potential sex/gender differences, how important they really were was an open question. Advocates, after all, weren't claiming that there were always differences, nor that they would always be so large that they'd impact medical practice, just that we should probably take a look and see.

It took a long time to convince the rest of the medical community that this was a worthy endeavor. "In my own area of cardiology, trying to convince them in the early nineties to reexamine the differences between the experiences of men and women with coronary disease took really the whole decade to achieve," says Dr. Marianne Legato, a cardiologist and founder of the Partnership for Gender-Specific Medicine at Columbia University. But over the last twenty-five years, as more and more research documenting sex/gender differences has accumulated, any lingering skepticism has become less and less justifiable.

Sex/gender differences have been observed in the prevalence, severity, symptoms, and risk factors of countless diseases. To take just a few examples: Women are two to ten times more likely to develop autoimmune diseases. Women are more likely than men to recover language ability after suffering a left-hemisphere stroke. Women who have lung cancer are more likely than their male counterparts to have never smoked. Women more commonly do not have any chest pain when experiencing a heart attack.

Differences have been found in the responses to many drugs, both in the pharmacokinetics (which is how the body acts on the drug) and the pharmacodynamics (which is how the drug acts on the body). Women have a greater risk than men of developing a potentially fatal heart arrhythmia that can be triggered by a variety of drugs, including antibiotics, antidepressants, and cholesterol-lowering drugs. Beta-blockers tend to have a more pronounced effect in women than in men. Women with depression generally respond better to selective serotonin reuptake inhibitors (SSRIs) than tricyclic antidepressants, while the opposite is true of men. Women tend to wake up from general anesthesia faster than men and suffer more side effects from it.

These sex/gender differences in drug response, it should be noted, are not all simply due to women's lower average body weight. Although that is one obvious difference, there's a complicated mix of other factors that affect pharmacokinetics, including percentage of body fat, hormonal fluctuations, enzyme levels, and speed of metabolism. One article on sex/gender differences in drug response notes that these are "often attributed solely to body weight differences and may therefore be dismissed as not being clinically significant, once corrected for these body weight differences." Except, they point out, it is not even standard practice to correct for body weight: "Paradoxically however, most drugs are not administered on a mg/kg basis but as a 'one size fits all' dose, leading to higher exposures in women due to their generally lower body weight."

While sometimes these differences may be small and irrelevant to clinical recommendations, sometimes they can matter. In 2013, the FDA announced that it was requiring the recommended dose of zolpidem, the active ingredient in the popular insomnia drug Ambien, which is prescribed to about 40 million Americans each year, to be slashed in half for women. Over the years, the FDA had received about 700 reports of patients getting into car accidents the morning after taking the drug. And new studies had found that because women take longer to clear the drug from their bodies, about 15 percent of women have a level of zolpidem in their blood that could impair driving eight hours after taking the pill, compared to about 3 percent of men.

The fact that there was a sex/gender difference in how zolpidem was metabolized was not actually news. Back in 1992, when the FDA first approved the drug, there was data showing that women's blood levels of the drug were 45 percent higher than those of their male counterparts. An FDA reviewer had, in fact, made this note on the drug's application: "The results suggest a gender-related difference." Yet back then, it wasn't thought to matter. Dr. Sandra Kweder, deputy director of the FDA's Office of New Drugs, acknowledged in a *60 Minutes* segment on the lower dose recommendation, "If I saw this today, in light of today's science, I think we would go back and try to tease this out a little bit further. But I think at the time . . . this was sort of business as usual for what you saw in clinical pharmacology studies."

There are countless other drugs on the market that were approved in the days when overlooking—even ignoring—sex/gender differences was just "business as usual." As ORWH director Clayton told *The New York Times*, "This is not just about Ambien—that's just the tip of the iceberg. There are a lot of sex differences for a lot of drugs, some of which are well known and some that are not well recognized." Given how many drugs weren't tested in women—or, even when they were, evidence of differences was ignored—it is perhaps not surprising that women are 50 to 75 percent more likely than men to have an adverse drug reaction.

In 2001, the IOM compiled the emerging knowledge in a report entitled *Exploring the Biological Contributions to Human Health—Does Sex Matter?* The short answer was yes: "Sex does matter," the report concluded. "It matters in ways that we did not expect. Undoubtedly, it also matters in ways that we have not begun to imagine." Noting that the study of sex/gender differences was "evolving into a mature science," the committee declared that "sex differences of importance to health and human disease occur throughout the life span"—from "womb to tomb"—and "should be considered when designing and analyzing studies in all areas and at all levels of biomedical and health-related research." Though somewhat focused on sex differences—that is, ones that seem to stem from biological factors like genetic or hormonal differences—the report also covered the ways that gender influenced health.

That raises an important point: while the concepts of sex and gender can be useful, when it comes to determining their effect on health and disease, it gets complicated. Since most people have a gender and sex that matches, it is often impossible to disentangle whether an observed average difference between men and women is rooted in sex or gender differences. In some cases, it's fairly clear. For example, men in the United States had higher rates of lung cancer than women for decades because men were more likely to smoke cigarettes. That's an obvious gender difference: men were not more biologically vulnerable to the disease; they simply had a differing level of exposure to a major cause. On the flip side, disorders that are caused by a genetic mutation on the X chromosome rarely affect women, since most of them are protected by having an additional X chromosome. That's an obvious sex difference.

But most medical conditions are not so clearly linked to a single biological or cultural cause. Instead, our health is affected by a complicated mix of genetic vulnerabilities and environmental factors. Within medicine, which has a tradition of overlooking the social factors that impact health, it is often assumed that any biological differences discovered between the genders are innate sex differences, but that's not necessarily the case. In a classic article, the feminist biologist Anne Fausto-Sterling explored how women's higher rates of osteoporosis—often portrayed as purely a sex difference—could also be the product of gender differences. Bone density in old age is affected by various factors, including diet, athletic activity, and vitamin D deficiency, throughout the life span.

In other words, our experience quite literally shapes our biology— even our seemingly solid and immutable skeleton—muddling attempts at divvying up the role of sex versus gender, biology versus culture, nature versus nurture. That's why in this book I generally use the term *sex/gender difference* when discussing these average differences between men and women.

Greenberger says that the IOM report marked a key turning point. "Before the IOM report, we were the only ones saying this," she says. "We were a women's organization, we were small; people said we were just being politically correct. We had these networks and a group of physicians who understood and supported us, but it certainly wasn't widespread. When the IOM report came out, it still took many years, but it was taken more seriously." Still, the "educational process" is ongoing. "On the one hand, we've made tremendous gains. On the other hand, I'd say we're about halfway there," Greenberger says. "Not even sure we're halfway there."

An attention to potential sex/gender differences matters to all of us. A few decades ago, when researchers were almost exclusively studying men and applying the results to women, while the latter were hurt, the former were sitting pretty; the medical knowledge emerging was, by design, applicable to them. But now that women are represented in studies—not always to parity but usually enough to influence the results—both women and men may be harmed when researchers aren't attuned to possible differences. Men, like women, might miss out on a treatment that's very effective for them, while completely ineffective for women, or be harmed by one whose side effects are significantly greater in them. Especially in diseases that are much more common among women, like osteoporosis or migraine, differences in men's experiences may be subsumed if women make up the majority of those studied. Legato says that's why she's "pushed the field like a boulder up a mountain" to stop talking about "women's health" and instead talk about gender-specific medicine. "Men have issues that are unique too."

More broadly, determining why these differences arise can offer important insights into how the human body works. Just as the point is not to include both men and women in studies out of some abstract sense of fairness but to actually analyze the results to see whether or not there are differences between the two, the investigation shouldn't end with a finding of a sex/gender difference; that should just be the jumping-off point. Figuring out why women or men have a better response to a drug, or why they're more likely to develop a certain disease, or why they're more resilient to another is all data that can further scientific knowledge to ultimately help improve the health of all. Indeed, even differences that are small and not directly relevant to medical care, the IOM report pointed out, "may provide clues than can be used to solve new biological questions." "Wanting to learn more about women and contrast it with our knowledge of men is not a matter of political correctness," writes Legato. "It is an intellectual imperative. Correctly used, the natural experiment of biological sex is one of the most powerful tools we have been given to help us understand the human condition."

Meanwhile, the increased research focus since the nineties on conditions unique to or more common in women has paid dividends too, underscoring the importance of careful scientific inquiry. The findings on hormone replacement therapy offer a good example of that: in the 1970s, a third of all postmenopausal women were taking estrogens because observational studies suggested it might help prevent heart disease. When the Women's Health Initiative was launched in 1991, it was the first time a controlled clinical trial looked at the safety and efficacy of hormone therapy (a full thirty-five years after the first randomized trial of estrogen's effect on heart disease in men). In 2002 and 2004, the two studies, one that looked at estrogen and another that looked at progesterone and estrogen in combination, were ended early after the researchers determined the health risks outweighed the benefits.

Federal funding for research on many conditions that mostly affect women has increased over the last few decades, in large part thanks to advocacy by patient groups that proliferated throughout the eighties and nineties. Yet we're still playing catch-up. In 2008, Congress asked the IOM to assess how much had been learned in the previous two decades about diseases that are specific to women, are more common or more serious in women, have distinct causes or manifestations in women, have different outcomes or treatments in women, or have higher morbidity or mortality in women. In its resulting report, *Women's Health Research: Progress, Pitfalls, and Promise,* the committee concluded that research had contributed to substantial progress in addressing breast cancer, cardiovascular disease, and cervical cancer, and that there had been "some progress" on depression, HIV/AIDS, and osteoporosis.

But the report also discussed areas in which the committee felt "little progress" had been made: unintended pregnancy; maternal mortality and morbidity; autoimmune diseases; alcohol and drug addiction; lung, ovarian, and endometrial cancer; nonmalignant gynecological disorders, including uterine fibroids, endometriosis, chronic pelvic pain, pelvic floor disorders, polycystic ovary syndrome, and sexually transmitted infections; and Alzheimer's disease. It also listed conditions that "affect many women's quality of life" that it didn't have room to review at all, some of which had "little research to discuss" anyway: arthritis, chronic fatigue syndrome, chronic pain, colorectal cancer, eating disorders, fibromyalgia, incontinence, irritable bowel syndrome (IBS), many pregnancy-related issues, melanoma, menopause, mental illnesses other than depression, migraine, sexual dysfunction, stress-related disorders, thyroid disease, and type 2 diabetes.

WHERE ARE THE FEMALE MICE?

In addition to pregnant women, the new inclusion paradigm hasn't extended to another group: female animals. During the hearings on the GAO report in 1990, Rep. Schroeder said, "If anyone thinks women are going to keep paying half the cost of health care and have researchers so elitist they won't even use female rats in the research, they're nuts." But the NIH Revitalization Act ultimately mandated only the inclusion of women in human studies, and for the past twenty-five years, most researchers have continued to largely use male animals and cell lines in preclinical research.

In 2011, in a study published in *Neuroscience & Biobehavioral Reviews*, researchers analyzed animal studies from ten biological disciplines—from pharmacology to endocrinology to neuroscience—published in 2009 and found a male bias in eight out of the ten fields. In neuroscience, the ratio of articles reporting on only males versus only females was skewed 5.5:1, in pharmacology it was 5:1, and in physiology it was 3.7:1. In neuroscience, physiology, and interdisciplinary biology journals, 22 to 42 percent of the articles didn't even mention the sex of the animals at all; in immunology, more than 60 percent didn't. When both sexes were included, only a third analyzed their results by sex.

Annaliese Beery, lead author of the study, explained to *HuffPost* that the default to studying male animals is deeply entrenched. "If you go to publish a study just on females, you always get asked, 'Why didn't you include males? If you go to publish a study on males, most people wouldn't bat an eye." In fact, the study found that the proportion of male-only studies not only hadn't decreased but had actually increased over the last several decades.

Researchers using human cells and tissues are even less likely to pay attention to whether the cells are chromosomally XY or XX. In 2014, a review of over six hundred studies published in prominent surgery journals recently found that among cell studies, three-quarters didn't specify the sex of the cell lines used and of those that did, over 70 percent used only male cells. This despite the fact that sex differences on the cellular level have been observed; as the 2001 IOM report put it, "every cell has a sex." For example, studies have found that skeletal muscle stem cells derived from females regenerated new tissue faster than those from males did, and only female bone marrow mononuclear cells have proven useful in preventing plaque buildup in the arteries of mice.

When it comes to animal studies, researchers can't justify their exclusion of females out of concerns about fetal harm. Beery said that she's heard a host of excuses, including that "female mice have smellier urine." But the widespread reliance on male animals seems to stem mostly from the assumption that females' hormonal cycle (a four-day cycle in rodents) complicates results. Researchers argued that to account for this variability, they'd need to use a larger sample of female animals and test them at each stage of their cycle, making their work more difficult and expensive. Of course, the same counterargument to the exclusion of women applies here: if the results of the study *do* vary significantly due to fluctuations in ovarian hormones, that's just all the more reason females need to be studied, no matter the cost.

Interestingly, however, it seems that the long-standing assumption that their hormonal cycle makes female animals inherently more variable than males is just that: an assumption. A 2014 meta-analysis of nearly three hundred articles found that female mice weren't more variable than their male counterparts on a range of behavioral, morphological, physiological, and molecular traits. And for several traits, it was the males that were more variable, perhaps, according to the researchers, largely because when male mice are housed together, they tend to fight among themselves for status, leading to differences in their levels of stress hormones and testosterone.

The persistence of male animal models is especially troubling when it comes to conditions that are more common among women. As the authors of a 2009 review of the male bias in basic pain research concluded, given that women are disproportionately impacted by chronic pain disorders, "one could argue that preclinical research that excludes females is incomplete at best or invalid at worst." Nevertheless, a 2005 study found that nearly 80 percent of animal pain studies published in recent years had used only males. That's "ethically indefensible," Dr. Jeffrey Mogil, director of the pain genetics lab at McGill University, has charged. "Even if you decide you should only be studying one sex, it damn well should be females." He recently called on his colleagues to get it together. "Most patients with pain are women. We fail in our duties if we conduct research using only male rodents, producing results that might serve only men."

And it's not just pain research. While women are twice as likely to be diagnosed with anxiety and depression as men, fewer than 45 percent of animal studies on these disorders used females. Women suffer more strokes than men and have worse outcomes when they do, yet 65 percent of studies based on animal stroke models included only males. Some autoimmune diseases, such as Graves' disease and systemic lupus erythematosus, are seven to ten times more prevalent among women (while others are found predominantly in men). But three-quarters of the immunity studies didn't specify subject sex. Meanwhile, a 2007 study found that roughly 80 percent of rodent drug studies used only male animals, even though there had been "repeated attempts to draw attention to sex-dependent drug effects."

In 2014, the NIH announced that, since there'd been no progress in correcting the male bias in preclinical research over the past two decades, "despite multiple calls to action," it would begin requiring all researchers seeking funding to report their plans for the balance of male and female cells and animals, unless they could offer a good reason for studying only one sex. "The overreliance on male animals and cells in preclinical research obscures key sex differences that could guide clinical studies," NIH director Francis Collins and ORWH director Clayton wrote in an editorial in *Nature*. "Publications often continue to neglect sex-based considerations and analyses in preclinical studies. Reviewers, for the most part, are not attuned to this failure." Ultimately, when the new policy went into effect in early 2016, it had been narrowed to require "the consideration of sex as a biological variable" only in preclinical research on vertebrate animals and humans, not cells and tissues.

The recent NIH focus on the issue has sparked some of the same kind of resistance that the inclusion of women in clinical research did twenty-five years ago, as well as more legitimate questions about how exactly it will be implemented. In addition, some feminist scientists and scholars have argued that differences between male and female mice or the cells in a petri dish can't really tell us much at all about differences between men and women, which arise from a complex interaction between genetics, hormones, and our environment. They worry that the policy could just reinforce a view that "men are from Mars, women are from Venus" and distract from more needed research on the social factors that lead to health disparities between the genders and among different groups of women. It's true: a human woman is definitely not a female mouse. But then, she's not a male mouse either. While there are certainly limitations to what animal studies can reveal about human health, nonetheless we do often rely on them to give us clues that help us understand disease mechanisms and develop new treatments. As long as that's the case, I'd rather be represented by the female mouse.

CHANGING MEDICAL EDUCATION

In a 1995 report, the Council on Graduate Medical Education concluded "that physicians have not been well prepared to meet the challenges of women's health. Fundamental changes are needed in the way physicians are educated and care is delivered to meet these challenges." Those changes have been slow in coming. Indeed, if convincing biomedical researchers to change the way they do research is hard, getting the knowledge that's emerged from that research to translate into the exam room may be even harder. It's a challenge that's not unique to women's health research. It takes a notoriously long time, often fifteen to twenty years, for any new scientific knowledge to make its way into medical education and, ultimately, change clinical practice: to go from "bench to bedside." But advocates working to get medical education to reflect the current state of scientific knowledge on women's health have faced a particularly daunting challenge.

In the midnineties, the Association of American Medical Colleges teamed up with federal agencies on the first comprehensive survey of what American medical schools were teaching students about women's health. Twelve percent of the schools reported that they had a curriculum on women's health—which often just meant a seminar on a single topic like domestic violence—and a quarter had a clinical rotation in women's health separate from the traditional ob-gyn clerkships. In terms of the topics taught in regular classes, most schools covered sexual and reproductive function, medical interviewing and examination skills, and diagnostic tests specific to women. But few of them included any information on sex/gender differences in the leading causes of death in women (heart disease, lung cancer, and stroke) or on health conditions that disproportionately affect them, such as osteoporosis or fibromyalgia.

Over the last two decades, as women's health research has accumulated, albeit slowly and haltingly, its integration into medical school curricula has been described as "uneven" at best. Subsequent medical school surveys have revealed some progress: The proportion of schools with an office or program charged with overseeing women's health curricula increased from 10 percent to 33 percent in 2000. A 2001 survey by the SWHR suggested that the number of schools with a women's health course had more than doubled. Residency programs and fellowships in women's health were established during the nineties. Between 1996 and 2007, federal funding flowed to dozens of National Centers of Excellence in Women's Health established at academic medical centers and community health organizations, with one of their goals being to address the gender gap in medical education.

During the nineties, some women's health advocates wondered whether a whole new specialty in women's health was needed. In 1996, several women physicians got together to create the American College of Women's Health Physicians. Modeling themselves on the specialty of pediatrics, which formed after decades of medicine treating children as "little adults," they hoped to establish themselves as specialists in all the nonreproductive aspects of women's health that had been so neglected. "But we got a huge amount of, I would label it, sexist backlash," says Werbinski, who was the founding president of the organization. Their hopes of becoming a certified specialty were quashed when the AMA passed a resolution against the idea. And the American College of Obstetricians and Gynecologists felt threatened by the move, according to Werbinski, concerned that the new specialty would "steal all their women patients."

Other women's health advocates, meanwhile, were staunchly opposed to the idea for different reasons. A separate specialty, they argued, would just further fragment the delivery of health care to women and marginalize their concerns. After all, a group that makes up the majority of the population is hardly a "specialty" patient base. Instead of having a minority of physicians who are well versed in, say, the sex/gender differences in the symptoms of a heart attack, or the prevalence of lupus, or the effects of general anesthesia, it would be far more beneficial for both women and men to ensure that all physicians, including cardiologists, rheumatologists, and anesthesiologists, are equipped to treat all their patients. "There should not be a department; it should not be sequestered," explains Legato. "The differences in men's and women's normal function and the differences in the experience of the same diseases by both sexes should be part of everything that we teach. And to isolate it as a subspecialty would be totally a wrong approach."

While Werbinski still thinks there'd be some benefits to having a women's health specialty, almost twenty years later she, along with most women's health advocates, has come around to the conclusion that integration is the way to go. Abandoning their dreams of being a specialty, the American College of Women's Health Physicians eventually teamed up with the American Medical Women's Association and the Society for Women's Health Research, and transformed into the Sex and Gender Women's Health Collaborative (SGWHC), which now serves as an online clearinghouse for sex- and gender-specific educational modules, training programs, and clinical practices. In the last several years, they've been focused on getting medical schools to fully integrate this information into their curricula, across every clinical arena, recognizing that while the ultimate goal is to get all doctors reeducated on these issues, medical students are "the most passive audience that would probably be easiest to tackle first."

The frustrating thing is that while the medical community resisted the formation of a separate specialty, they've also resisted integration. While most everyone agrees these days that the former route would just further marginalize women's health, the truth is that in the current system women's health remains marginalized. In a sad testament to this, the SGWHC is planning to vote this year on whether to drop the word "Women's" from its name out of concern that it leaves "everybody else off the hook," according to Werbinski. "Because as soon as you label yourself as a women's organization, there are doctors, like rheumatologists and orthopedic surgeons, who say, 'Oh well, that doesn't affect me, I don't have to learn anything there, because that's about women.'" To many physicians, "women's health" remains synonymous with "reproductive health," a topic that can be left to ob-gyns.

Changing medical education is a very slow and difficult task in general. "Every medical school has its own curriculum. And everything is changing the field," Greenberger explains. And somewhat ironically, given how medicine portrays itself as continually on the scientific cutting edge, the institutions responsible for educating the next generation of physicians are conservative. "They hate to change things," Legato says. "They are used to operating in one mode: 'It works well enough.'" It's even harder to change the curricula when the new content needs to be added not in a single course or department but across *all* of them.

Legato remembers when she realized how long the road ahead would be. It was 2004 and she'd just published the first textbook on gender-specific medicine: *Principles of Gender-Specific Medicine.* "When I published the first two-volume edition, which was filled with contributions from over fifty-five experts, I took it to the dean of curriculum at Columbia and I said, 'Here's this new science,' and he actually looked up at me and said, 'Very interesting, but who will we find to teach it?' I never forgot that comment," she says. "My own university certainly has not integrated in any formal way gender-specific medicine in each of the courses that it teaches in medical school. Yes, it makes reference to it, but there is no overall effort to make it a systematic part of everything that we now teach."

And Columbia is not alone. According to a 2011 survey of forty-four medical schools in the United States and Canada, 70 percent of schools indicated that they did not have a formal sex- and gender-specific integrated medical curriculum. Between 45 and 70 percent rated their coverage of areas where evidence of sex/gender differences exists as minimal. A 2006 study took a different approach to assessing the problem. Mining the Association of American Medical Colleges' centralized online curriculum database, they found that about 10 percent of the ninety-five schools that had entered data on their required courses offered a separate interdisciplinary women's health course, which, in most cases, was an elective class that only a small number of (usually women) students took. Coverage of topics of particular concern to women had improved somewhat: more than half the schools reported sessions on topics that disproportionately affect women—for example, migraine, domestic violence, or hormone therapy. But coverage of sex/gender-specific information about conditions that affect both women and men was still minimal; fewer than 30 percent of the schools reported sessions discussing the sex/gender differences in areas like cardiovascular disease, mental health disorders, or substance abuse.

Hopefully that may be changing soon. In October 2015, the SGWHC helped convene an invitational summit on the topic at Mayo Clinic School of Medicine, which brought together curriculum representatives from nearly every American medical school, as well as experts from around the globe. The response, Werbinski says, was really positive, but it was also a reminder of how little has changed. "To many of them it was their first introduction to what we're doing—to thinking that medicine in men and women could be different," she says. One indication of just how far off the radar it was: a number of the participants admitted that they'd come to the conference, which was called the Sex and Gender Medical Education Summit, assuming that it was going to be focused on LGBT health, which was a part, to be sure, of what was covered in the sessions but not the whole thing. "A lot of schools and doctors still have no idea," she says.

Medical students, for their part, are eager for the information. A 2012 case study assessed how well sex/gender-specific knowledge had infiltrated the curriculum at Mayo Clinic School of Medicine, which ranks among the top quarter of medical schools in the country. Surveys of second- and fourth-year students suggested there's wide variation across different clinical areas when it comes to covering these topics. More than half the students indicated sex/gender differences were covered in gynecology, cardiology, and pediatrics; on the other end of the spectrum, less than 20 percent said they were included in nephrology, neurology, and orthopedics. The survey also included a quiz to test the students' own knowledge of such differences, based on an evaluation developed by the European Curriculum in Gender Medicine. For only about half the questions could a majority of students provide the correct answer.

In their comments, many students said the quiz was eye opening. "This test is quite revealing [about] how much I don't know. Thank you," wrote one fourth year, while another said, "My understanding of the effect of sex on biology's pharmacology is less than it should be considering my future career." A second year noted, "Most of the questions in this test were not covered in the curriculum in my memory and I would be interested to learn more." Some had ideas about what it would take for such information to be fully integrated across the curricula: "Surprising to see how few of these concepts were emphasized in our present curriculum. If the national board exams emphasize material, the medical schools will teach it."

It's true: medical schools tend to teach to the test. "But the problem is the sex and gender differences aren't addressed in those exams yet either, because more research needs to be done first, and even in areas where the research is done, it's still not on the radar of the people who write the exams," Werbinski explains. The SGWHC is working to change that too. It convened a group of thirty experts to review all three of the board exams given to medical students to identify the key gaps and propose revisions. They finagled an invitation to discuss its concerns and recommendations with the National Board of Medical Examiners (NBME), which writes the exam questions.

"Their first response to us was, 'We do ask sex and gender questions because we have a whole section on reproductive health,' and we had to educate them that it's not just about reproductive health," Werbinski reports. However, the SGWHC was able to get one of its members on one of the NBME question-writing groups. Unfortunately, they placed her on the "women's health writing group," which, Werbinski explains, is basically just reproductive health, so she's still not in a position to affect the questions on, say, kidney health or immunology. "Because again, everything is siloed in those exams"—and "women's health" is still too often equated with "reproductive health."

While medical students are the most captive audience, and changing the formal education they receive is important, there are other routes to take in the digital age. "The information is at our fingertips and so you don't necessarily have to go to a course to learn it," Werbinski says. The SGWHC is working to influence the content in UpToDate, a popular app used by medical students and doctors that provides evidence-based, physician-authored information on possible diagnoses and treatment options. "If we could influence some of those educational materials, that would be a big coup for us."

KEEP THE PRESSURE ON

Where does this leave women today? To some extent, the slow pace of changing research norms and medical education means that the knowledge gap is destined to close as the seeds planted in the early nineties continue to bear fruit. "We're really talking about a very short period of time that we have now begun to seriously study women and seriously look at sex differences," Mazure has said. "We're just at the beginning of understanding what we need to study, what's important about the findings that we're generating, and where to go from here."

But it would be a mistake to think that continued progress is completely inevitable. A 2012 IOM report concluded that fully integrating an attention to sex/gender differences into biomedical research would require a "culture shift within science." That's a shift that still hasn't fully happened—and may not without ongoing demand from the public. "From my standpoint, we've made progress," Pinn says, "but we still have many gaps in knowledge related to women's health." And she worries that the urgency to close these gaps has waned since the nineties. Without the headline-grabbing examples of all-male studies, complacency can set in. "Continued attention is needed because I'm not sure the thrust is still there as it once was."

It's important to remember the role that grassroots advocacy played in getting the knowledge gap on the radar to begin with, Pinn says. "It was advocacy by individual women, groups of women, and then women in positions of power"—within the biomedical community and Congress—"who really brought forward the concept of women's health." They challenged women's exclusion from clinical research, demanded greater attention to neglected women's conditions, and raised the concern that there may be important sex/gender differences that "hadn't been considered important enough to study." In many ways, this effort was enormously successful, leading to a change in federal law and many reforms that have percolated throughout the medical system.

That, Pinn says, should be a lesson in the power of women's activism. "If you don't have the answers—especially to questions about your health—ask for them. And if the answers don't exist, ask, 'Well, why don't they exist?' And what is being done to ensure that scientific research is still looking to expand what we know, so that we have more knowledge about the conditions that affect the health of women?"

Advocates say individual patients can also create some bottom-up pressure for change by becoming informed themselves and bringing up these issues with their own doctors. Women should "bring the data, which is solid and extensive, to their physicians when they go for treatment," Legato says. "Any attempt of the doctor to say 'I don't have time for this, or I don't believe in that,' should be challenged." Pinn agrees that women, as health care consumers, need "to keep the pressure on" by asking questions of their doctors: "Do I know that this medication really is going to help me? Am I getting the right dosage? Do I know that you're really taking the right tactics in treating me? Is this the right way to prevent a disease in me—or was it studied more in men than in women?"

It's worth pointing out that this is ridiculous. Women should not be required to be more knowledgeable about women's health than their doctors are, and the ultimate goal, of course, is that they no longer need to be. "Hopefully, as the years go by, there'll be more information and women won't have to ask those questions," Greenberger says. "A woman will walk into the office, and the doctor will know whether this test is going to work for her. At some point, the doctors will know this and the patient won't have to."

FROM OBSESSING OVER WOMEN'S POOR HEALTH TO IGNORING IT

There was a real irony to the charge leveled in the early nineties that medicine overlooked biological differences between men and women. For most of its history, that was one of the very last things you could have said about Western medicine. On the contrary, for centuries, medicine had been obsessed with differences—between genders, races, and classes—and had invoked them to justify everything from women's oppression to slavery to eugenics. As sociologist Steven Epstein writes, "Until recently, medical emphases on differences—such as those between women and men or between black people and white people—were closely linked with social notions of superiority and inferiority. By treating variations between genders and races as something fixed in the body, medical theorists helped to reinforce the perception that social inequalities were a straightforward reflection of the natural order of things."

Certainly, the history of Western medicine is littered with examples of treating the male body as the norm—the most perfect representative of the species—but definitely not because it was assumed that women were so alike; women were their own special inferior subgroup. Women were portrayed as dissimilar to men—weaker, abnormal, inherently sickly—in inalterable ways that stemmed from their obviously different reproductive organs but went far beyond them. "The essence of sex is not confined to a single organ but extends, through more or less perceptible nuances into every part," the French physician Pierre Roussel wrote in 1775. Soon doctors were measuring women's skulls and pelvises and concluding that women were lower than men on the evolutionary ladder.

While men may have been the norm, it was women who were imagined as the "typical patient." In the nineteenth century, according to medical historian W. F. Bynum, "more often than not, the abstract patient was referred to as female." And medicine was greatly concerned about her health. "In contrast to the current view that medicine ignores or neglects women," Carol Weisman pointed out in her 1998 book *Women's Health Care: Activist Traditions and Institutional Change*, "the recruitment of women patients was critical, historically, to physicians' practices, and the development and control of medical treatments for women played a key part in the professions' attempts to establish itself both economically and socially."

The roots of this shift within medicine—from obsessing over women's poor health to ignoring it—can be found in the history of hysteria. For centuries it was a label for pretty much everything that went wrong in women's bodies, but by the beginning of the twentieth century, hysteria had come to be considered a mental disorder. The legacy of this transformation has been a persistent assumption that women's symptoms are "all in their heads"—until proven otherwise. This assumption has had incredibly long-lasting effects on what is known about women's health and diseases and how women are treated when they enter the medical system.

CHAPTER 2

THE TRUST GAP

THE PAIN STARTED ON a Friday morning early in Maggie's senior year of college. She'd been fine when she woke up, fine when she went for a run, but about thirty minutes after eating breakfast, she suddenly felt a horrible pain—"the worst I'd ever experienced in my entire life," she says. Within an hour, almost as quickly as it had started, it stopped, so she went about her day. But the pain—in her left abdomen and radiating up into her left shoulder—returned again, once after she hung out with some friends on the quad, and then in her afternoon class. This time, "it was worse than the first two times." Leaving class to take refuge in the bathroom, Maggie fainted in the hallway.

When she came to, the on-campus health services emergency team that had been summoned first asked if she might be pregnant. When she said no, their second question was whether she was on her period. Unsure of what was wrong and about to close for the weekend, the campus clinic sent Maggie on to the emergency room, where the doctors did a couple of tests and told her they could admit her and run some more—it was up to her. Since the pain had completely abated once again, Maggie, famished and stressed about missing her a cappella group's auditions, opted to leave. But that night, after she ate a bag of chips and some pretzel M&M's, the pain returned again. And when it came back the next morning, after she ate a bagel, even the slightest movement triggered such excruciating spasms that she could hardly draw a breath. "That's when I knew something was really wrong."

Her roommate drove her back to the ER, wheeling her into the waiting room because she couldn't walk through the pain. "At this point, there were tears streaming down my cheeks, and I was still gasping for air. The nurse asked, completely unfazed by my appearance, 'What seems to be the problem?' In between gasps, I said that I was in so much pain that I couldn't breathe." Noting that her vitals were normal, he told her, "You need to calm down. I think you're having a panic attack." She said emphatically that she wasn't. She called her mom and handed the phone to the nurse. She heard him say, 'She's a Brown University student and a twenty-one-year-old girl—this is anxiety talking.'"

Maggie would spend the next forty-eight hours in and out of that hospital before the doctors finally figured out what was wrong with her. Until they did, her report of terrible pain would alternately be blamed on being a stressed-out student, a "dramatic" personality, and, finally, a drug seeker looking for prescription painkillers. "I can't even count the number of times I was told to stop 'being hysterical.'"

———

When I first began hearing stories like this—of women whose symptoms were not taken seriously by health care providers, women whose symptoms were brushed off as normal or attributed to depression, anxiety, or "stress," women who were treated as if they were hypochondriacs or being overly dramatic—I initially put it down to women's general lack of authority in a sexist culture.

After all, feminist progress has been an ongoing fight for women's voices—their ideas, their opinions, their accounts of reality—to be taken seriously. Women are still interrupted more in professional settings. They're still quoted less as experts by the media. And forget the authority to speak about the world; some of the most urgent feminist battles have been over women's ability to speak to the conditions of their own lives.

Women still struggle to be believed when they say that their husbands may kill them, or their bosses sexually harassed them, or their classmates raped them. They're still told by everyone from lawmakers to strangers on the Internet that they'll regret their abortions. It's no coincidence that "believe survivors" is a rallying cry of the anti-rape movement and that the slogan "trust women" adorns pro-choice signs.

But the more I thought about it, the less sure I was that I understood why women's accounts of their symptoms so often were not trusted by health care providers. Women seemed to be stereotyped as hypochondriacs whose symptoms were often all in their heads, but I didn't know any women who were hypochondriacs, nor did I see any reason why women would be more hypochondriacal than men. Stereotypes aren't based in fact, but they have usually emerged for some reason, and it wasn't clear to me exactly where this particular stereotype had come from.

My research to figure it out took me all the way back to the root of that word that Maggie's doctors and nurses kept throwing around. When they told her to stop being hysterical, they likely meant it in the modern meaning of the word—to stop being so emotional. But their treatment of her was also informed by the original meaning of word. Before *hysterical* became an adjective, it was a disease.

A BRIEF HISTORY OF HYSTERIA

The word *hysteria* derives from the Greek word for uterus, *hystera*. Although it's a modern myth that ancient Greek medicine described a single distinct disease called hysteria, early Western medical texts did attribute an array of physical and mental symptoms—from menstrual pain to dizziness to paralysis to a sense of suffocation—to the effects of a restless uterus roving about the body; treatments were aimed at either enticing or driving the organ back into its proper place in the pelvis. Since a womb that "remains barren too long after puberty" was especially prone to wandering, the philosopher Plato explained, prompt marriage was another recommended cure. Even as later writers began to doubt the anatomical possibility of a "wandering womb," they continued to see the organ as the source of many mysterious complaints. One of the Hippocratic medical texts from the fifth century BC put it simply: "The womb is the origin of all diseases" in women—a hypothesis that would remain influential in Western medicine for millennia.

During the medieval period, the uterine theory of hysteria gave way to a demonological one. Between the fifth and thirteenth centuries, symptoms that might have previously been blamed on a wandering womb were often seen as *stigmata diaboli*—marks of the devil. "The hysterical female was interpreted alternately as a victim of bewitchment to be pitied and the devil's soul mate to be despised," writes historian Mark S. Micale. Early in the period, she might have been treated with prayer, incantations, and exorcism. But as witch hunts swept the continent in the late medieval and Renaissance periods, she may have been tortured and executed. With the arrival of the scientific revolution in Europe, physicians began to argue that mysterious symptoms "which in the common opinion, are imputed to the Devil, have their true natural causes" as signs of a genuine disease that should be treated medically, as the early seventeenth-century English physician Edward Jorden wrote.

When medical men began resurrecting ancient Greek and Roman medical texts in the seventeenth century, they initially echoed their predecessors' focus on the uterus as the source of nearly all female maladies. As prominent English physician Thomas Willis noted, "When at any time, a sickness happens in a woman's body, of an unusual manner . . . so that its Cause [lies] hid . . . presently we accuse the [evil] influence of the womb . . . and in every unusual Symptom, we declare it to be something hysterical." But by the end of the century, some, including Willis, were laying the blame on a newly recognized system in the body. He argued that "the chief disorder is in the nervous system" in which "animal spirits" released by the brain were carried through the body.

In the eighteenth century, hysteria was increasingly lumped together with various different "nervous disorders." No longer linked directly to the possession of a uterus, they were diagnosed in both sexes. Still, women were considered more vulnerable since, as one British physician put it, they tended to have "a more volatile, dissipable, and weak Constitution of the Spirits, and a more soft, tender and delicate Texture of the Nerves." Since hysteria was stereotyped as a women's disease, male hysterics were often portrayed as effeminate, sensitive, and sometimes homosexual. Doctors also simply created a different label for male sufferers of nervous disorders. Loosely, the male equivalent of hysteria—also known as "the vapors"—was hypochondria, or "the spleen." The two, according to the British physician Thomas Sydenham, were as alike "as one egg is to another."

A plethora of theories and treatments of hysteria proliferated during the nineteenth century, but eventually, an influential theory married the ancient focus on the female reproductive system with the emerging interest in the nervous system. One doctor explained, "The functions of the brain are so intimately connected with the uterine system, that the interruption of any one process which the latter has to perform in the human economy may implicate the former." In short, women were inherently prone to nervous disorders because their reproductive functions—menstruation, pregnancy, lactation, menopause—took a great deal of energy away from their relatively small brains.

The new specialty of gynecology—which emerged in the middle of the nineteenth century—was especially fond of this theory, though opinions differed on which specific reproductive organ was to blame. Some maintained that the uterus was "the controlling organ in the female body," while others thought that it was the ovaries that "give woman all her characteristics of body and mind." Whichever was blamed, the treatments gynecologists offered during heroic medicine's reign were brutal. Almost any symptom in women would get a "local treatment" of the reproductive organs, including injections of various concoctions into the uterus, leeches placed on the vulva, and cauterization of the cervix. For a good decade leading up to the twentieth century, an estimated 150,000 oophorectomies—the removal of perfectly healthy ovaries—were performed in the United States for such afflictions as "troublesomeness, eating like a ploughman, masturbation, attempted suicide, erotic tendencies, persecution mania, simple 'cussedness,' and dysmenorrhea." The trend came to an end mainly because doctors became uncomfortable sterilizing women—or, as one put it, being "the destroyer of everything that makes a woman's life worth living."

In the later part of the nineteenth century, another new specialty was competing with gynecologists for the treatment of hysteria and other nervous disorders: neurology. Disdainful of gynecologists' methods, early American neurologists experimented with electrotherapy, drugs—arsenic, opiates, and others—and Dr. Silas Weir Mitchell's infamous "rest cure." The writer Charlotte Perkins Gilman, who was a former, unsatisfied patient of Mitchell's, gave an unflattering depiction of his regime in her well-known short story "The Yellow Wallpaper." For several weeks, the patient would be confined to bed in a dimly lit room, allowed to see only the doctor and a nurse, and forbidden from reading, writing, or doing anything else besides eating fattening foods and receiving a daily massage. The theory went that the cure was such "bitter medicine" that when Mitchell commanded the patient to get better at the end of it, she would bend to his will.

The French researcher Jean-Martin Charcot, considered the "father of modern neurology," on the other hand, felt that nothing could be done to treat hysteria, which he believed was a degenerative neurological disease. In the 1870s he gave a series of packed public talks demonstrating the bizarre contortions and fits his hysterical patients would have while they were under hypnosis. Another prominent American neurologist, George Beard, was responsible for coming up with a respectable, new label for men's nervous symptoms: *neurasthenia*—or weakness of the nerves. ("Hypochondria" no longer sufficed since it had gradually come to take on its broader, contemporary meaning.) Neurasthenia's primary symptom was fatigue, accompanied by seventy other possible symptoms—which overlapped with hysteria's wide array of possible symptoms—and it was eventually diagnosed in women and men with about equal frequency. While women continued to be seen as prone to nervous disorders because of "something fundamental in their nature, something innate, fixed or given," among elite gentlemen, the same symptoms were often attributed to overwork and the stresses of urban, industrial modern life.

The uterine-nerve theory of hysteria proved especially useful for keeping women in their proper place; one might even suspect it was designed to. The precarious balancing act between the reproductive organs and brain meant that great swaths of a woman's life—puberty, menstruation, pregnancy, and menopause—were all considered periods of "ill health" when her body could easily be thrown into dangerous disorder—by any activity, really, but especially by mentally taxing ones. So, Mitchell warned, "It were better not to educate girls at all between the ages of fourteen and eighteen, unless it can be done with careful reference to their bodily health." In the midst of debate over allowing women to attend Harvard, Dr. Edward H. Clarke, a professor at the school, published *Sex in Education; or, A Fair Chance for the Girls*, in which he reviewed the medical literature and concluded that higher education would cause women's uteri to atrophy. As for pursuing a career, another doctor noted, "One shudders to think of the conclusions arrived at by female bacteriologists or histologists at the period when their entire system, both physical and mental, is, so to speak 'unstrung,' to say nothing of the terrible mistakes which a lady surgeon might make under similar conditions."

The scientific "fact" of a zero-sum tug-of-war between women's reproductive functions and their brains was transparently self-serving for the young male-dominated medical profession—doubly so. "The theory of female frailty obviously disqualified women as healers," Ehrenreich and English write. "At the same time the theory made women highly qualified as patients." The economic self-interest driving doctors' growing concern about women's health was not lost on some of the few female doctors who'd broken into the profession by the end of the nineteenth century. As Dr. Mary Putnam Jacobi wrote drily in 1895, "I think, finally, it is in the increased attention paid to women, and especially in their new function as lucrative patients, scarily imagined a hundred years ago, that we find explanation for much of the ill-health among women, freshly discovered today."

But, of course, many women *didn't* make lucrative patients. Conveniently enough, nineteenth-century "science" showed that black women and working-class white women were magically resistant to the health problems that plagued well-off white women. One physician noted, "The African negress, who toils beside her husband in the fields of the south, and Bridget, who washes, and scrubs and toils in our homes at the north, enjoy for the most part good health, with comparative immunity from uterine disease." In a remarkably lucky boon to the new medical profession, it was only those women who had the time and the money to be treated who were prone to perpetual illness and in need of their services. And it was only women trying to push into professional work—those aspiring bacteriologists, histologists, and surgeons—who faced such dire health consequences from working.

As the nineteenth century wore on, though, doctors' accounts of hysteria and other female nervous disorders were increasingly marked by a note of suspicion and frustration. In part, this attitude stemmed from a sense that women were bringing ill health upon themselves by denying their prescribed roles. Historian Ann Douglas Wood explains, "One finds an underlying logic running through popular books by physicians on women's diseases to the effect that ladies get sick because they are unfeminine—in other words, sexually aggressive, intellectually ambitious, and defective in proper womanly submission and selflessness." Mitchell, for example, though convinced hysteria was a physical disease, admitted the hysterical woman was the "hated charge" of his specialty, a "self-made invalid" who was "like a vampire, slowly sucking the blood of every healthy, helpful creature within reach of her demands."

There were also some concerns that hysterical women were just faking their symptoms—for attention or sympathy, or to avoid their domestic duties. One British doctor described the typical hysterical woman as a "performer" who must be convinced through "shame and humiliation" to accept that "she has nothing at all the matter with her, and is, in reality, in perfectly good health: her ailments being, one and all, fraudulent imitations of real disease." While earlier in its history, the profession may have welcomed wealthy chronically ill women as a cash cow, the public increasingly expected their doctors to actually help them; patients who didn't get better were a reproach to medicine's confidence in its growing knowledge.

And growing it was. Thanks to advances in anatomy, physiology, pathology, and microbiology over the course of the nineteenth century, the field was starting to have some success in matching laboratory findings to patients' symptoms. Gradually, it was adopting the view that all symptoms could be traced back to a particular visible, measurable pathology—a shift that was solidified with the acceptance of germ theory in the 1880s. The discovery that infectious diseases were caused by specific microbes strengthened the growing belief that all diseases had a specific cause. This was a new idea. Previously, diseases were defined as collections of symptoms; "fever" or "pains" were disease categories in their own right. As historian of medicine Charles Rosenberg writes, "Recognizably modern notions of specific, mechanism-based ailments with characteristic clinical courses were a product of the nineteenth century."

This transformation led to an important change in the way medicine thought about symptoms. Before, doctors had no choice but to take patients at their word about what they were experiencing in their bodies; after all, without any tools to see within the body and without the foggiest notion, really, about what caused most diseases, they usually didn't have anything else to go on. But as diseases came to be categorized based on the physiological disturbance at their root, symptoms were transformed into clues that could help the doctors uncover their source. The patients' subjective reports of what they felt—pain, dizziness, nausea, et cetera—were becoming "complaints" that became symptoms of a disease only once the doctor—assisted by the ever-growing arsenal of laboratory tests and technologies he'd begun accumulating by the beginning of the twentieth century—found an objectively observable cause that explained them.

It's within this context that the final phase in hysteria's history occurred. In the late 1800s, Sigmund Freud abandoned the neurological theory of hysteria in favor of a psychological one. In his famous case studies of hysterical women, he argued that psychological conflict—or "strangulated affect"—was "converted" into physical symptoms. Describing this process as "the puzzling leap from the mental to the physical," he left it to others to fill in how it actually worked. Initially, Freud suggested that hysteria arose when traumatic memories—usually of sexual abuse—that had been repressed deep into "the unconscious" found expression in the body in a symbolic manner. Later, backing off from the implications of that assertion, he decided that it wasn't actual sexual abuse—just fantasies of it—that converted into hysterical symptoms. The symptoms would disappear, he believed, if the patient consciously recalled the psychological distress, through a technique of "free association" of his invention: psychoanalysis. As historian Carroll Smith-Rosenberg puts it, psychoanalysis is "the child of the hysterical woman."

For millennia, hysteria had been considered a physical ailment that could cause a wide array of mostly physical symptoms. But in the post-Freud era, it came to be seen as a mental disorder that caused physical symptoms.

After alternately tracing all of women's unexplained aliments back to a wandering womb or demonic possession or sensitive nerves, medicine finally punted them over to the psyche. As Ehrenreich and English write, "Under Freud's influence, the scalpel for the dissection of female nature eventually passed from the gynecologist to the psychiatrist." And medicine's view of women "shifted from 'physically sick' to 'mentally ill.'"

The psychologization of hysteria, arriving just as medicine increasingly defined "real" diseases as those it could see with its current technologies and explain by a known physiological mechanism, introduced the idea that any symptoms it *couldn't* yet see and explain—particularly those that occurred in women—could be blamed on the unknowable "unconscious mind," a theory that medicine has liberally utilized whenever it comes up against the limits of its knowledge. It has led to the persistent distrust of women's subjective reports of their own bodies—until those reports are backed up by objective evidence.

THE DISORDERS FORMERLY KNOWN AS HYSTERIA

One of the biggest myths about hysteria is that it disappeared in the first part of the twentieth century. That's what scholars concluded when they first began writing histories of the condition. As one French historian wrote, "Hysteria is dead, that it is certain. It has taken its secrets with it to the grave." But few provided hypotheses about how and why exactly this disease, once supposedly so common, mysteriously disappeared in a matter of decades. To the extent that they did, most offered explanations that largely accepted Freud's theory of the condition: one common conclusion was that before the twentieth century, people in the West were more psychologically "primitive," prone to expressing their mental distress through physical symptoms, but as the public became more knowledgeable about psychological concepts, they were more likely to simply develop depression or anxiety disorders instead.

Even many second-wave feminist accounts of hysteria left something to be desired. They tended to highlight the fact that by the end of the nineteenth century, doctors seemed to be labeling as "hysteria" any behavior in women they disliked—particularly rebellious claims to autonomy and equality. In other words, women weren't actually sick; doctors were just saying they were. Other feminist accounts of hysteria, largely accepting a psychological theory of the condition, have portrayed nineteenth-century hysterical women's "flight into illness" as an unconscious protest against their oppression in a patriarchal culture. In this telling, the decline of hysteria was the result of feminist progress: women got closer to equality and got better.

But while there's no doubt some truth to these accounts, they tend to leave out the most mundane explanation for hysteria: that most of the women lumped into this broad diagnostic category were indeed sick. Sick with a multitude of physical ailments that a medical profession in its infancy—that didn't accept germ theory until the 1880s and didn't have the X-ray until 1895—was not yet capable of differentiating. After all, it is not as though physicians were diagnosing "hysteria" *in addition* to the thousands of diseases we recognize today. As Micale writes, the term "came to mean so many different things that, by around 1900 it ceased to mean anything at all."

It's understandable that second-wave feminists would be reluctant to focus on that explanation for hysteria. After all, for centuries, medicine had been insisting that women were sick, that they were sick because women were *inherently* sick, and that this justified their inferior social status. But one needn't accept the second and third conclusions to accept the first. Indeed, if women were in poor health, that could just as easily be taken as an indictment of the medical system that was treating them. Harriot Hunt, one of the earliest women doctors in the United States, pointed out in 1856, "Man, man alone has had the care of us [women], and I would ask how our health stands now. Does it do credit to his skill?"

So to the extent that hysteria seemed to become less common during the first half of the twentieth century, it was because this bloated diagnostic category inevitably shrunk as medical knowledge grew. In a process that Micale called "diagnostic drift," what would have been called hysteria a generation ago was likely to instead fall into one of numerous newly recognized diagnoses, creating only "the retrospective illusion of a disappearance of the pathological entity itself." For example, during the time that "hysteria" was on the decline—particularly the dramatic fits and paralysis that had so captured the medical imagination—doctors were getting much better at diagnosing neurological conditions like epilepsy, multiple sclerosis, and the neurological effects of syphilis. Many scholars have hazarded retrospective diagnoses of the women that Freud (mis)diagnosed with "hysteria": Anna O. perhaps would today be diagnosed with temporal lobe epilepsy—a condition that wasn't diagnosable until the electroencephalogram became widely available in the 1940s—or perhaps tuberculous meningitis; Frau Emmy von N., Tourette's syndrome; Elisabeth von R., pelvic appendicitis.

But even as many conditions drifted out of the hysteria category as they were recognized as distinct diseases, the psychological concept of hysteria remained. One of the innovations of Freud's theory was that it transformed hysteria from a single disease category (though one with a suspiciously long list of potential symptoms) into a theoretical process—the "conversion" of psychological distress into physical symptoms. And another likely reason for hysteria's apparent decline post-Freud is that once the condition wasn't considered an organic disease, physicians no longer considered "hysterical" symptoms to be their problem. "A generation ago," one American doctor wrote in the late 1970s, "a diagnosis of hysteria meant a patient with a conversion reaction (a symptom with no evident physical cause). Either placebos were prescribed or the patient was shipped off to an analyst for psychotherapy. Neither approach benefited the patient much, but both helped the physician rid his practice of 'crocks' so he could concentrate on 'treating sick people.'"

As the term *hysteria* gradually entered the popular lexicon with its modern meaning of excessive, uncontrollable emotionality, a less pejorative term was needed. By the 1960s, a few new euphemisms had started to take its place.

Though the idea of hysteria as a single disease marked by an incoherent multitude of symptoms had briefly disappeared, in the 1960s, a group of American researchers resurrected it and rechristened the condition "Briquet's syndrome," after a nineteenth-century French physician who had studied hysteria. According to their diagnostic criteria, a patient would qualify if she—and it was almost always a "she"—had a lifetime history of at least twenty-five of fifty-nine possible symptoms in nine of ten different symptom areas before the age of thirty-five and no diagnosis of an organic disease that could explain them. Its possible symptoms included essentially every possible symptom under the sun: headaches, blindness, paralysis, fits, fatigue, a lump in the throat, fainting spells, dizziness, chest pain, visual blurring, weakness, abdominal pain, vomiting, diarrhea, menstrual disorders, changes in sexual interest, pains in various parts of the body, nervousness, fears, depressed feelings, and difficulties with breathing, weight, and eating.

Meanwhile, the concept of *somatization* was also taking hold. First coined in the 1920s by Viennese psychoanalyst Wilhelm Stekel, who defined it as the "process by which neurotic conflicts appear as a physical disorder," it was expanded in the late sixties by American psychiatrist Zbigniew J. Lipowski. Acknowledging that the idea was "related to, if not identical with" the Freudian concept of conversion, Lipowski described it as "the tendency to experience and communicate psychologic distress in the form of somatic symptoms that the patient misinterprets as signifying serious physical illness." "Somatizing" mental distress was considered common, but it became a psychological disorder when patients kept insisting they were sick though doctors had concluded that they were not. "Patients with persistent somatization relentlessly seek medical diagnosis and treatment despite repeated reassurance that physical illness is either absent or insufficient to account for their symptoms and disability."

As Freudian theory's influence on American medicine peaked during the middle of the century, a new subspecialty of "psychosomatic medicine" was born. At the height of its popularity, the field was looking for the "mental states" and "personality factors" involved in a wide range of organic diseases, including cancer and heart disease. Still, it considered some diseases to be more influenced by the mind than others—such "psychosomatic disorders" included asthma, ulcers, and hypertension—and they tended to be those that medicine didn't yet know much about in biological terms. As Susan Sontag argued in her famous 1978 book *Illness as Metaphor*, psychological theories of illness "are always an index of how much is not understood about the physical terrain of a disease." (The field suffered a blow to its reputation when stomach ulcers, long believed to be caused by stress, were linked to the bacteria *Helicobacter pylori*.)

And despite the more narrow definition of *psychosomatic* used by experts in the specialty, in general medicine—as well as in popular culture—it often came to be used as a synonym of *psychogenic* (having its origin in the mind) in contrast to *organic* (having its origin in bodily organs). Another euphemism for *hysterical*.

"DOES THE PATIENT ACCEPT HERSELF AS A WOMAN?"

By the 1970s, women were beginning to complain that they seemed to be particularly vulnerable to this kind of medical psychologizing. They were more likely to have their physical symptoms dismissed as psychogenic when they presented to their doctors, and medicine seemed especially fond of blaming conditions unique to them on psychological factors. As scholar Shari Munch notes, "there was remarkable agreement among both scholars and lay community that this problem existed," and in the late seventies studies began to document it.

In explaining this "gender-biased diagnosing," some pointed to differences in how men and women tended to communicate with their doctors. A 1981 study hypothesized, "The open and emotional behavioral style used by women in reporting their illnesses may prompt physicians to react to women's complaints as though they were expressions of emotional problems, whereas the more stoic style found in men reporting a similar complaint does not elicit a psychosomatic diagnosis from the physician." But their study offered only partial support for the theory. "Even non-expressive female patients were judged to have psychosomatic problems," the authors wrote, "as though women were *a priori* more emotional creatures than men." Another study on the problem concluded that doctors "might be responding to current stereotypes that regard the male as typically stoic and the female as typically hypochondriacal."

But medicine wasn't just "responding to" a stereotype that was in the air; it was also perpetuating it. If doctors believed women's symptoms were likely to be "all in their heads," the most immediate reason for that was that their medical education was teaching them so.

Though there were still very few women physicians at the time, they helped expose the problem. In a 1974 article entitled "What Medical Schools Teach About Women," Dr. Mary C. Howell, the first woman dean at Harvard Medical School, wrote, "Following traditional linguistic convention, patients in most medical-school lectures are referred to exclusively by the male pronoun, 'he.' There is, however, a notable exception: in discussing a hypothetical patient whose disease is of psychogenic origin, the lecturer often automatically uses 'she.' For it is widely taught, both explicitly and implicitly, that women patients (when they receive notice at all) have uninteresting illnesses, are unreliable historians, and are beset by such emotionality that their symptoms are unlikely to reflect 'real' disease."

According to a 1973 survey of over a hundred female students in forty-one American medical schools conducted by Howell, their lectures were filled with references to women as "hysterical mothers," "hypochondriacs," and "old ladies" whom doctors must "manage." One student described being told by a surgeon that a young woman with abdominal pain "was by definition an 'unreliable historian.'" Another explained, "Often women are portrayed as hysterical or as nagging mothers or as having trivial complaints. Men are almost never pointed to as having a psychological component to their illnesses—this is generally attributed to women." In fact, another noted, "Women's illnesses are assumed psychosomatic until proven otherwise."

The portrayal of women as particularly prone to psychogenic symptoms was formally taught as scientific "fact" in textbooks too. A 1971 gynecology text warned that "many women, wittingly or unwittingly, exaggerate the severity of their complaints to gratify neurotic desires." It advised doctors to be on the lookout for psychological and "personality factors" that contribute to everything from urinary problems to infertility to back pain, and suggested that the surest way to tell whether the source of the symptom was physical or psychological was to consider the question, "Does the patient accept herself as a woman?"

If a woman attempted to resist her feminine role, this mental conflict could emerge in a number of symbolic ways—particularly in disorders affecting her reproductive system. According to the textbook, in cases of dysmenorrhea (painful menstruation) "a thorough study of the woman's

attitudes toward femininity is often necessary." Nausea during early pregnancy—the morning sickness experienced by the vast majority of pregnant patients—"may indicate resentment, ambivalence and inadequacy
in women ill-prepared for motherhood." Just as in the nineteenth century,
women were still thought to bring illness upon themselves by failing to be
properly womanly—only now their symptoms were all in their heads.

MEDICALLY UNEXPLAINED . . . BY WHOM?

The concept of hysteria has an impressive ability to adjust to changing times.
Freudian theory fell firmly out of favor in American medicine in the 1970s.
The feminist movement radically expanded the roles available to women.
Yet medicine retained the idea that unexplained physical symptoms could
be attributed to the mind. When the third edition of the *Diagnostic and
Statistical Manual of Mental Disorders (DSM)* was published in 1980, hysteria had been removed, but there was a new section: the "somatoform disorders." For the next two decades these disorders described patients whose
physical symptoms were "not explained by a general medical condition"
and were judged to be caused by psychological factors. As Lipowski wrote,
"The somatoform disorders have been mostly derived from the wreckage of
what used to be called hysteria."

A simplified criteria for Briquet's syndrome—now renamed "somatization disorder"—was included, requiring a lifetime history of fourteen of
thirty-seven possible symptoms. (In a subsequent revision, it was further
streamlined to require just eight of thirty-two symptoms distributed among
four symptom groups.) "Conversion disorder" applied to unexplained neurological symptoms, like paralysis, seizures, and amnesia. "Psychogenic
pain disorder" (eventually revised to just "pain disorder") described unexplained chronic pain in any part of the body. "Hypochondriasis" was
reserved for patients with "medically unexplained symptoms" who also
had an intense fear of having a serious illness. A couple of residual categories, "undifferentiated somatoform disorder" and "somatoform disorder
not otherwise specified," covered any unexplained symptoms that didn't fit
neatly into any of the other labels.

With the exception of hypochondriasis, all the somatoform disorders were described as more common among women. They were also reported to be more prevalent among patients with less education, those with lower incomes, and people of color. Somatization disorder, like its immediate predecessor Briquet's syndrome, was considered to be almost exclusively a female ailment—ten times more common in women than men. In the mideighties, a couple of researchers came up with a screening test for the disorder. While technically the *DSM* criteria required fourteen of thirty-seven possible symptoms at that time, they argued that just three or more of seven "highly suspicious" ones indicated a high probability of the disorder: shortness of breath, dysmenorrhea, burning in sex organs, lump in throat, amnesia, vomiting, and painful extremities. The mnemonic aid they offered for remembering them: "Somatization Disorder Besets Ladies and Vexes Physicians."

Meanwhile, more euphemisms have popped up over the last few decades. The term *functional* initially did not imply a psychogenic cause—only the lack of a discernible organic one—but it has come to be used that way in practice. As Dr. David Edelberg wrote in a 2012 article in *AMA Journal of Ethics*, "'Functional' [is] the contemporary term for what was 'psychosomatic' 50 years ago and 'hysterical' a century ago." Or as Lipowski wrote, "The symptoms of somatizing patients have been called 'functional,' 'psychosomatic,' 'psychogenic,' and 'somatoform.' All these terms imply that however strongly such symptoms suggest physical illness, they belong to a different realm and are but an imitation of the 'real' thing."

In recent years, the phrase *medically unexplained symptoms*—often abbreviated as MUS—has also been added to that list of terms. While on its face a neutral description, it is also often used to imply a psychogenic origin. In an analysis of seventy-five articles on "medically unexplained symptoms," Annemarie Goldstein Jutel, author of *Putting a Name to It: Diagnosis in Contemporary Society*, found that half of them used the phrase interchangeably with psychiatric terms such as *somatoform disorder* and *somatization*. Less than a quarter of the articles critiqued that tendency. Again, "following a frequently challenged but nonetheless surprisingly resilient dualistic perspective," one article explains, "if no disease is found in the body, it is assumed that the disease is 'all in the mind' and that symptoms that are medically unexplained are considered, by default, to be 'psychiatrically explained.'"

Though these terms—*somatoform, functional, MUS*—are used by researchers and doctors among themselves, they often aren't used with patients. Physicians are in the unenviable position of trying to explain to patients why they are having symptoms that they believe to be, by definition, unexplained, and ideally to do so without implying that the symptoms are "all in their heads," despite the fact that, by and large, that's exactly how medicine thinks of them. In one 2009 study, doctors reported that they most commonly reassured patients with "medically unexplained symptoms" that "nothing's wrong" because diagnostic tests had come back negative. They also used metaphors to explain why they might be feeling poorly. Often, they normalized the patients' complaints, telling them that having symptoms is just a part of life. Almost invariably patients do not find these explanations reassuring.

Patient accounts suggest that unexplained symptoms are frequently attributed to depression or anxiety, causing no small amount of confusion for patients who were under the impression that to have a mood disorder one needed to actually *feel* depressed or anxious. And, perhaps above all else, patients have their "medically unexplained symptoms" attributed to "stress." In an afterword to his influential 2007 book *How Doctors Think*, Dr. Jerome Groopman, chief of experimental medicine at Beth Israel Deaconess Medical Center, wrote that, based on the many stories he'd heard from patients since its publication, "It seemed that 'stress' had become a catchall term to explain problems that were not readily unraveled." To be sure, depression, anxiety, and prolonged stress can cause specific physical symptoms, but these symptoms are not limitless, nor are they actually unexplained. When doctors invoke these labels for symptoms as diverse as vomiting, paralysis, and severe, unending pain, it is the concept of the somatoform disorders—hysteria dressed up in modern garb—that allows them to do so.

Meanwhile, when the fifth edition of the *DSM* was published in 2013, the somatoform category had been revamped significantly. Somatization disorder, hypochondriasis, pain disorder, and undifferentiated somatoform disorder had been replaced with a single disorder, somatic symptom disorder (SSD), characterized by one or more "symptoms that are either very distressing or result in significant disruption of functioning, as well as excessive and disproportionate thoughts, feelings and behaviors regarding those symptoms." Freud's old conversion disorder is still there, now with the subtitle "functional neurological symptom disorder." While previously, the somatoform disorders had involved only symptoms that were "medically unexplained," in the new SSD, the symptoms may or may not be explained by a medical problem. Now the disorder hinges on whether the patient's concern about them is judged—by a doctor—to be "excessive."

In a biting critique in *BMJ*, Dr. Allen Frances, chair of the *DSM-IV* task force, argued that without even a reminder to attempt to "rule out other explanations" before concluding that a psychological disorder is present, the new label would lead to missed diagnoses of underlying medical causes, as well as risk "casually mislabeling the physically ill as also mentally disordered." A trial study suggested that 15 percent of cancer patients, 15 percent of patients with heart disease, 26 percent with IBS, and 26 percent with fibromyalgia would qualify for a diagnosis of SSD, as would 7 percent of healthy people. Particularly women: "Millions of people could be mislabeled, with the burden falling disproportionately on women," Frances wrote, "because they are more likely to be casually dismissed as 'catastrophizers' when presenting with physical symptoms."

It is convenient that "medically unexplained symptoms" has become the latest label to be applied to allegedly hysterical symptoms since the term itself—and the way medicine uses it—highlight the problems with the whole concept. Studies have estimated that up to a third of patients in primary care, and up to two-thirds of those in specialty clinics, have "medically unexplained symptoms." Approximately 70 percent of them are women. But, of course, symptoms are not explained or unexplained per se; symptoms are explained by individual doctors when they make a diagnosis. Some patients with "medically unexplained symptoms" then are those whose symptoms simply haven't been explained *yet*. Many millions of people in this country experience long delays and see multiple health care providers before getting correctly diagnosed: Four years, on average, for patients with autoimmune diseases. Seven for patients with rare diseases. As many as ten for those with endometriosis. Yet most of the medical literature on "medically unexplained symptoms" seems to take place in an alternate reality where diagnoses are always made accurately on the first try.

And on the collective level, diseases are explained by scientific research, and what science can explain is changing all the time. At this point in medical history, the pattern has repeated itself again and again: a step forward in medical knowledge and yesterday's mysterious, psychogenic-by-default conditions suddenly become medically explained. Nearly all the diseases mentioned in this book were at one point attributed to women's neuroses or repressed anger or hidden traumas. The dynamic that's all too familiar to individual women—of symptoms dismissed as "all in your head" until objective tests confirm that the symptoms are real and correspond to a specific disease—is a mini-drama of the story that's played out collectively throughout history. As Jutel writes, "It is not unusual for physical diseases to be incorrectly attributed to psychiatric disorder either early in the disease history of an individual or in the history of the disease itself."

Yet despite this record, each generation of medical practitioners has remained remarkably confident in the theories and technologies of the current era, treating what is currently "medically unexplained" as if it is, in fact, unexplain*able*—even to a doctor in the future with greater knowledge and more precise tests. In treating "medically unexplained symptoms" as if it is a unified condition, Jutel points out, medicine resorts to "creating a catch-all diagnostic category in which it can place the unexplained." And in attributing a psychogenic cause to "medically unexplained symptoms," medicine "presumes the infallibility of the physician and the omniscience of medicine."

Hysteria, in its many modern-day labels, remains, as French physician Charles Lasègue wrote in the mid-1800s, "the wastepaper basket of medicine where one throws otherwise unemployed symptoms."

"A DISGUISE FOR IGNORANCE AND A FERTILE SOURCE OF CLINICAL ERROR"

Maggie's mother had managed to convince the nurse that Maggie, who didn't have a history of anxiety, wasn't having a panic attack. But once a chest X-ray, blood tests, and a CT scan came back normal, the ER doctor was ready to discharge her. First, though, she wanted to see whether Maggie could eat something without pain. She couldn't; the pain came back worse than ever. The doctor admitted her for observation overnight but said she doubted further testing would reveal anything really wrong. In the morning, once again, Maggie was given graham crackers and saltines. "Once again, the pain returned with such intensity that I could not stand up or move." But a nurse reported that the doctor had already discharged her, without waiting for the results of the cracker test. As the pain worsened, Maggie begged the nurse to call a doctor. "She refused, said that my tests were normal, that I should stop being dramatic and told me, 'You were not in pain until you were told you were being discharged.'"

Figuring they had no choice, she and her mom, who'd gotten on a plane and joined her in the hospital by this point, left. Once discharged, Maggie spent the next fourteen hours in so much pain she couldn't speak, stand up, or eat. "According to my mother, at times I was silently rocking back and forth, totally withdrawn—as if in a trance. I only remember being certain I was going to die soon and what a shame that would be, but I didn't have the energy to explain or fight or even be afraid."

———

For a long time, critics have pointed out that there's a high risk of misdiagnosis inherent in the concept of psychogenic illness—whether it's called hysteria, somatization, or "medically unexplained symptoms" due to stress. In one of the most influential discussions of the problem, the British psychiatrist Eliot Slater warned in a 1965 editorial that too often a label of hysteria just allowed doctors to believe they'd solved the mystery when, in fact, most of the time they hadn't. After following up with eighty-five patients who'd been diagnosed with hysteria at the National Hospital in London throughout the fifties—including by Slater himself—he discovered that, nine years later, more than 60 percent had been found to have an organic neurological disease, including brain tumors and epilepsy; a dozen of them had died. "The diagnosis of 'hysteria,'" he concluded, "is a disguise for ignorance and a fertile source of clinical error. It is, in fact, not only a delusion but also a snare."

The reason it is such a dangerous "snare" is that there's a stark imbalance in the burden of proof needed to make a psychogenic diagnosis versus an organic one. To attribute a symptom to a physical disease, observable evidence of pathology is required, but to label it psychogenic, all you need—indeed, since there's no test for psychogenesis, the best you'll ever have—is a strong suspicion. As medical journalist Laurie Endicott Thomas points out, this is a uniquely low bar: "The lack of an objective test for psychological disorders is something that hampers the whole field, but the somatoform disorders are the only mental health diagnosis that are based not on a description of symptoms but instead on speculation about their cause." Once symptoms are suspected of being psychogenic and the doctor starts looking for a source of stress that might be to blame, it's usually not hard to find one.

Worse still, a patient doesn't even have to show any signs of being stressed, depressed, anxious, or otherwise emotionally distressed at all to get a psychogenic diagnosis. According to theories of conversion and somatization, psychogenic symptoms are thought to be produced when the psychological distress causing them is repressed, pushed deep into the inaccessible unconscious, precisely in order to avoid consciously feeling psychological distress. Lipowski explained that consequently, "a patient with somatization will often deny being depressed or anxious or will assert that any emotional distress he or she is experiencing results from physical suffering and disability. Neither such explicit denial nor the patient's causal interpretation needs to be accepted as necessarily correct, as either may be misleading." A psychogenic diagnosis thus most frequently involves a doctor telling a patient that there is no physical ailment even though her body feels sick and that there is a mental disorder even though she doesn't feel emotionally distressed.

In practice, then, a psychogenic diagnosis tends to be what's known as a "diagnosis of exclusion." As Jutel explains, "It is a diagnosis made not on the basis of what it is but on the basis of what it is not. The absence of explanation, rather than the presence of a well-defined feature, defines the condition." But, of course, the doctor could prematurely decide the symptoms are "medically unexplained" and therefore miss the correct diagnosis for a great many reasons, including but not limited to the disease being rare and/

or difficult to diagnose, the patient having an atypical presentation, a test being inaccurate or misread, or the doctor simply making a mistake—as human beings inevitably do on occasion—and not thinking of the correct diagnosis.

Despite these risks, incredibly, there is more discussion in the medical literature on somatoform disorders on the risks of *doing* a thorough investigation into medical causes than of not. The American Academy of Family Physicians, for example, advises doctors to consider the possibility of a somatoform disorder "early in the evaluation process" in order to limit "unnecessary diagnostic and medical treatments." The worry, as one article explained, is that "out of a fear of overlooking a serious disease, many physicians give their patients full physical examinations and interventions, thereby incorrectly confirming the somatic nature of their condition." To be sure, there are real risks to overtesting that should be minimized in any patient, but the idea that doctors could determine whether symptoms are "medically unexplained" before attempting to explain them would seem to be a contradiction in terms.

And yet, many doctors do apparently believe that they can somehow intuit whether a patient's symptoms will turn out to be "medically unexplained"—and do so quite quickly. In a 2016 Dutch study, family physicians reported that they suspected patients' symptoms were MUS if they had many symptoms and had had lots of previous doctor's visits and referrals. They also considered the "subtle feelings" the patients provoked in them to be a clue. One of those feelings was confusion. One doctor explained, "I believe I know what is going on within 30 [seconds], like many of us. When I think within 2 [minutes] 'I do not have a clue of what is going on here,' then I start to think 'This can be [MUS].'" The other feeling was "irritation" at the patient. Most of the respondents "stated that when they did not feel empathy for their patients, they were more often inclined to recognize symptoms as [MUS]." A 2000 British study found a similar pattern: of the cases that the doctors had initially diagnosed as "unexplained," 17 percent were later found to be "explained," and the single biggest factor that increased the likelihood of misdiagnosis was if the physician felt the interaction with the patient had been negative.

The danger here is just compounded by the fact that a psychogenic diagnosis, while easy to make, is very difficult to overturn. All misdiagnoses are vulnerable to confirmation bias (the tendency to see new evidence only if it's in line with your existing theory), but a psychogenic diagnosis is a particularly sticky one because the only exonerating evidence that could show it to be false—proof of an organic pathology—is exactly what doctors have now ceased looking for. Once doctors have settled on the conclusion that "nothing's wrong," further investigation halts, making it all the more unlikely that they will uncover anything wrong. And once you have been labeled an unreliable reporter, it becomes all but impossible to get your credibility back.

Indeed, there's a circular logic built into psychogenic theories that ensures that once a doctor has decided the symptoms are psychogenic, pretty much anything the patient does will just reinforce that perception. According to the medical literature, some of the "red flags" that suggest patients may be suffering from a somatoform disorder include repeatedly seeking medical care—described as "doctor shopping"—despite assurances that they have no organic disease and denying that their symptoms are psychogenic. In fact, according to one prominent British proponent of psychogenic explanations for "medically unexplained" syndromes, "The vehemence with which many patients insist that their illness is medical rather than psychiatric has become one of the hallmarks of the conditions."

Of course, there's another group of patients who tend to insist their illness is medical and "doctor shop" until they get a diagnosis: people suffering from yet-to-be-diagnosed physical diseases. That such behavior could be considered a "hallmark" sign that there is in fact no organic disease at all is an absurd and very dangerous logic. The possibility of a psychogenic diagnosis creates a system in which trying to get an explanation for persistent or worsening symptoms puts a patient at risk of acquiring a mental health diagnosis right up until the moment the correct diagnosis is made. In fact, the actions that are often *required* to get a diagnosis in a fragmented and inefficient medical system may be seen as "abnormal illness behaviors" until, finally graced by the legitimacy afforded by a medical diagnosis, they retrospectively become the perfectly rational actions of a sick—and no doubt increasingly desperate—patient. As one patient with chronic fatigue syndrome put it, "The difference between a crazed neurotic and a seriously ill person is simply a test."

There is remarkably little concern about the possibility of missed diagnoses in discussions of the somatoform disorders or "medically unexplained symptoms." "In medicine, resistance to the notion of error in somatoform diagnoses is so thoroughly pervasive that there exist no precautions of any kind, no protocols, and no forms of oversight to ensure that as few patients as possible are mistakenly diagnosed," writes Diane O'Leary, a bioethicist and former director of the Coalition for Diagnostic Rights. The criteria for the somatoform disorders call for "appropriate medical evaluation" before concluding the symptoms aren't explained by a medical condition. But in a medical landscape in which there are currently over 10,000 known diseases, over 5,000 diagnostic tests, and over 120 medical specialties and subspecialties, it's entirely an individual doctor's subjective opinion when the search for a medical explanation can be exhausted and symptoms attributed to the patient's mind by default.

I soon learned that this disconnect is reflective of a bigger problem. According to experts like Dr. Mark Graber, founder and president of the Society to Improve Diagnosis in Medicine, diagnostic errors are a "large and silent problem" that has begun to be acknowledged only in the last decade or so. In 2015, an IOM report concluded, "For decades, diagnostic errors—inaccurate or delayed diagnoses—have represented a blind spot in the delivery of quality health care" and "continue to harm an unacceptable number of patients." The Society to Improve Diagnosis in Medicine estimates that each year, 40,000 to 80,000 people die due to diagnostic errors in the United States. A 2014 study concluded that 12 million Americans who see their primary care doctor each year experience a diagnostic error. According to a *conservative* estimate published in *The BMJ* in 2016, medical errors in general are the third leading cause of death in the United States, after heart disease and cancer.

Experts in diagnostic errors provided an answer to the puzzle that had been nagging me: How was it possible for missed diagnoses to be so common and yet not perceived by doctors as a major problem? The problem is that physicians, while generally aware that mistakes happen, greatly underestimate how often *they* make them. In his talks to doctors on the topic, Graber often asks how many have made a diagnostic error in the past year; typically, only about 1 percent of the hands go up. "The concept that they, personally, could err at a significant rate is inconceivable to most physicians," he writes. In short, they think it's the other guy. This overconfidence is not necessarily their fault: doctors simply do not get the feedback needed to gain an accurate sense of their batting average. They assume their diagnoses are correct unless they hear otherwise. Since there are few, if any, health care organizations that systematically measure diagnostic error rates, they typically learn of their mistakes only from the patients themselves.

And that's especially unlikely when it comes to patients whose symptoms were dismissed as being all in their heads. In the case of a patient incorrectly diagnosed with another disease, the patient *may* stick with her original doctor long enough for the mistake to come to light. But if a doctor has concluded that it's "just stress," a patient with persistent symptoms will almost invariably simply move on to another doctor—if she doesn't give up entirely. Indeed, she has no other option. And the first mistaken doctor usually doesn't get a memo if, down the road, her symptoms finally are "medically explained" by someone else. Consequently, to him, she remains the somatizing stressed-out woman he concluded she was, and diagnostic error remains a mistake that only *other* doctors make.

"WOMEN'S ILLNESSES ARE ASSUMED PSYCHOSOMATIC UNTIL PROVEN OTHERWISE"

To many of the doctors and advocates who were calling for a greater attention to women's health in the nineties, the fact that so many women were finding their symptoms brushed off as "all in their heads" was a clear indication that there was a knowledge gap that needed to be closed. As feminist disability scholar Susan Wendell, reviewing the epidemiological research on somatoform disorders, wrote in 1999, "It seems a remarkable coincidence that men of higher socioeconomic backgrounds from the developed Western countries are, in all the world, the people least likely to 'somatize,' given that they also happen to be the people who are accorded the most believability and authority in Western scientific settings." If women and other socially disadvantaged groups have more "medically unexplained symptoms," that is probably because medicine has been less interested in explaining their symptoms.

Not only that, but medicine hasn't been interested in explaining women's "medically unexplained symptoms" largely because it has believed that it *already* has an explanation for them. As a young ob-gyn in the late eighties, Werbinski recalls, she began to realize that many of her patients were reporting symptoms for which she didn't have an explanation. Apparently other doctors *were* offering an explanation, though. "Whenever medicine gets into a brick wall that it can't explain, it says, 'Well, it has to have a psychological component.' So a lot of my patients were telling me, 'My doctor told me that this symptom is all in my head.' And the doctor may or may not have said that directly, but the training was telling us that the things we couldn't explain—just put them into that wastebasket. And then we would clap our hands and say, 'Okay, I'm done with that; that's not my problem.'"

As Angela Kennedy points out in her book, *Authors of Our Own Misfortune? The Problems with Psychogenic Explanations for Physical Illnesses,* this is the dangerous paradox about psychogenic theories of "medically unexplained" conditions: by providing an explanation for them—but one that can't be scientifically proved or disproved—they thereby discourage further investigation into their causes. Psychogenic explanations slip in "wherever there is a vacuum of medical and/or scientific knowledge about somatic conditions." But in continually filling in these knowledge gaps, they relieve any need to fill them with actual scientific knowledge.

This is as self-fulfilling on the collective level as it is on the individual one—perhaps more so. An individual woman can at least go to another doctor if the first, deciding her symptoms are psychogenic, stops looking for a medical explanation. But if medicine has collectively concluded that a condition is sufficiently explained by the long-standing medical "fact" that women are prone to somatizing their emotional distress, then there is no reason to do the scientific research needed to provide a medical explanation for it. There is, in fact, not much reason to study it at all. When the same biomedical community that's decided—as that medical student in the seventies put it—that "women's illnesses are assumed psychosomatic until proven otherwise" is in charge of doing the research that would prove otherwise, the proof simply never comes—or at least takes decades to accumulate.

This is the maddening trap that functional somatic syndromes have been caught in for decades. By the eighties and nineties, some physicians— often spurred by patient advocacy—had begun carving specific "functional somatic syndromes" out of the wastebasket of the "medically unexplained" and arguing that these conditions shouldn't be considered the random symptoms of "somatizing" patients but rather physical conditions whose underlying mechanism was simply not yet understood. In other words, they suggested that medicine should treat these conditions as if they were truly medically unexplained and attempt to explain them. Diagnoses like fibromyalgia, interstitial cystitis, IBS, idiopathic low back pain, vulvodynia, and chronic fatigue syndrome—to name a few—awkwardly straddled the gray area at the "borderland between psychiatry and medicine," known in the former as somatoform disorders and in the latter as functional somatic syndromes.

These functional somatic syndromes are sometimes called "contested diseases," a reflection of the disagreement over how they should be understood. Over the last few decades, thanks to the efforts of individual clinician-researchers and patient advocates, there has been—to greater and lesser degrees—progress made in explaining these conditions. So these days there is often a large discrepancy between how they are viewed by experts who study them—namely, as poorly understood diseases whose biological mechanisms medicine will eventually unravel—and how they are viewed by the profession at large, where they remain shrouded in an air of psychosomatic suspicion, lacking the legitimacy and acceptance afforded to diseases whose underlying pathology is more fully understood.

As much of the rest of this book will show, the progress made toward understanding these conditions has been greatly hampered by medicine's tendency to consider the "medically unexplained" psychiatrically explained by default. The assumption that these conditions are psychogenic—just modern labels for women's age-old hysterical tendencies or, as one article put it, "old wine in new bottles"—means there isn't much interest in studying them within the biomedical community. But only scientific research to uncover their biological mechanisms could rescue them from the wastebasket of the "medically unexplained." As one researcher on multiple chemical sensitivity lamented in the nineties, "we are in a catch-22 situation. It is difficult to attract research money for a controversial condition and it is difficult to resolve the controversy without the necessary research." In the meantime, skeptical doctors would point to the absence of consistent biological abnormalities as proof that there was "nothing wrong" with these patients, never mind that finding such abnormalities would have required research to *look* for them.

Meanwhile, a good deal of what little research has been done on functional somatic syndromes has been focused on trying to confirm their psychological roots. On the whole, the evidence marshaled to attribute a psychogenic cause to such conditions is as speculative on the collective level as it is on the individual level. Countless studies have been done showing that patients with functional somatic syndromes have higher rates of depression and anxiety than healthy people. But this is true of patients with "explained" chronic diseases too. Rarely do such studies include a control group of patients that are similarly debilitated by an organic disease or pay more than lip service to the possibility that being sick—particularly with a poorly understood and therefore poorly treated condition—could be the cause, not the consequence, of mental distress. Research also points to higher rates of childhood sexual abuse or other early-life stresses among patients with functional somatic syndromes to imply a psychogenic cause. But, again, such findings are common in a range of diseases.

Indeed, one reason that the evidence that has been used to back up psychogenic theories looks so weak is that there is an ever-growing body of research showing how mental and physical health is utterly intertwined. We know that chronic stress—from everything from living in poverty to experiencing discrimination—is linked to a higher risk of conditions as diverse as heart disease and viral infections. We know that not solely sexual abuse but "adverse childhood experiences" of many kinds are associated with higher odds of poorer health—from autoimmune diseases to type 2 diabetes to depression—later in life. These connections aren't due to an abstract theoretical process like "conversion" but to the physiological effects of elevated stress hormones on a great many bodily systems.

But medicine has a tendency to highlight these mind-body links most when it comes to "medically unexplained" syndromes that affect mainly women, and, further, assign them a causal status that it simply can't back up. In a 2016 article, for example, two researchers from New Zealand's Victoria University of Wellington reviewed the evidence in favor of psychogenic explanations of two functional neurological syndromes: so-called psychogenic movement disorders and psychogenic nonepileptic seizures, which are both about three times more common in women. Noting that they saw "no reason why a lower standard of evidence should apply to a psychological than to a medical explanation," they decided to evaluate the evidence just as rigorously "as one would demand for any other causal explanation" and concluded it wasn't sufficient. They suggested that the medical community "may need to retire those overworked psychological explanations that are commonly invoked in the face of un-certainty and instead adopt a completely fresh perspective." It appeared that medicine had simply accepted psychogenic theories of these disor-ders by "default."

"One of the great puzzles of the psychogenic literature," writes Dr. Martin Pall, a researcher on functional somatic syndromes, "is how do so many bad papers get published?" Calling the publication of research with such shoddy scientific standards "by far the largest failure of the peer-review system that I am aware of," he notes, "I cannot help wonder-ing whether it is based on the fact that most victims of these illnesses are women. There is a long history of sex discrimination in medicine, and while I would like to think we are more enlightened in the twenty-first century, this pattern suggests that perhaps we are not."

WOMEN DISMISSED: A SELF-FULFILLING PROPHECY

If doctors are going with their gut instincts about whether patients are likely to have "medically unexplained symptoms," it is no wonder that women, who've been considered the typical patients with psychogenic symptoms for a century, so often find their symptoms dismissed as all in their heads. In a 1986 study, for example, researchers looked at a group of patients who'd been diagnosed with "hysteria" or a "functional disor-der" and were subsequently found to have a serious organic neurologi-cal disorder. Concluding that a "diagnosis of hysteria is usually wrong," they identified the characteristics that seemed to make patients especially vulnerable to a hysteria misdiagnosis: being a woman, having a prior di-agnosis of a psychiatric disorder, offering a plausible psychological expla-nation for the problem, and embellishing their symptoms—which, the researchers suggested, stemmed from patients' fear that their doctors would not believe them.

With two strikes against them, women who have previously been di-agnosed with mental health problems have an especially hard time getting their physical symptoms to be taken seriously. Indeed, the fact that women have higher rates of common mental health conditions is, itself, likely one reason that women are more vulnerable than men to psychogenic misdiag-noses. Women are about twice as likely to have a diagnosis of depression or an anxiety disorder as men. About one in five women in the United States take a psychotropic medication, compared to one in eight men. And it's estimated that four out of five prescriptions for antidepressants are now written by physicians who aren't psychiatrists.

But this gender disparity in mental health diagnoses and psychiat-ric medication use may also be in part a *result* of the tendency to dismiss women's symptoms as "all in their heads." While women may truly have a higher risk of depression and anxiety disorders—for cultural or biological reasons or some combination of the two—many have argued that the dif-ference in prevalence rates is at least partly a consequence of overdiagnosis in women and underdiagnosis in men. Studies in the nineties suggested that as many as 30 to 50 percent of women diagnosed with depression were misdiagnosed.

Since mood disorders are stereotyped as women's conditions, doc-tors may be more likely to attribute the physical symptoms that can ac-company these conditions—like heart palpitations, shortness of breath, fatigue, and insomnia—to anxiety and depression in women rather than consider the many physical conditions that can cause such symptoms too. Furthermore, depression and anxiety are themselves *symptoms* of other diseases. In their 1997 book *Preventing Misdiagnosis of Women: A Guide to Physical Disorders That Have Psychiatric Symptoms,* Elizabeth Klonoff and Hope Landrine reviewed dozens of conditions—including endocrine, neurological, and autoimmune disorders—that are more common among women whose primary symptoms are psychological. They warned their fellow mental health professionals that "the misdiagnosis of these physical disorders as psychiatric in part accounts for women's higher rate of depression, anxiety, and somatization disorders." And just to really complete this self-fulfilling circle: the stress of suffering from an undiagnosed—and therefore untreated—disease often takes its mental toll. As one article points out, "Ironically, medical misdiagnoses of physical conditions may induce depressive reactions in female patients."

Whether women truly do have a primary psychological disorder or have been misdiagnosed with one, once listed in their chart, it heightens the risk that any other physical symptoms they have in the future will be automatically dismissed as psychogenic. Dr. Pat Croskerry, director of the Critical Thinking Program at Dalhousie University and a leading expert on diagnostic errors, has dubbed this particular type of mistake a "psych-out error," in which medical conditions may be "overlooked or minimized" in patients with psychiatric diagnoses.

I heard from one woman, a middle-aged Italian immigrant with a history of depression, whose worsening abdominal pain was dismissed as menstrual pain for three years. It wasn't taken seriously even when she brought up the fact that she had a family history of colon cancer. And it wasn't taken seriously even when she began having rectal bleeding. When she finally pushed for a colonoscopy, it revealed stage-three colon cancer. Just a few months longer and it would have been at stage four and incurable. Another woman I spoke to had been on antidepressants on and off since she was a teenager. For several years, she'd brought up concerns—dizziness, fatigue, vision problems, unexplained weight gain—to different doctors: "But the second my antidepressants came up, it was always brushed off as 'stress,'" she says. The first doctor who decided to do a thorough workup to get to the bottom of it discovered she had thyroid cancer. She adds, "I'm troubled by the fact that a cancer diagnosis almost felt like good news because it validated the more mysterious symptoms and made me feel less 'crazy.'"

And it's not just women with clear-cut mental health diagnoses, like depression, who are vulnerable to the psych-out error. Since many physicians assume any "medically unexplained symptoms" are psychogenic, patients with functional somatic syndromes may find that doctors don't take their reports of new, unrelated symptoms seriously, assuming that they must be "unexplained" as well. To many doctors, a diagnosis like fibromyalgia or IBS listed in a patient's chart signals a propensity to somatization, predisposing them to view the patient as an unreliable reporter, prone to "medically unexplained symptoms" unlikely to indicate organic disease. In *How Doctors Think*, Groopman tells of a young woman with IBS, who nearly died of a ruptured ectopic pregnancy after three doctors missed it, assuming it was a flare-up of her IBS, even as she insisted the pelvic pain she was suddenly experiencing was different from her usual IBS symptoms.

The psych-out error may have played a role in Maggie's experience too, though she didn't realize it at the time. Maggie had fainted once during her freshman year, which the doctor she saw at the campus clinic afterward blamed on an alleged eating disorder. Maggie didn't have an eating disorder and switched to another clinic doctor who focused on her physical symptoms. For the next three years, she'd been healthy, returning to the clinic only to get treated for the occasional sinus infection and strep. But she later saw in her chart that the intake instructions that the campus clinic had sent along with her to the ER included a note from the first campus doctor saying she still suspected Maggie had an eating disorder and that the cause of her pain may be "trying not to eat." "I think that colored some of the views that the doctors had toward me in the beginning," she says.

At this point, women seem to be caught in a self-fulfilling prophecy. On the collective level, since medicine has failed to explain many of our symptoms, women are, in reality, more likely to have "medically unexplained symptoms"—whether those symptoms are side effects of drugs that haven't been tested in women, or atypical symptoms of diseases that have been largely studied in men, or symptoms of functional somatic syndromes that are more common among women and that medicine, assuming they must be psychogenic, has hardly researched at all. And since the tendency to see any "medically unexplained symptoms" as psychogenic has become deeply entrenched in medicine, this knowledge gap creates the stereotype that women are hysterics and hypochondriacs with a tendency to soma-tize. This stereotype, in turn, affects how all women patients—whether their symptoms are explained or unexplained—are perceived when they enter the medical system. Profiling them as patients prone to "medically unexplained symptoms," doctors more quickly settle on the conclusion that women's symptoms are "just stress," offering antidepressants instead of doing a more thorough workup to find a medical explanation, which just exacerbates this endless cycle.

THE GIRL WHO CRIED PAIN

In an influential 2001 article entitled "The Girl Who Cried Pain: A Bias Against Women in the Treatment of Pain," Diane E. Hoffmann and Anita J. Tarzian reviewed a number of studies that had accumulated showing gen-der disparities in the treatment of pain. The gap could be seen in a wide range of clinical contexts. In the hospital setting, one study showed that women received less pain medication than men after abdominal surgery. Another found that after a coronary artery bypass graft, men were more likely to receive narcotics, while their female counterparts were more likely to get sedatives. The difference started early: in a study of postoperative pain in children, more codeine was given to boys than girls, and the girls were more likely to be given the less heavy-hitting acetaminophen. And the same pattern persisted when it came to more long-term pain management too. Studies of metastatic cancer and AIDS patients found that women were overrepresented in the disturbingly large proportion of patients who were undertreated for their pain.

As Hoffmann and Tarzian pointed out, this differential treatment could be justified if, on average, women reported less pain than men, but in fact, the opposite was true. In the late eighties and early nineties, pain researchers—spurred by the calls for greater attention to sex/gender differ-ences in all areas of biomedical research—had begun exploring differences in pain perception between men and women. The research suggested that women tend to be more sensitive to pain and/or more likely to report it.

Given that, they wrote, "it seems appropriate that they be treated at least as thoroughly as men and that their reports of pain be taken seriously." At the very least, they shouldn't get *less* treatment. "The data do not indicate that this is the case. Women who seek help are less likely than men to be taken seriously when they report pain and are less likely to have their pain adequately treated."

They considered various potential reasons for this bias, ultimately concluding that the main one was that women's complaints of pain are less likely to be trusted. "The subjective nature of pain requires health care providers to view the patient as a credible reporter," and women are "more likely to have their pain reports discounted as 'emotional' or 'psychogenic' and, therefore, 'not real,'" they wrote. "These biases have led health-care providers to discount women's self reports of pain at least until there is objective evidence for the pain's cause. Medicine's focus on objective factors and its cultural stereotypes of women combine insidiously, leaving women at greater risk for inadequate pain relief and continued suffering."

In the years since, the research on gender disparities in pain treatment has been somewhat more mixed. Some studies have found women are undertreated; some have not. One reason for the inconsistency may be that while pain is always subjective, a willingness to trust the patient's report is more important in some clinical contexts than others. As Hoffmann and Tarzian pointed out, women are at greatest risk of having their pain reports discounted before the pain's source is discovered. And research continues to suggest that many women, like Maggie, find their pain isn't taken as seriously when they first enter the ER. A 2008 study of nearly a thousand people who arrived in a Philadelphia emergency room with acute abdominal pain found that while men and women had similar pain scores, the women waited longer to get pain medication: sixty-five minutes, on average, compared with forty-nine minutes for men. They were also significantly less likely to get any kind of pain medication and were 13 to 23 percent less likely than men to get opioids. And when it comes to chronic pain, which is often "unexplained" or at least poorly correlated with objective abnormalities, women also face barriers to getting adequate treatment.

The way women's reports of pain are received seems to be at least as influenced by cultural stereotypes about *men* as about women. The stoicism expected of men is cited as one of the reasons that their pain is taken more seriously; their reports of pain are less likely to be doubted, because it's assumed they're more reluctant to make them in the first place. But there's no rational reason that men's assumed stoicism should result in women's pain *not* being taken seriously. As Hoffmann and Tarzian pointed out, if men are indeed more reluctant than women to admit they're in pain, "this reluctance on the part of men does not lead to the conclusion that women, as not reluctant, must therefore be less in need of adequate treatment." If women, spared from the cultural pressure put on men to tough it out, are more free to express their pain, their reports would seem to be not overreports but simply more *accurate* reports. Instead, women are treated as if *they're* the unreliable reporters.

The stoic male stereotype extends to an assumption not only that men are less likely to admit they're in pain but also that they're less likely to seek medical attention for their symptoms at all. Public health researcher Kate Hunt and her team point out that an assumption that men are reluctant to seek medical care has become "deeply entrenched" in both medicine and the public at large. And it seems to come with a corollary assumption that women are *not* reluctant, which "may result in health care providers assuming that women have a lower level of symptom severity" when they enter the medical system. But these contrasting stereotypes, so thoroughly unquestioned that they've been accepted as "commonsense" facts, aren't actually that well supported by evidence.

There is certainly research based on interviews with men to suggest that they commonly *say* that they're reluctant to see a doctor—and that damaging masculinity norms that discourage admitting vulnerability and asking for help often play a role in that—but few studies have directly compared men's and women's thinking on the matter. In other words, men may indeed be reluctant, but women may be just as reluctant—perhaps for different reasons. And, as we'll see, one of the common reasons women give for delaying getting medical care is a fear of being seen as a hypochondriac. It seems that these stereotypes may drive us all to a similar spot: in attempting to *adhere* to the stoic male stereotype, men may hesitate to get the care they need; in attempting to *avoid* playing into the hypochondriacal female stereotype, women may do the same.

Indeed, when it comes to studies that look at what patients actually *do*, women are not, as a general rule, any quicker to seek medical care. There is relatively little research that has explored whether men and women with the same condition or the same similarly debilitating symptom differ in whether and how quickly they seek medical care, and the research that does exist has yielded mixed results: for some conditions, gender isn't a factor; for others, men delay longer; and for others, women do. (For example, women tend to wait *longer* than men to get help when they're having a heart attack.) As Hunt and her colleagues concluded in a 2011 review of studies on help-seeking for two common symptoms—headache and back pain—the evidence that women sought medical attention more readily than men was, given the strength of the stereotype, "surprisingly weak and inconsistent."

But, again, even if women were, on average, more willing to seek medical attention than men are, it wouldn't justify not taking their symptoms seriously when they do. Yet, Hunt and her colleagues point out, the assumption that men are more reluctant than women to see a doctor seems to lead, unconsciously, to an assumption that women seek care not only more readily but *too* readily—"sometimes for trivial symptoms which are self-limiting or amenable to self-management." These stereotypes operate, illogically, as if they're necessarily on a seesaw: if men are stoic, women must be overly emotional; if men underreport their pain, women must exaggerate theirs; if men are reluctant to seek help, women must be too quick to.

A DOUBLE BIND: EITHER YOU'RE HYSTERICAL OR NOTHING'S WRONG

It is always tempting to imagine that women can avoid sexism by acting more like men. In this case, it's easy to think that perhaps women would be taken more seriously if they were just a little more stoic, if they bit their lips and held back their tears; if their voices betrayed no hint of emotion that could be used against them. In short, if they weren't so hysterical in the colloquial sense of the word, then maybe they wouldn't be treated as if they were hysterical in the medical sense of the word.

That's certainly how Maggie felt. "Being told to 'calm down' is just the most infuriating thing when something is actually really wrong," she says. But she nevertheless attempted to do so. "I tried really, really hard with all the doctors to act very serious and even-toned and to temper my voice, but as soon as the pain would start, it was hard to maintain that." She even felt as though her mom's display of emotion would be held against her. "She was getting so worked up and starting to cry. I remember thinking that I needed to be even *more* serious because now they weren't going to take me seriously because she was freaking out."

But gender stereotypes have a tendency to put women in double binds, and this one is no exception. Since women are *expected* to have an overly emotional response to pain, they are at risk of having their reports not taken seriously whether they adhere to the stereotype or break with it. Dr. Vicki Ratner brings a unique dual perspective to the problem as an orthopedic surgeon and an advocate for patients with interstitial cystitis. She's blunt about the dilemma women patients face: "It's very difficult for a woman to present in a doctor's office. Because if she's very stoic—if she talks about the problem in the tone that I'm talking to you—then the doctor's going to think, 'Oh, there's nothing really wrong with her.' And then if she gets very emotional, he's going to blame it on, 'Oh, she's a psychological mess blah blah blah.' You get judged right away because you're female: you're either stoic and nothing's wrong or you're crying and you get labeled hysterical."

Conversely, the expectation that men keep a stiff upper lip when they're in pain serves to ensure that they're likely to be taken seriously no matter what: if they're stoic, they're just being a typical "macho" guy, and if they're emotional, well, then it must be really, *really* bad. However, just how much leeway men have to break with the stoic male stereotype and still be taken seriously may depend on how closely they adhere to masculine norms in other ways. In a 2014 study that found female heart attack patients weren't tested and treated as quickly as their male counterparts in the emergency room, the researchers also gave the patients a personality test gauging how closely they conformed to gender stereotypes. They found that both men and women with more traditionally "feminine" traits experienced a greater delay than patients with more "masculine" traits.

Take Lauron's experience. At first the twenty-six-year-old figured it was food poisoning—those fried clam strips at Red Robin, perhaps?—but after a few days of terrible abdominal pain, no appetite, and a slight fever, she knew she should get checked out. Having just aged out of her parents' health insurance to her own limited plan, she found the one urgent care center that was in-network. The doctor she saw assured her she probably just had the stomach virus going around. She told him the pain was excruciating and asked if she could get something to alleviate it. But he said no, explaining that, if it turned out it actually was appendicitis, the pain would get much worse and she would need to notice that and seek treatment right away. In retrospect, Lauron says, it was a little concerning that he hadn't done much of a physical exam besides briefly feeling her abdomen. But at the time Lauron figured, "Okay, he's the doctor—someone I'm supposed to be able to trust. And I didn't want to be hysterical. I assumed that if he had given me the okay, then it was probably okay." She went home intending to take his advice to go to the ER if it got worse.

What Lauron didn't know then was that if it was appendicitis and she was *already* at the peak pain level—a possibility the doctor apparently discounted completely—then the pain would actually first lessen when the appendix ruptured and then get really bad. A couple of days later that's what happened. "All the pressure that I had been feeling—the pain from it being inflamed—was relieved because it finally burst. I didn't know that I was in a dangerous situation." Then the pain returned with a vengeance. After Lauron spent a night throwing up with a high fever, her partner sent her to the ER. Her ruptured appendix had formed an abscess and was infected.

The ER staff told Lauron that if she had waited just three hours more before coming in, she probably would have died. "The infection was so bad that they couldn't operate; they could only insert a drainage tube and fill me with painkillers and antibiotics." Several delirious days and one collapsed lung later, she was released from the hospital. Over the next several months, she was in and out of the hospital as the tube was removed and then reinserted when the infection returned twice. It was months before she was finally well enough to have surgery to remove what was left of her appendix.

Lauron says this nightmare has made her less trusting of doctors. "Now I see how fallible doctors are. If I have a serious situation like that again, I'd be more willing to seek out a second opinion, and if something didn't feel right about an interaction with a medical professional, I'd be more likely to trust myself about why that is." Still, she knows that she was as firm as she could have possibly been with that urgent care doctor about how much pain she was experiencing—he simply didn't seem to think it could be as bad as she said it was. "I was really honest—like, 'This is a pain level that I have never experienced before in my life.'" With a mom who worked in health care, she felt especially well equipped to communicate with doctors; she'd learned how important it is to not downplay your symptoms. "But I wasn't hysterically sobbing." And she thinks because of that, he didn't believe her account. "Because I'm a woman he didn't think I had that pain tolerance, so he probably thought I was overexaggerating the level of pain I was actually in. I could not have done more to advocate for myself in that moment because I was really clear about it. That's the frustrating thing—even if you do know the words to say, you're not always heard."

HEARTSINK PATIENTS

There's one final thing that is important to know about patients with "medically unexplained symptoms": doctors do not like them. "Patients with persistent somatization are not only well-known to physicians but also singularly disliked by them. Their widespread unpopularity is reflected in the mostly derogatory labels they have acquired, such as 'crocks,' 'gomers,' 'turkeys,' 'hypochondriacs,' 'hysterics,' and 'the worried well,'" Lipowski explained. "These labels express the frustration of doctors faced with patients who claim to be physically ill, clamor for medical diagnoses and treatment, tend to be dissatisfied with any therapy they get, and are inclined to 'doctor shop.'" Women with "medically unexplained symptoms" also featured prominently in an influential article from the late eighties that coined the term "heartsink patients" to describe patients who "exasperate, defeat, and overwhelm their doctors by their behavior."

It's understandable that doctors would feel frustrated when they cannot explain a patient's symptoms. As Dr. Lisa Sanders, who pens the Diagnosis column for *The New York Times Magazine*, writes in her book *Every Patient Tells a Story: Medical Mysteries and the Art of Diagnosis*, "Nobody likes not knowing, but doctors, perhaps, find this state of being even more intolerable because it utterly thwarts their ability to alleviate suffering, which is often the fundamental motivation for their entire career." But, as the derisive labels suggest, all too often, doctors' "discomfort in the face of the unexplained" leads them to project the frustration they feel onto the patient. As one article on "medically unexplained symptoms" noted, doctors tend to adopt strategies "deflecting the threat to medical competence posed by medically unexplained symptoms" by "shifting the blame from the limits of medicine to some characteristic of the patient."

There's another reason for this attitude, though. In theory, medicine considers psychogenic symptoms to be *un*consciously produced and no less real to the sufferer than organic ones. But in practice, those with unexplained symptoms are often treated as though they're *willfully* staying sick. This is probably because Freud's theory of hysteria introduced the notion of "secondary gain," which has been part of theories of conversion and somatization ever since. The "primary gain" patients got from unconsciously "converting" their psychological conflict into physical symptoms was to avoid consciously feeling mental distress. But the symptoms were thought to be perpetuated by the "secondary gains" they received from being ill. Lipowski explained, "The communication of somatic complaints may also represent an attempt by the patient to attain certain personal objectives, such as release from social obligations or an excuse for failure to meet them, resolution of an inner or an interpersonal conflict, securing of support from others, or financial benefit. Any one or any combination of these factors may foster illness behavior and adoption of a sick role."

This theory has, at times, led to punitive therapeutic strategies that seem to borrow directly from Mitchell's nineteenth-century rest cure for hysteria. In one 1978 article on the "often thankless challenge of the hysteric patient," an American physician described his approach to "managing" patients with Briquet's syndrome, who made up 6 percent of the adult women in his practice. Since "symptomatic behavior persists only as long as it continues to be reinforced," he explained, "withdrawal of the reinforcement must be accomplished to extinguish the symptom." The patient should not be referred to other doctors to avoid "the secondary gain—attention—the patient experiences each time she retells her story." Her family should be advised to ignore her symptoms, rather than "cater[ing] to the patient's wishes." In a hospital setting, she could be isolated in a locked room and "given privileges contingent upon symptom reduction."

Chloë Atkins's experience offers a chilling illustration of just how far this thinking will sometimes be taken. As a young woman she began experiencing episodes of paralysis that, over the course of a decade, worsened until she was eventually quadriplegic and frequently had to be hooked up to life support because she was unable to breathe on her own. With inconclusive test results, her doctors had decided early on that she was suffering from conversion disorder, a diagnosis they clung to even after evidence began to suggest that she might have an atypical form of the autoimmune neuromuscular disease myasthenia gravis. And even as her mystery disease threatened to actually kill her, she was treated as if she were to blame. "Clinicians behaved as though I wanted to be ill and that I conspired to confuse and frustrate them," she writes in her book *My Imaginary Illness: A Journey into Uncertainty and Prejudice in Medical Diagnosis*. "I was treated as though I were a criminal or a juvenile delinquent. Instead of my illness being the problem, I became the problem."

The notion of secondary gain also inevitably results in some conflation between psychogenic symptoms and those that are simply made up entirely. According to the *DSM* criteria for the somatoform disorders, they must be differentiated from two other diagnoses: factitious disorder and malingering. While a patient with a somatoform disorder is thought to *unconsciously* produce symptoms, the factitious disorder patient *consciously* fakes symptoms in order to achieve some *internal* benefit (e.g., a sense of victimhood). And the malingerer *consciously* fakes symptoms for an *external* benefit (e.g., disability compensation, painkillers). Since doctors cannot read patients' minds—conscious or unconscious—it's not surprising that anyone with "medically unexplained symptoms" is liable to be viewed with suspicion.

It's long past time for medicine to abandon the notion that anything it can't currently explain can be blamed on the psyche. The only reason it has this idea to begin with is that at the end of the nineteenth century, the same year the X-ray was invented, a German nerve doctor suggested that "hysteria"—a label that undoubtedly covered hundreds of yet-to-be-recognized diseases affecting mostly women—could be attributed, through some mysterious occult process, to "the unconscious mind." This concept was passed down, grandfathered into each successive generation of medicine, even as more and more conditions previously believed to be "hysterical" were removed from the category as medical knowledge grew. As Atkins puts it, the idea of psychogenic illness appears to be "a cultural artifact masquerading as a medical truth." It has led to the neglect of millions of mostly women patients suffering from conditions that medicine doesn't yet understand, and leaves all women patients, like Maggie, at risk of dangerous missed diagnoses when doctors can't readily crack the case.

———

By the time Maggie returned to the hospital yet again near dawn on Monday, she'd been moved into the malingering category. In the ER for the third time in just a few days for pain and no diagnosis to show for it, the doctors clearly suspected she was inventing her pain to get prescription painkillers. "No one would give me any pain medication, despite my complaint that my pain was, on a scale of one to ten, a 'bazillion.' In the hallway, the ER doctor told my mother that she thought I must be 'narco-savvy.'" In fact, Maggie had had a terrible reaction to the opioid medication she'd received while she'd been admitted before. "It was awful. The implication seemed to be that I wanted more of that, even though I definitely did not."

Maggie just wanted them to figure out what was wrong with her. Unfortunately, the only clue they had to go on was her "own claims of indescribably horrific pain." And yet none of the doctors had asked for more information about the nature of that pain—like the fact that it had shifted from the left to the right shoulder or that she felt as if there were a sandbag shifting about in her abdomen when she moved—information that might have led them to the right diagnosis. At this point, they no longer seemed to believe in her pain at all.

But as the day wore on, tests finally started coming back supporting what Maggie, readmitted to the hospital but still denied pain relief, had been saying: something was really, really wrong. A high white blood cell count pointed to an infection somewhere in her body. And then another chest X-ray showed a telltale blob that meant there was air in her abdomen that shouldn't be there. The switch was flipped: before she'd even been told of the new development, a nurse was in her room, administering pain medication. The health care providers' entire attitude toward her changed immediately. "The nurses and doctors began treating me with compassion and sympathy."

It was clear that an organ had ruptured, but since Maggie was starting to go into septic shock, there was no time left to find out which one; she was rushed into emergency exploratory abdominal surgery. There the doctors discovered and repaired a hole in her stomach, caused, she would later learn, by an especially fast-growing ulcer. The pain she'd been experiencing for the last seventy-two hours—the final six of which she'd spent in the hospital without pain medication—was from air and fluid leaking into her diaphragm.

Unlike in many nonacute cases, Maggie's doctors did ultimately learn what was actually wrong with her. She heard that her doctors were asked to answer questions and justify their decisions to their colleagues at a hospital morbidity and mortality conference. Someone who was there reported that they would be "kicking themselves for the rest of their lives" for taking so long to determine the correct diagnosis. Every doctor who'd been on her case visited her room as she recovered from surgery, often offering up this defense: a perforated ulcer is just so rare, especially in someone her age. "For them, considering a perforated organ as the explanation for my pain was nearly inconceivable." But, as Maggie points out, in the interest of not putting lives at risk, for doctors, particularly in the emergency room, there should probably not be any diagnoses that are considered "outside the realm of the possible."

Indeed, the unjustifiable error was not in failing to more quickly determine a very unlikely diagnosis but in not taking Maggie's report of extreme pain seriously—and eventually deciding it must not be real at all—until they did. There is always a gap between when a symptom begins and when it is "medically explained." It is unreasonable to expect that doctors, who are fallible human beings doing a difficult job, can close this gap instantaneously—and, given that medical knowledge is, and probably always will be, incomplete, they may at times not be able to close it at all.

But it shouldn't be unreasonable to expect that, during this period of uncertainty, the benefit of the doubt be given to the patient, the default assumption be that their symptoms are real, their description of what they are feeling in their own bodies be believed, and, if it is "medically unexplained," the burden be on medicine to explain it. Such basic trust has been denied to women for far too long.

PART 2

INVISIBLE WOMEN IN
A "MALE MODEL" SYSTEM

CHAPTER 3

HEART DISEASE AND OTHER LIFE-THREATENING EMERGENCIES

ON A SPRING MORNING in 2008, Carolyn Thomas was out for an early morning walk in her Victoria, British Columbia, neighborhood, when a pain—"a cross between crushing heaviness and a severe burning sensation"—hit her smack in the center of the chest, then wandered up into her lower throat. Suddenly sweating profusely, she felt as though she was going to vomit. A prickling sensation traveled down her left arm. For about twenty minutes, she clutched a tree trunk and, frightened, fruitlessly scanned the empty block for any passersby who could help. Eventually her symptoms let up enough for her to slowly continue walking toward home.

It was the arm that convinced Thomas to stop by the local emergency room; she vaguely remembered hearing that left-arm pain could be a symptom of a heart attack. And she'd literally be passing the hospital on her route anyway, so she might as well make sure it wasn't her heart. In the ER, she was whisked through the standard diagnostic protocol for patients with chest pain. But when an electrocardiogram (EKG) and cardiac blood tests came back normal, the ER physician told Thomas, an active public relations professional who had celebrated her fifty-eighth birthday the day before, that she was "in the right demographic for acid reflux." When she asked, "But doctor, what about this pain down my left arm?" he brushed her off, assuring her that it was definitely not her heart. Later, as Thomas was being discharged, a nurse scolded her for "questioning" him: "He is a very good doctor, and he does not like to be questioned."

Flushed with embarrassment, Thomas apologized to the ER staff for wasting their time and went home. But over the next two weeks, despite popping Tums like candy, her symptoms only got worse. Soon she'd have to pause to rest after just five steps. "But hey," she says, "at least I knew it wasn't my heart!" Finally, her symptoms became so severe on a five-hour flight home from a family visit back east that, upon landing, she went straight back to the ER. Even then, she didn't think it could be her heart; the doctor, after all, had been quite confident on that point. But this time, Thomas was told she'd had two heart attacks on the flight. She was diagnosed with a 95 percent blockage in her left anterior descending coronary artery, the type of heart attack so deadly that doctors—tellingly—call it "the widowmaker."

HOW THE LEADING KILLER OF WOMEN CAME TO BE A "MAN'S DISEASE"

In 1964, the American Heart Association (AHA) held its first official conference on women and heart disease. Advertised "for women only," it was called Hearts and Husbands: The First Women's Conference on Coronary Heart Disease. Ten thousand women gathered to get tips on how to keep their husbands from developing heart disease and how to care for them if they did. It would be another twenty-five years before the AHA held a conference that was actually about heart disease *in* women. In 2016, the association released its first official scientific statement on the topic; over fifty years after that first conference, it declared that despite some progress over the last two decades, heart disease "remains understudied, underdiagnosed, and undertreated in women."

Given this history, you could be forgiven for thinking that heart disease is rare in women. In fact, cardiovascular disease, which along with coronary artery disease—the cause of most heart attacks—includes conditions like stroke, heart failure, arrhythmias, and heart valve problems, has been the leading cause of death for women in the United States for over a century. About one in three deaths among women each year is from heart-related causes, significantly more than from all kinds of cancer combined.

And yet heart disease had become so thoroughly imagined as a "man's disease" in the middle of the twentieth century that, back in 1964, nobody really batted an eye when that first conference geared toward women was all about preventing their husbands from getting it. The stereotype hadn't come out of nowhere. Rates of coronary artery disease, the most common cause of cardiovascular death, had spiked dramatically by the fifties, particularly among middle-aged men. Women, by comparison, seemed to be relatively protected until after menopause, when their rates of heart disease began to climb. Combating premature heart attacks that were striking down men in the prime of their lives was the growing concern. And the biomedical community responded with urgency, launching a concerted effort to study, prevent, and treat the disease.

By the late eighties, though, experts were beginning to warn that, as Dr. C. Noel Bairey Merz, director of the Barbra Streisand Women's Heart Center at the Cedars-Sinai Heart Institute, has put it, the "diagnostic and therapeutic strategies, which had been developed in men, by men, for men, for the last 50 years . . . weren't working so well for women." While cardiovascular deaths among men had been steadily declining, among women, they were rising. The result was that since 1984, more women than men have been dying of cardiovascular causes each year. And while women are at relatively lower risk for developing coronary artery disease than their male counterparts for most of their lives, they tend to have worse outcomes when they do get it: 26 percent of women versus 19 percent of men die within the first year after a heart attack—a myocardial infarction, in the medical lingo. Within five years, nearly half of all women, compared to about a third of men, have heart failure, suffer a stroke, or die.

Meanwhile, the fact that heart disease had become so associated with men seemed to lead physicians to underestimate women's cardiovascular risk. In 1991, Dr. Bernadine Healy described this problem as the Yentl syndrome. Reviewing new research showing that women with symptoms of a heart attack were undertreated, receiving fewer diagnostic tests and lifesaving treatments, she compared their dilemma to that of the heroine of Isaac

Bashevis Singer's short story "Yentl the Yeshiva Boy," who disguised herself as a man to attend school and study the Talmud. "Being 'just like a man' has historically been a price women have had to pay for equality," Healy wrote. "Decades of sex-exclusive research have reinforced the myth that coronary artery disease is a uniquely male affliction and have generated data sets in which men are the normative standard." To get equal care, women first had to prove that they were as sick as their male counterparts. "Once a woman showed that she was just like a man, by having severe coronary artery disease or a myocardial infarction, then she was treated as a man would be."

Twenty-five years later, there's more knowledge about sex/gender differences in heart disease than perhaps any other area of medicine. At the same time, there is a wealth of research documenting the gender disparities that stubbornly persist in diagnosing, preventing, and treating it.

————

Since 2000, the number of women dying from cardiovascular disease has been declining significantly—a few decades after men started seeing improvements. Experts attribute the progress to an increase in awareness, among the public and health care providers alike, a greater focus on reducing women's risk factors, and the better application of evidence-based treatments. In 1997, only 30 percent of American women surveyed were aware that cardiovascular disease was the leading cause of death in women; by 2009, that figure was up to 54 percent.

Still, as recently as 2005, only 8 percent of primary care physicians, 13 percent of ob-gyns, and 17 percent of cardiologists surveyed in one study knew that cardiovascular disease kills more women than men every year. And according to a 2017 survey, only 22 percent of primary care physicians and 42 percent of cardiologists said they felt well prepared to assess women's cardiovascular risk.

Meanwhile, a 2015 meta-analysis of forty-three studies since the early nineties on women's experiences of heart disease concluded that the myth that heart disease is a "man's disease" remains pervasive. "The women described feeling invisible within a medical context that frames coronary symptoms within a dominant (male) paradigm," the authors wrote. "They thought physicians treated them differently than men and believed researchers paid little attention to heart disease in women. Women felt their risk factors and symptoms were not taken as seriously as men's."

The research backs up these women's perceptions. In a 2008 experiment, just one of many studies documenting gender bias in the diagnosis of heart disease, 128 primary care physicians in the United States, Germany, and the United Kingdom watched videotaped patients, played by actors, presenting with symptoms of heart disease. They were then interviewed about what follow-up questions they would ask the patient, what test they would order, what diagnosis they felt was most likely, and what, if any, referrals or treatments they'd recommend. The doctors gave the women patients less attention than the men: they asked them fewer questions, were less likely to give them a possible diagnosis of cardiovascular disease, and were less certain about their diagnosis. "Although patients with identical symptoms were presented," the researchers concluded, "primary care doctors' behavior differed by patients' gender in all 3 countries under study. These gender differences suggest that women may be less likely to receive an accurate diagnosis and appropriate treatment than men."

Gender disparities persist even when it comes to patients with the same actual calculated risk of the disease according to traditional risk factors for the disease. In 2005, the AHA tested five hundred physicians (three hundred primary care physicians, a hundred ob-gyns, and a hundred cardiologists) on how well they could assess patients' cardiovascular risk and apply the association's new evidence-based prevention guidelines. The study found that, across all three specialties, when presented with male and female patients who, on paper, both had an intermediate risk based on various factors like age, smoking history, family history of heart disease, et cetera, they were more likely to incorrectly judge the women as low risk. Because of this underestimation, they recommended fewer prevention measures to the women compared to the men. One of the few exceptions to that rule: among the patients judged to have an intermediate risk, the women were significantly more likely than the men to be advised to lose weight.

Even women with family histories of heart disease tell of meeting resistance from their health care providers when they attempted to be proactive about monitoring their heart health. A woman in one study asked her doctor for a cholesterol test and was told, "But a young and healthy woman like you can't have raised cholesterol." Another recalled, "I talked to the nurse practitioner and told her about my mother's history of heart disease and she just looked at me real funny, and I said, 'You think this is all in my head, don't you?' She said, 'I'm not saying it's all in your head, but your mind can make your body do things.'"

"SHE IS TOO YOUNG AND SHE IS A WOMAN"

Middle-aged women with heart disease are especially likely to be overlooked. The stubborn myth that younger women don't get heart disease lingers, it seems, because of the sex/gender difference in rates of the disease according to age: women are typically older than men when they suffer a first heart attack (seventy-two years compared to sixty-five years for men), and at every age up until seventy-five, men have greater odds of having a heart attack than women.

Still, about 40,000 women under age fifty-five are hospitalized for a heart attack each year in the United States, and about 16,000 of them die. Heart disease, in fact, kills more women at every age than breast cancer does. And, as with heart disease more generally, those women who do get heart disease early fare more poorly than do men. Studies in the nineties showed that younger female heart attack patients were about twice as likely to die in the hospital as their male counterparts—a mortality gap that has just recently begun to narrow. In fact, despite the overall downward trend in heart disease mortality, in recent years, there's been a striking *increase* in cardiovascular deaths among women age forty-five to fifty-four.

Too often, health care providers' perception of their middle-aged women patients' risk of heart disease appears to be overly influenced by how it compares to *men's*, as if the fact that it's even *more* common in men somehow means it's nonexistent in women—rather than being one of their leading causes of death. In one study, a fifty-one-year-old woman described being told her heart attack was categorically impossible—while it was happening. "I can clearly remember the distress I felt when they phoned the ambulance from the hospital and asked them to turn round, because they were so busy: 'She is too young and she is a woman,' they argued."

After she recovered from her own close call, Thomas attended the WomenHeart Science and Leadership Symposium, a leadership training program for women with heart disease put on by specialists from the Mayo Clinic, and started a blog called *Heart Sisters*. (When we spoke she was at work on her book *A Woman's Guide to Living with Heart Disease*, which was published in 2017.) As an advocate who now speaks regularly about women's heart health, she's learned that her experience is not as uncommon as she'd assumed. "I thought my story was pretty dramatic at the time, until I met so many women who, like me, had been misdiagnosed mid–heart attack and sent home." Of the forty-five other women in her WomenHeart class, a full third of them had the same experience.

Indeed, in a study published in *The New England Journal of Medicine* in 2000, researchers analyzed the records of thousands of patients who had come into ten American emergency rooms with symptoms of a heart attack, and determined the characteristics that were linked to a patient being mistakenly discharged. According to their calculation, the rate of misdiagnosis translated into at least 11,000 missed heart attacks per year in the United States. And women under fifty-five years old were seven times more likely to be sent home than the average patient. The consequences of the mistake were dire: being released from the hospital nearly doubled the patient's odds of dying.

THE CHALLENGE OF OVERCOMING "KNOWLEDGE-MEDIATED BIASES"

The myth that "younger women don't get heart disease" points to the danger of what Dr. Katarina Hamberg of Sweden's Umeå University has called a "knowledge-mediated bias." While an awareness that men or women have, on average, greater or lesser risks of certain diseases is important and useful up to a point, this awareness can lead to diseases becoming so stereotyped as a "man's disease" or a "woman's disease" that doctors are blinded to the individual in front of them—to the extent that the stereotype actually becomes self-fulfilling: knowing a condition is more common in one gender tends to result in its underdiagnosis in the other gender.

The history of chronic obstructive pulmonary disease (COPD) illustrates this dynamic well. The fourth most common cause of death in the United States, COPD is closely linked to cigarette smoking. Accordingly, for decades the typical COPD patient was the typical smoker: an older white man. But beginning in the sixties, as tobacco companies began targeting women, the gender gap in smoking rates began to close—and the gap in COPD rates soon followed suit. Between 1980 and 2000, women's mortality rates from COPD tripled. Since 2000, more women than men have died from COPD each year. In a 2001 study, researchers suggested that COPD was being underdiagnosed in women due to the entrenched stereotype associated with the disease. They asked 192 primary care physicians to consider the case of a middle-aged patient, either a man or a woman, with a chronic cough and a history of smoking. On first pass, 49 percent of the women patients received a COPD diagnosis compared to 64.6 percent of the identical male patients. Once test results pointing to COPD were offered, the gender gap narrowed but still didn't disappear completely.

As the researchers noted, some would argue that the bias demonstrated in the study wasn't entirely inappropriate given that "the risk of COPD is truly higher in men than in women given the historically higher tobacco consumption rates in men." But they point out that this is a circular argument: the accuracy of the epidemiological data that tells us how common diseases are in different groups is dependent on doctors making accurate diagnoses. If COPD was underdiagnosed in women—as the study suggested it was—how would anyone know whether it was still actually more prevalent among men? And even if it was somewhat more common among men, that's irrelevant to whether an individual woman has it. Yet the image of the male "typical patient" was so strong that the doctors in the study overlooked COPD in female smokers, even though the only reason for men's historically higher rates of COPD to begin with was their higher rates of smoking. Today, despite now officially having higher rates of COPD than men throughout most of their lifetime, women continue to face delays in getting diagnosed.

"Knowledge-mediated" biases do affect patients of both genders. Studies have suggested that men are underdiagnosed with some conditions that are more common among women, including depression, migraine, fibromyalgia, and breast cancer. Still, this type of bias seems to be especially difficult for women to overcome. After all, when the diagnosis goes against what's statistically expected, a willingness to listen to the individual patient's symptoms—to trust that she is a reliable reporter even when the symptoms she reports seem unlikely—becomes even more important to making the correct diagnosis. Many women with other diseases stereotyped as "men's diseases," like autism and attention deficit disorder, report that doctors were absolutely resistant to the possibility—even when the women suggested the correct diagnosis themselves.

It took Mae six doctor's visits and eighteen months to get someone to listen when she described her cluster headaches. Considered one of the single most painful medical conditions, cluster headaches are nicknamed "suicide headaches" for a reason. When Mae's attacks started, her husband, then a medical student who'd just learned about headache disorders, suggested she keep a spreadsheet of when they happened and her symptoms. The level of pain and the pattern suggested that they might be cluster headaches, which, as the name suggests, tend to strike at the same time every day in episodes of a few weeks or months at a time. Mae also had the watering eye and droopy eyelid on one side that are typical of the disorder; she never had the aura that's common with migraines.

"But the doctors wouldn't listen to me," she says. "They heard the word 'headache' and immediately determined I was suffering from hormonal migraines 'like all women.'" While cluster headaches are certainly rarer than migraines and women are less likely than men to have them, the male–female ratio is not as high as previously thought: in the sixties, it was estimated at 6:1 but is now put closer to 2:1. And even if it were 99:1, there would still be the one, whose only hope of getting the correct diagnosis would be for doctors to notice that her symptoms matched those of cluster headaches.

Mae showed her longtime primary care physician her spreadsheets, but it didn't matter—she was prescribed treatments for migraine. She pushed to get a referral to one neurologist, then another. By this point, she was having multiple headaches per day; the migraine medications clearly weren't helping at all. "When I talked about the symptoms I was experiencing, two prominent neurologists, one from each major teaching center in our city, used a nearly identical phrase: 'You couldn't be experiencing that.'"

To Mae, it seemed clear that the fact that *she'd* suggested the diagnosis was part of why the doctors wouldn't even consider it. "The first two neurologists were just like, 'That's not what you're feeling; you need to get off WebMD.' They were looking for *brain cancer* before they would take my word that I had these headaches that followed this pattern." The sheer frustration of not being heard was almost as bad as the pain itself. "It was infuriating to be told I wasn't capable of even knowing what I felt. It was more infuriating than the headaches."

Finally, Mae went to yet another neurologist and presented all the same information. "He just sat there listening to me and then said, 'You're right—this sounds a lot like cluster headaches.'" He offered an immediate solution that would both determine if they were indeed cluster headaches and, if they were, relieve her unbearable pain: an oxygen tank to breathe from when an attack began. "That was a miracle pill. By finally having somebody—my third neurologist—actually listen to me, I had an immediate treatment that worked."

Mae had ninety-two untreated headaches while trying to get her diagnosis. She says she doesn't know what would have happened if she hadn't had a partner in the medical profession, if she hadn't lived in a major medical mecca, or if she hadn't had excellent insurance that gave her the financial ability to keep going to specialist after specialist. "I would probably still not have a diagnosis. And I don't know how I could've lived through five-plus years of that. I don't think I could have."

DIVERGING FROM THE TEXTBOOK

The stereotyping of heart disease as a "man's disease" is not the only reason for women's undertreatment. It's not just that doctors too often fail to follow evidence-based standards of heart care for women; it's also that the evidence base itself is skewed. In short, medicine developed a model of heart disease based on research conducted almost exclusively on men. The inevitable result is that women's experiences—from their risk factors to their symptoms to the very definition of what qualifies as a heart attack—are less likely to neatly fit into this model.

Even when properly applied, traditional risk scores aren't as accurate at predicting women's odds of getting heart disease to begin with. While the major risk factors are the same for both men and women, there are some sex/gender differences in their relative importance. For example, while high total cholesterol is a key predictor of future heart disease in men, low levels of HDL cholesterol—the "good" cholesterol—and high triglyceride levels are far more important in women. Having type 2 diabetes increases the risk of heart disease in women more than it does in men, as do stress and a history of depression.

Meanwhile, new research is starting to identify previously overlooked "nontraditional" risk factors for women. In 2011, the AHA declared for the first time that pregnancy complications, such as preeclampsia, gestational diabetes mellitus, and pregnancy-induced hypertension, can serve as warning signs that a woman is more likely to develop heart disease, a link that many physicians still aren't aware of. When Thomas had her heart attack, she was repeatedly asked if she had been a smoker or had high cholesterol or had a family history of heart disease—but she had none of the "traditional" risk factors. She had, however, developed preeclampsia when she had her first child decades ago, which gave her double the risk of developing cardiovascular disease, a fact she was neither warned about at the time nor asked about after her heart attack. In the future, women's risk scores may also incorporate whether they have disruptions in ovulation, inflammatory biomarkers, or a history of autoimmune disorders.

When it comes to the symptoms of a heart attack too, women are more likely to diverge from the textbook. The "classic" symptoms, derived from research on men, are relatively well known: crushing chest pain and shooting pain down the left arm. An image of an older, slightly overweight white man suddenly clutching his chest and slumping over in his chair has made its way into the cultural consciousness as the "Hollywood heart attack" and has, quite literally, illustrated the medical textbooks for decades.

But women, premenopausal women especially, are more likely to have other "atypical" symptoms during a heart attack and often in the days or even weeks leading up to it: pain in the neck, throat, shoulder, or upper back; abdominal discomfort; shortness of breath; nausea or vomiting; sweating, anxiety, or a sense of impending doom; light-headedness or dizziness; and unusual fatigue or insomnia. Yet in 1996, a national survey revealed that two-thirds of doctors were completely unaware of any sex/gender variations in symptoms. And a 2012 survey of American women found that less than a fifth knew the atypical symptoms like nausea and fatigue.

This difference in symptoms contributes to the longer delays in getting treated that women experience during a heart attack. Certainly, it's clear that not having the hallmark symptom of chest pain at all can lead doctors astray. A 2012 study that tracked more than 1.1 million heart attack patients from 1994 to 2006 concluded that a lack of chest pain helped explain why 15 percent of the women died in the hospital, compared to 10 percent of the men. Patients who never experienced chest pain were nearly twice as likely to die, due in part to delays in getting lifesaving interventions. And women, particularly younger women, were overrepresented in this group: 42 percent of the women didn't have chest pain, compared to only 31 percent of the men.

Perhaps the most glaring example of how a lack of attention to sex/gender differences contributes to women's undertreatment is the fact that the standard test currently used to diagnose a heart attack—which measures the level of troponin, a protein released from the heart into the blood when it's damaged—is less sensitive in women. In recent years, newer "high-sensitivity" troponin tests have been developed that are able to detect the protein at much lower levels and have suggested there should be different cutoffs for men and women. "It's becoming increasingly clear with the high-sensitivity troponins now that are coming out that the standard troponin level that we've used for years and years and years—which is the male standard again—misses about one in five heart attacks in women," Bairey Merz says.

A study published in *The BMJ* in 2015 looked at hundreds of patients with symptoms suggesting a heart attack and found that when the high-sensitivity troponin test with sex-specific thresholds was used, the proportion of women diagnosed with a heart attack doubled from 11 percent, according to the standard test, to 22 percent. In contrast, among men, the two tests didn't yield different results. The consequence: with the standard test, twice as many men as women were judged to have had a heart attack; with the new test, the rates for both genders were the same. The one-size-fits-all test, in other words, has been systemically underdiagnosing women's heart attacks.

From one perspective, these are some of the more understandable reasons for the gender disparities evident in heart disease care. It is, after all, unsurprising that women are less likely to be treated for a heart attack if they are less likely to qualify as having had one in the first place. As Bairey Merz says of the troponin test problem, "There are good and bad reasons why women are less aggressively treated. That's kind of a 'good' reason in the sense that we can fix it. It's just a lack of recognition that here's an important variable where women and men differ and it's making a difference in the diagnosis." But, of course, it's not a coincidence that women's presentations are less likely to be "textbook" cases; the only reason their risk factors are considered "nontraditional" and their symptoms are called "atypical" is that the norm has been a male one.

"DOCTORS THINK THAT MEN HAVE HEART ATTACKS AND WOMEN HAVE STRESS"

But the knowledge gap when it comes to women's symptoms doesn't explain everything here. For example, in the study above that suggested atypical symptoms and the absence of chest pain contribute to women's higher mortality rate, gender played a role independent of symptoms among the patients under age fifty-five: with or without chest pain, younger women had a higher mortality rate than younger men with similar symptoms. Indeed, most studies have found that while, on average, women do seem to have *more* symptoms, which may confuse the diagnostic picture, the majority of people having a heart attack, including women, do have chest symptoms. And those women are *also* more likely than men to be misdiagnosed.

In a 2015 qualitative study out of the Yale School of Public Health exploring the experiences of younger female heart attack patients, for example, while the interviewees had a range of symptoms, the vast majority of them (93 percent) had chest pain. And yet, they told stories of unresponsive health care providers and delays in getting timely workups when experiencing both atypical and typical symptoms. One woman, for example, called her doctor to report chest pain and was told to schedule a regular appointment—for five days later.

Even some women, like Thomas, suffering a picture-perfect "Hollywood heart attack," report that their symptoms were initially brushed off. "I often say if that emergency room doctor had only googled my symptoms at the time, there's only one diagnosis that would have popped up, really," Thomas says. "Had I been a man who had presented with central chest pain, nausea, sweating, and pain down my left arm, there is no doubt I would have been admitted for observation"—even with normal cardiac test results, just to be safe.

In addition to finding their symptoms blamed on other, more minor physical conditions—acid reflux, ulcers, gallstones, and arthritis—many women were told they were the result of stress, anxiety, depression, or "worry." In one study, 44 percent of women with heart disease said they felt health care providers trivialized their complaints and attributed them to psychological causes. As one woman put it simply, "Doctors think that men have heart attacks and women have stress."

A series of studies led by psychologist Gabrielle R. Chiaramonte in 2007 vividly illustrated this problem. In one version, 230 family doctors and internists were asked to read two vignettes of hypothetical patients: a forty-seven-year-old man and a fifty-six-year-old woman with the same probability of having heart disease according to their ages, identical risk factors, and "textbook" heart attack symptoms: chest pain, shortness of breath, and an irregular heartbeat. Half of the vignettes included a note that the patient had recently experienced a stressful life event and appeared to be anxious. In the vignettes without that note, there was no difference between the doctors' recommendations to the woman and the man. Despite the popular conception of the quintessential heart attack patient as male, in this quiz at least, the doctors seemed perfectly capable of making the right call in the female patient too.

But when the note about stress was added, an enormous gender gap suddenly appeared. Only 15 percent of the doctors diagnosed heart disease in the woman, compared to 56 percent for the man, and only 30 percent referred the woman to a cardiologist, compared to 62 percent for the man. Finally, only 13 percent suggested cardiac medication for the woman, versus 47 percent for the man. The presence of stress, the researchers explained, seemed to spark a "meaning shift" in which women's physical symptoms were reinterpreted as psychological, while "men's symptoms were perceived as organic whether or not stressors were present." The male patient's stress not only didn't detract from a heart disease diagnosis but actually seemed to support it; stress is, in fact, linked to greater odds of suffering a heart attack and, in the men, it was "viewed (rightly so) as a risk factor."

That was when the patients *did* experience the "classic" heart attack symptoms. In the next twist on the study, the researchers asked 142 family physicians to assess a male and a female patient presenting with atypical symptoms, including nausea and back pain. This muddied the picture further: the woman was slightly less likely than the man to receive a heart disease diagnosis, but neither was likely to get one at all. And when stress was added to the mix, both men and women became even more likely to be diagnosed with a gastrointestinal problem instead.

If even a single line about the patient appearing to be anxious can spark such a dramatic "meaning shift," it's a wonder that women with diagnosed anxiety disorders are ever promptly and accurately diagnosed with heart disease. As Thomas says, "It's too tempting. As soon as they hear that, it's very tempting for physicians to say, 'Oh, that's what it is.'" In fact, she heard from one woman who felt that her anxiety diagnosis was such a barrier to adequate care that she successfully fought to get it scrubbed from her medical records. "Women know that it is the label that follows you around from doctor to doctor and from diagnosis to diagnosis—that it's always going to be a 'problem list,' as doctors call it, on that chart."

This bias is obviously most dangerous during the acute emergency of a heart attack, when, as cardiologists like to say, "time is muscle." A 2014 study that tracked over a thousand heart attack patients under fifty-five at twenty-six hospitals in Canada, the United States, and Switzerland found that less than half of all patients got access to cardiac testing and care within the benchmark times set by experts, and women experienced longer delays. The median time it took for men to get an EKG was 15 minutes, compared to 21 minutes for women; the gender gap was 28 compared to 36 minutes for fibrinolytic therapy to break up a clot and 93 compared to 106 minutes to implant a coronary stent. The researchers noted that while some factors—like an absence of chest pain—contributed to a delay for both men and women, there was one that seemed to pose a problem in women only:

anxiety. Women with high scores on a scale measuring anxiety symptoms were less likely to meet the 10-minute benchmark for an EKG than women without anxiety; in men, it didn't matter.

And it's not just women who have been diagnosed with an anxiety disorder or who seem to be anxious or who mention a recent stressful event that are at risk of having their symptoms dismissed as psychological; simply being a middle-aged woman may be sufficient. That's what was suggested by a 2009 study in which 128 internists, family practitioners, and general practitioners viewed different versions of a video of an actor presenting with signs and symptoms of coronary artery disease. The doctors were least confident in their diagnosis of heart disease in the fifty-five-year-old women patients, and those patients were twice as likely as their middle-aged male counterparts (31 percent compared to 16 percent) to receive a mental health diagnosis instead. The combination of their gender and age, the researchers concluded, "misled physicians, particularly toward mental health alternative diagnoses." They warned that "physicians should be aware of the potential for psychological symptoms to erroneously take a central role in the diagnosis of younger women."

"HYSTERICAL FEMALES WHO COME TO THE EMERGENCY ROOM"

The tendency to misdiagnose women's, especially younger women's, heart symptoms as anxiety, particularly in the ER setting, is often explained by pointing to the relative probabilities. Chest pain is the second most common complaint that brings patients to the emergency room, accounting for 8 million visits in the United States each year, but only about 20 percent of those who are admitted are found to be having a heart attack or other cardiac problem. Meanwhile, there is symptom overlap between a heart attack and a panic attack, and younger women are at relatively lower risk for the former and higher risk for the latter. Given this reality, "triage personnel might initially dismiss a cardiac event among young women with anxiety," as the 2014 study discussed above concluded. One cardiologist put it more bluntly in a media interview: "In training, we were taught to be on the lookout for hysterical females who come to the emergency room."

It's not entirely clear who all these mythical "hysterical females who come to the emergency room" actually are, though. Certainly, many people experiencing their first panic attack do go to the ER, convinced it's their heart, but trained professionals can differentiate between a genuine panic attack and a heart attack. Instead, the perception that women's chest pain is likely to be anxiety or stress seems to stem from a more general sense that women are hypochondriacs prone to blowing minor ailments—like, say, acid reflux, as in Thomas's case—out of proportion and talking themselves into believing they're having a heart attack.

And there's no reason to think that women do that. Exactly the opposite, in fact: research has pointed to women's tendency to delay going to the ER when they're actually having a heart attack as one factor that may contribute to their worse outcomes compared to men. Chest pain is one of the symptoms for which the assumption that women seek care more readily than men do just doesn't hold up. While survival rates increase by half if patients are treated within an hour after their symptoms begin, few patients, of either gender, get to the hospital that quickly, and multiple studies have shown that women wait longer than men do before seeking treatment. According to a 2014 study by researchers at Harvard School of Public Health, when chest pain struck, men and women went through a similar progression of stages, starting with uncertainty and denial, before finally reaching a "symptomatic tipping point" that compelled them to seek out medical treatment. But women were one and a half times more likely than men to wait for their symptoms to become worse or more frequent before seeing a doctor.

Of course, one reason for women's delay in seeking treatment may be that, either misled by the myth that heart disease is a "men's disease" or confused by "atypical" symptoms, they simply dismiss the possibility that they could be having a heart attack. That certainly seems to be part of the story, according to the 2015 study from Yale School of Public Health. Some of the women under the age of fifty-five interviewed by the researchers explained that they had hesitated before coming in to the ER because they had figured that they were too young to be having a heart attack or they had attributed their atypical symptoms to other health problems. In other words, having internalized the male stereotype of the disease, they misdiagnosed themselves in much the same way their doctors very well might have.

But the study identified another worrying trend: some of the women had, in fact, immediately suspected they were having a heart attack but had waited until they were sure because they were worried about being seen as hypochondriacs if they were wrong. "Not wanting to make a fuss, or not wanting to be embarrassed 'in case it turns out to be nothing and I would feel like a fool'—that's hugely pervasive in women's reasons" for delaying care, Thomas says. "Even in the middle of very severe symptoms, we talk ourselves into thinking that it's probably nothing."

Of course, all too often this fear of being labeled a hypochondriac proves to be entirely justified. Once they finally sought help, many of the women in the Yale study encountered health care providers who treated them precisely like the hypochondriacs they feared they were—until they overcame the Yentl syndrome and proved they really were sick.

Indeed, while there are many factors that may contribute to women's reluctance to "make a fuss," previous experiences with health care providers are often a big one. Many of the interviewees reported having had "poor physician-patient relationships, feeling rebuffed or treated with disrespect, and being denied care." And it had discouraged them from seeking medical attention even before their heart attack; they reported having "limited and sporadic" routine doctor's visits—preventive care that may have helped prevent them from getting heart disease to begin with—because they didn't want to be "perceived as complaining about minor concerns."

Patti is one woman whose fear of being *that* woman, that "hysterical female" clogging up the ER, nearly cost her her life. A concussion after tripping on an uneven step had marked the beginning of two months of "nothing but health care—just one thing after the other." Two weeks after the fall, she'd suddenly developed blinding double vision while driving. A month after that, she'd woken up to severe vertigo that kept her from working for weeks. "I'd never experienced anything like it in my life. The room was completely spinning around me." Then there was a "hard, hot burning" in her leg that her husband thought might be a blood clot—and yet another trip to the emergency room revealed it was indeed.

The ER doctors had instructed her to follow up with her regular doctor in a few weeks, so now she was, this time with a new worrisome symptom to report: for the last couple of days, the slightest exertion would bring chest pain and shortness of breath. "I was so winded just getting up and going to the kitchen. It felt like one of my lungs had collapsed."

Her doctor had a medical student shadowing him that day, so after Patti relayed the last months' events, she got to hear him spell out his thinking about her case to his trainee. As if she weren't in the room, Patti recalls, he explained to the student why he thought they were likely dealing with anxiety: "It is anxiety that would take her to the ER on a Saturday with what might be a blood clot. Most people would wait until Monday and call here to get an appointment, but she went to the ER. We can tell from that that she's overwrought about her health and all she needs is anxiety medication."

It was not the first time Patti had felt like this particular doctor didn't take her symptoms seriously, nor was he the first in the long line of health care providers she'd seen during this recent saga to suggest that it was all in her head. The ER doctor who had examined her when she came in with sudden double vision put down "anxiety" in her chart—even as she told Patti to follow up with a neurologist about an abnormality on her brain scan. Similarly, the fact that Patti's "anxiety" about a blood clot had been warranted—she actually *did* have one—somehow didn't detract from her primary care physician's analysis. Neither did the fact that Patti had no history of an anxiety disorder, which her doctor, who'd been her regular physician for years, knew. Patti says she can't imagine her doctor saying the same thing to a male patient. "My husband would have gotten very different care. He would have immediately been hooked up to an EKG machine in my doctor's office—I'm sure of it."

Two days later, as a snowstorm engulfed her home in the North Carolina mountains, Patti was hoping a hot shower might make it easier to breathe. Minutes later, she yelled for her husband to call 911. Taken by ambulance to the ER, she was diagnosed with a heart attack and eventually had a stent placed. Like Thomas, she'd had a widowmaker; the artery was 90 percent blocked. "I was lucky that I paid attention to my own intuition. Had I not told my husband to call 911, I'm not sure I would be alive; I probably wouldn't be." She trusted her gut, in part, because her father had died of a heart attack when he was just fifty-three—three years younger than she was at the time. "Because of my dad, I'm perhaps more aware of heart attacks—with good reason, it turns out."

But there was still a part of her that hesitated before telling her husband to make the call. "In the back of my mind, I was thinking about what my doctor had said," she recalls. Laid up for a week in the hospital recovering from a complication from the stent procedure, she wrote a *HuffPost* piece about what had happened: "The sad fact is that I waited. I waited because I felt shamed into feeling like a hysterical female, shamed into feeling like I was just anxious. JUST anxious. Like anxiety is something to be ashamed of or embarrassed by." In fact, a healthy dose of anxiety had saved her life. "This was not something to be calm about. Calm people are dead people, when you're dealing with a heart attack or anything life-threatening."

UNDERTREATMENT IN THE ER

Though it's been the focus of the most research, a heart attack is certainly not the only acute, life-threatening condition for which women are treated less aggressively in the ER. Dr. Alyson McGregor, an associate professor of emergency medicine and director of the Division of Sex and Gender in Emergency Medicine at the Warren Alpert Medical School of Brown University, recently coauthored a new medical textbook, *Sex and Gender in Acute Care Medicine*. "It's amazing and really alarming to see that cardiac arrest, stroke, conditions of sepsis—in almost all of these conditions, women receive less intense care," she says.

Indeed, in 2014, the first large-scale study of the misdiagnosis of stroke in the United States, based on medical records of 187,188 patients in over a thousand hospitals nationwide, found that up to 12.7 percent of people later admitted for stroke had been erroneously sent home from an ER in the thirty days prior. At that rate, the researchers estimated that there are between 50,000 and 100,000 missed stroke diagnoses each year, the consequences of which could be significant: prompt treatment can lower the risk of a repeat stroke by as much as 80 percent. Typically, the misdiagnosed patients had come in complaining of dizziness or a headache and left with a diagnosis like inner ear infection or migraine, or no diagnosis at all. Women were a third more likely than men to be misdiagnosed.

Each year, over 300,000 people suffer a cardiac arrest in the United States. A cardiac arrest, though it can be caused by a heart attack, is not the same thing: it occurs when a malfunction of the heart's electrical system causes it to suddenly stop beating, and death can occur within minutes if CPR isn't started. Few people even make it to the ER, and of those who do, nearly two-thirds still aren't saved. Though in-hospital survival rates have been increasing for cardiac arrest patients of both genders in the last fifteen years, this improvement has been smaller in women. A 2016 analysis of the records of a sample of cardiac arrest patients in over a thousand United States hospitals between 2003 and 2012 suggested that's at least partly because women are treated less aggressively than men. After adjusting for other factors, women were 25 percent less likely to have an angiography to check for blocked arteries, 29 percent less likely to undergo angioplasty to open them, and 19 percent less likely to be treated with hypothermia to lower body temperature, which increases odds of recovery.

"What we've done over the past couple years is really gather this type of health disparity data," McGregor says. "Our next step is to identify why, then to educate people and health care providers to improve and to decrease this gap." As with heart attacks, the reasons why may include both bias and biology; perhaps women have more "atypical" symptoms or are less likely to test positive on the diagnostic tests to detect certain conditions. But surely part of the reason is they're just not taken as seriously. When I asked McGregor why she thought women's symptoms in an urgent care setting often didn't seem to be met with the same level of, well, urgency, she suggested that the fact that women might be more open in displaying the emotions that pain—or any sudden alarming symptom—often provokes may mislead doctors. "Women may be more likely to express that they are anxious that they're in pain, so oftentimes physicians translate that to 'this patient is anxious,' when they're actually anxious because they're in pain." But, as we've seen, sometimes women are perceived as anxious regardless of whether they express that they are, while men are perceived as in pain regardless of whether they're anxious.

"FEMALE-PATTERN" HEART DISEASE

When women's heart disease experts say that our knowledge of heart disease has been based on a "male model," they're not just talking about how women's symptoms or risk factors may differ, or how tests and treatments—from troponin tests to stents—were designed for a male norm. One of the most important findings to come out of sex/gender-specific research in the last two decades has been the discovery of a whole new form of ischemic heart disease—that is, heart disease that causes reduced blood flow to the heart. Previously unrecognized and, to this day, largely undiagnosed, it is more common in women. In a 2014 AHA scientific statement, cardiologist Dr. Jennifer H. Mieres explained, "For decades, doctors used the male model of coronary heart disease testing to identify the disease in women, automatically focusing on the detection of obstructive coronary artery disease. As a result, symptomatic women who did not have classic obstructive coronary disease were not diagnosed with ischemic heart disease, and did not receive appropriate treatment, thereby increasing their risk for heart attack."

Here's how the classic (read: male) model of coronary artery disease is thought to work: over time, plaque builds up in the arteries that deliver blood to and from the heart (a process called atherosclerosis) and causes them to narrow. If a patient begins to experience chest pain, they might be given a stress test that indicates they're getting reduced blood flow to their heart (known technically as ischemia). If that's positive, they might get an angiogram: an X-ray image of the heart's arteries. If one of the major arteries of the heart is revealed to be more than 50 to 70 percent blocked, they'll be diagnosed with obstructive coronary artery disease (CAD). Treatment is focused on preventing further narrowing of the arteries and, if they're already severely blocked, reopening them with procedures like an angioplasty, a stent, or, in the worst cases, bypass surgery. The hope, of course, is to detect the disease before it causes the life-threatening event of a heart attack. Under the classic model, a heart attack happens when a plaque obstruction suddenly ruptures and causes a blood clot that completely cuts off blood flow to a part of the heart, which, deprived of oxygen, rapidly begins to die.

For the first few decades that we were studying coronary heart disease, it was this form of the disease—obstructive CAD—that we were focused on. However, it's long been known that a large proportion of patients have chest pain that suggests heart disease and an abnormal stress test, but when an angiogram is done, it shows that they don't have obstructive CAD. In some cases, their arteries appear to be perfectly "normal," with no visible narrowing. In others, there is some mild narrowing, but it doesn't reach the greater than 50 percent blockage that typically qualifies as obstructive CAD; this condition has been labeled "nonobstructive CAD." In men, this is the exception, but in women, it is actually the norm. Studies suggest that 60 to 70 percent of women undergoing an angiogram because of symptoms and signs suggesting reduced blood flow to the heart are found to have normal or nearly normal arteries, compared to just 30 percent or less of men.

These patients posed a baffling dilemma. They seemed to have reduced blood flow, yet in the classic model of the disease, if there wasn't a visibly blocked artery, it wasn't clear what was to blame. So initially, they were considered "false positives." If the angiogram showed their arteries were clean, perhaps the stress test was wrong. Instead of taking the existence of these perplexing patients as evidence that the model wasn't adequate and needed to be adjusted in order to explain their symptoms, some of the evidence was simply thrown out so that they would fit into the existing paradigm. This despite the fact that these women had not only the subjective symptoms—namely, chest pain—but also objective signs of ischemia measured by a variety of different technologies, including electrocardiogram, PET imaging, and contrast cardiac MRIs.

Eventually, the evidence of ischemia in the absence of obstructive CAD was accepted, but the poorly defined condition (sometimes called cardiac syndrome X) was thought to be a fairly harmless one. Small observational studies since the sixties had suggested that these patients were not at increased risk of suffering a heart attack or other life-threatening cardiovascular conditions. So while they often continued to have ongoing and debilitating symptoms, they were offered nothing more than reassurance that they did not have heart disease.

In 1996, the National Heart, Lung, and Blood Institute launched the Women's Ischemia Syndrome Evaluation (WISE) study, a groundbreaking research project to correct the decades-long focus on men's heart disease. It confirmed that the mysterious condition was hardly a benign one in terms of quality of life and economic costs: about half of women sent home "reassured" that they had "normal" or "nonobstructive" arteries still had chest pain five years later; many returned repeatedly for diagnostic testing and largely ineffective treatment, and one in five had been rehospitalized. Over the course of a lifetime, the researchers estimated, the health care costs of women with nonobstructive CAD were over $750,000, not that far below the $1 million price tag that women with obstructive CAD faced.

Furthermore, by the mid-aughts, results from the WISE project began to reveal that, contrary to the conclusions of those earlier small studies, which experts now believe were poorly designed and didn't have a long enough follow-up period, these patients actually *do* face increased cardio-vascular risks, having two to four times higher odds of suffering a heart attack, heart failure, or stroke within five years. Yes, that prognosis is better than that of those with obstructive CAD, but only marginally. After ten years, 6.7 percent of the symptomatic patients with "normal" arteries, 12.8 percent of those with nonobstructive CAD, and 25.9 percent of those with obstructive CAD had died from heart-related causes or had a heart attack.

Indeed, while most people who have a heart attack have obstructive CAD, a minority of them—more of them women—don't. The WISE study found that 10 to 25 percent of women who experienced a heart attack didn't have evidence of obstructive CAD, versus 6 to 10 percent of men. Autopsy studies also show that while about three-quarters of fatal heart attacks in men are due to plaque ruptures, only 55 percent of women's heart attacks are explained by ruptures; instead they have more evidence of plaque erosions. Turns out the classic model, in which a heart attack is caused by a rupture of an obstruction, doesn't tell the whole story for a significant number of women.

Research like the WISE study has now identified several other abnor-malities that can cause ischemia in the absence of obstructive CAD. The most common one seems to be coronary microvascular disease (CMD). Undetectable by traditional angiogram, it's a condition that affects the small arteries or the inner lining of the main arteries leading to the heart. Among the WISE women, nearly half of them had evidence of microvas-cular dysfunction.

Despite this emerging knowledge, at this point, a comprehensive search for other causes of ischemia, once obstructive CAD has been ruled out, is still not the norm. McGregor explains, "When you come to the emergency department with chest pain, all of the protocols that we undergo—what happens to you, what tests we do, whether you get admitted, whether you get further testing, what medications you're on—they're all designed based upon a male pattern of disease, the obstructive disease." If you have non-obstructive heart disease, there may be a delay in getting put on the "rule out heart attack protocol," because your symptoms may be more "atypical." And once on that protocol, "none of those tests are designed to test for it, so you might go through this entire medical system and be discharged, and we'd never detected the type of heart disease that you actually have. That's what's happening to women more often than men."

When I learned about this "female-pattern" heart disease, the puzzle of why doctors seemed to have the impression that there were countless hypochondriacal women rushing to the ER for every slight chest pain, despite the fact that, in reality, women are *more* reluctant to seek care when having a heart attack, suddenly got a whole lot clearer. *Here*, finally, were those mythical "hysterical females" coming into the ER: the millions of mostly women patients—perhaps 3 million in the United States, by the WISE researchers' estimate—who have heart disease and all its symptoms but have, for decades, been told that they do not.

No wonder doctors might unconsciously come to take women's chest pain a bit less seriously when the reality is that women make up the majority of the patients they see whose symptoms can't be explained by obstructive CAD. That's not, primarily, because women are more prone to anxiety but because of medicine's own failure to recognize and detect the forms of heart disease they do have. A 2015 study of patients with chest pain but no obstructive CAD, 77 percent of whom were women, found that over three-quarters had other coronary abnormalities, such as CMD. According to a 2016 article by emergency room physicians, in their experience, CMD may account for the symptoms of as many as 40 percent of patients, the majority of them women, coming into the ER with recurrent chest pain, yet "applying the current standard of care, most patients with microvascular angina remain undiagnosed."

Just as "male-pattern" obstructive CAD is not unique to men, CMD, while more common in women, doesn't affect only them. And it's not an either-or scenario: the same person may have both. In fact, the growing appreciation that alternate mechanisms may cause ischemia is helping to explain a number of other previously perplexing realities about heart disease, including the fact that nearly a third of patients with obstructive CAD who've undergone procedures that successfully opened up their blocked arteries find that their symptoms, inexplicably, persist.

That's what happened to Thomas. After her "male-pattern" widow-maker heart attack, she had a stent implanted in her clogged main artery. But her chest pain, shortness of breath, and crushing fatigue didn't go away. At first, her cardiologist suspected a blockage inside the new stent, but another angiogram showed that her arteries were "pristine." "I actually cried when I heard that—and not happy tears," she remembers. "If it wasn't stent failure, what the hell was causing these debilitating symptoms?" Thankfully, her doctor was familiar with CMD and suspected it might be the culprit.

Many others aren't so lucky. As Bairey Merz, who is lead investigator for the WISE study, said in a 2011 TED talk, "We've been working on this for fifteen years, and we've been working on male-pattern disease for fifty years. So we're thirty-five years behind." That thirty-five-year knowledge gap means awareness of "female-pattern" abnormalities like CMD in the medical community is currently variable. "I think more physicians are paying attention to it. I'm getting more referrals," Bairey Merz says. "Is it widespread? I would say not quite yet." Indeed, Thomas recalls hearing from a reader of her blog whose cardiologist had told her, " 'I don't believe in microvascular disease.' Like it was Santa Claus or something."

"LIKE CHANGING THE DIRECTION OF THE *TITANIC*"

Despite findings like this that clearly illustrate the importance of looking at sex/gender differences in heart disease, recommendations for preventing, diagnosing, and treating the condition continue to be largely extrapolated from research conducted on middle-aged white men, and women are *still* underrepresented in current clinical trials. A review of the AHA's 2007 prevention guidelines for women, for example, found that they drew on studies in which women made up only 30 percent of the subject population. Only one-third of the studies even broke down the results by gender. Women made up about one-third of participants in seventy-eight clinical studies of cardiovascular devices between 2000 and 2007.

Bairey Merz explains that the focus on men's disease has become somewhat self-perpetuating because so many of the clinical trials use obstructive CAD as part of the entry criteria. "It's a little bit like 'no women need apply.'" It's not as if investigators did it intentionally to exclude women, she says. "It's just that for fifty years we've pretty much only recognized the male pattern, and women get male pattern but it's more like 70 percent men, 30 percent women." Furthermore, the fact that clinical research doesn't often include the elderly leaves women, who tend to get the disease later, doubly disadvantaged. "If the trial excluded anyone over the age of sixty-five or seventy-five, they also excluded women."

"It's like changing the direction of the *Titanic*," Bairey Merz says. As the science catches up, she urges women to advocate for themselves and not accept it if your physician says there's nothing wrong with you—to try, as difficult as it can often be, to quell that fear of being seen as a hypochondriac. "Women know their bodies well. If you think something's wrong, get a second opinion."

Or as many as it takes. In her talks, Thomas always tells the story of another woman, whom she calls her "hero," as a counterpoint to her own. She was also sent home from the ER while having a heart attack, not once, not twice, but three times. "And every time, she said, 'I don't care what you say. Something is wrong with me.' Whereas I was too embarrassed; having been sent back once, I was so humiliated that I'd made a fuss over nothing that there was no way I was gonna go back to the hospital. She was saving her own life by going back and going back and going back. The third time she went back, they suggested she might want to consider taking antidepressants, and the fourth time was for double bypass surgery."

CHAPTER 4

AUTOIMMUNE DISEASE AND THE LONG SEARCH FOR A DIAGNOSIS

JACKIE WAS SIXTEEN THE first time she fell ill. One minute, she was at orientation for her first job at Banana Republic; the next, she was coming to on the floor. Rushed to the hospital with a raging fever, she was diagnosed with a bad kidney infection. "That was pretty much the start of ten years of me being in and out of hospitals," she recalls.

Throughout the rest of high school and into college, she had chronic kidney problems, fevers, and terrible joint pain. She continued to pass out randomly. Her menstrual periods brought heavy bleeding and pain so severe she sometimes blacked out. She was tired all the time—a fact that, for years, she attributed to just being "a lazy person." In college, she'd joke to friends about how she couldn't schedule a class before noon, never thinking that the reason she was unbearably exhausted was because of a medical issue. She saw a primary care doctor, a urologist, and a pulmonologist. Test after test revealed nothing amiss. "Everybody was telling me there was nothing wrong with me."

Autoimmune diseases encompass a diverse range of conditions that result ·
from the same basic underlying problem: the immune system is mistakenly
attacking a part of one's own body as if it were a foreign invader. In my own
case of RA, for example, the immune system mobilizes against the lining of
the joints, making them inflamed and painful and eventually, if untreated,
leading to the erosion of bone and cartilage. In type 1 diabetes, the immune
system destroys the beta cells in the pancreas that produce insulin, leaving its sufferers without the ability to control their blood sugar levels on
their own. In Hashimoto's thyroiditis, it's the thyroid gland that's attacked.
In multiple sclerosis, it's thought to be the myelin sheath surrounding the
nerve cells. In Sjögren's syndrome, it's the glands that make tears and saliva.
In systemic lupus erythematosus, it's a part of the nucleus of cells, which
means that any part of the body, including the joints, skin, kidneys, blood
cells, brain, heart, and lungs, can be affected.

Many autoimmune diseases are quite rare, but several of the most
common ones, including all those mentioned above, each affect a million
or more Americans. And collectively, autoimmune disease is up there
with heart disease and cancer as one of the top three most prevalent
disease categories. According to the NIH, up to 23.5 million Americans
have an autoimmune disease. But experts and advocacy groups, like the
AARDA, put the figure at more than twice that—50 million—since the
NIH's estimate is based on only a couple dozen of the diseases for which
solid epidemiology studies have been done. By comparison, 28 million
Americans have heart disease, and 21 million have been diagnosed with
cancer. At this point, researchers have identified between eighty and a
hundred different autoimmune diseases, and another forty that are suspected of having an autoimmune basis and may eventually be added to
the growing list.

Overall, about three-quarters of people with autoimmune diseases are
women. As many as one in four women in the United States suffer from one
or more of these conditions. The gender disparity varies from disease to
disease. For example, RA and multiple sclerosis affect about twice as many
women as men, while women make up 90 percent or more of those with
lupus and Hashimoto's thyroiditis. On the other hand, a few autoimmune
conditions are more common in men. In the United States, autoimmune

disease makes the top ten list of causes of death in women and girls under sixty-five. It is the fourth leading cause of disability in women in general, and is likely the number one cause among young and middle-aged women. Because unlike many chronic diseases, autoimmune diseases often strike during the prime of adulthood, leaving sufferers with debilitating symptoms and reliant on treatment with drugs that have side effects that can often rival the diseases themselves for the rest of their lives.

By any measure, autoimmune disease is a major women's health threat—and a major health threat in general. And it is a growing one: rates of many autoimmune diseases are on the rise—in some cases, tripling over the last few decades—which experts attribute largely to the impact of environmental pollutants and toxic chemicals on our immune systems. Yet in the early nineties, only 5 percent of Americans could name an autoimmune disease. Today, that's increased only slightly to 15 percent. In the medical community too, autoimmune diseases have only recently been recognized as a disease category, which, experts say, has been a huge barrier to recognizing them as the epidemic they have become.

THE GREAT IMITATORS

One of the key reasons for the lack of awareness is that the whole concept of an autoimmune disease has been around for only a little over half a century. In fact, for the first half of the twentieth century, the possibility that the immune system could attack the body's own healthy tissue and cells was explicitly discounted. In the early 1900s, German immunologist and Nobel laureate Paul Ehrlich put forth the theory of horror autotoxicus (literally "the horror of self-toxicity"), which posited that the immune system simply could not turn against itself, and the field adopted it as dogma.

The theory held sway until 1956, when Dr. Noel Rose, considered the father of autoimmunity, published results of a study that suggested Hashimoto's thyroiditis was driven by an autoimmune attack against the thyroid. Researchers began to uncover autoantibodies (immune cells directed against the body's own tissue) in other previously "idiopathic" diseases. But so entrenched was the horror autotoxicus theory that it took until the seventies for the possibility of autoimmunity to be fully accepted in the medical community. And it wasn't until the midnineties, when Rose and the AARDA teamed up to produce the first-ever estimate, that we started to have any idea just how prevalent these diseases really are in the United States: they put the estimate at 22 million. As journalist Donna Jackson Nakazawa writes in her book *The Autoimmune Epidemic,* "Twenty-two million, for a set of diseases no one was looking at, was a startling statistic."

Though their relationship to the immune system was unknown, some autoimmune diseases were first described and recognized as distinct diseases in the nineteenth century or even earlier. Indeed, some—like type 1 diabetes, which, before insulin was discovered in 1921, killed its sufferers when they were young—would have been hard to miss. But many nonfatal autoimmune diseases would likely have fallen into the catchall categories of hysteria, neurasthenia, and other nervous disorders, their typical symptoms (fatigue, muscle and joint pain, fevers, weight loss, weakness, neurological symptoms, rashes) often waxing and waning inexplicably for years on end. It's easy to hear echoes of hysteria, a malady that could supposedly "mimic all the physical diseases to which man is heir," as Sydenham wrote back in the seventeenth century, in the modern knowledge that autoimmune diseases can affect every organ and system in the body. Lupus, considered the prototypical autoimmune disease, is often described, like hysteria was, as "the great imitator" since it can affect so many parts of the body.

————

Perhaps one of the clearest examples of an autoimmune disease carved out of the wastebasket of hysteria is multiple sclerosis (MS). In 1868, Jean-Martin Charcot, the noted hysteria researcher, named the disease after finding distinctive lesions after cutting into the brain of his deceased housekeeper. For the next half century, however, American neurologists believed the disease to be rare. In the early twentieth century, this perception started to change, first gradually, then very rapidly, and by 1950, neurologists considered MS among the most common neurological diseases in the country. This shift, as researcher Colin L. Talley has shown, likely didn't reflect an actual increase in prevalence of the disease. Instead, between the twenties and the fifties, there were growing numbers of neurologists who were becoming more skilled at making the diagnosis of MS.

Some of the "new" MS cases were likely those that would have previously been misdiagnosed as Parkinson's, various spinal cord diseases, or neurosyphilis. But the most significant source for the increasing MS cases during this time was likely "hysteria." "As hysteria gradually declined as a neurological diagnosis in the first half of the 20th century," Talley explains, "physicians interpreted increasing numbers of these patients, especially women, as having MS." But even decades after MS was recognized, doctors were struggling to differentiate the two. At a 1917 AMA meeting, one physician pointed out "the frequent mistaking of this condition [MS] for hysteria," noting that he was often forced to revise the misdiagnoses of other physicians. It was a problem that continued to be lamented into the fifties.

Another clue that it was lots of women who'd formerly been labeled hysterics swelling the ranks of MS patients: the gender breakdown of MS diagnoses also changed during this time. From the 1870s to the 1910s, there was no consensus among American doctors about whether MS was more common among men or women. In 1921, the first large survey of patient records concluded that male MS patients outnumbered women by nearly three to two. But in tandem with the rising prevalence, the numbers flipped over the next few decades. By the 1950s, the disease was thought to affect both genders equally. Larger epidemiological studies questioned that, until finally, by the early nineties, the medical literature was asserting that MS affects twice as many women as men.

It took about that long for another long-standing misperception about MS to be put to rest. Throughout the first half of the twentieth century, it was thought that while MS caused a wide array of neurological symptoms, pain was rarely one of them. So entrenched was this "fact" that when MS patients reported pain to their doctors, they were often told it was simply impossible for them to be experiencing what they claimed to be—a response that caused "considerable resentment on the part of the patients," as one study put it. Finally, in the mideighties, various researchers decided to survey patients on the subject and concluded that, indeed, anywhere from half to three-quarters of them suffered from ongoing pain as part of their disease.

MS remains at risk of being mistaken for "hysteria" just as it was 150 years ago. There's still no one definitive test for the disease. Instead, physicians make the call by listening carefully to the patient's history and performing various tests that can suggest the disease. When patients are given a diagnosis of MS, it is only ever a probable one. Consequently, there's still ample room for the disease to be misdiagnosed as "conversion disorder" or "functional neurological symptom disorder" if the patient's symptoms are atypical or if, for whatever reason, the doctor simply doesn't do that first step: listen. A 2003 Israeli study found that men and women eventually diagnosed with MS were equally likely to be initially misdiagnosed, but the women were more likely to get psychiatric referrals, while the men received orthopedic workups.

These days overdiagnosis of MS is also a problem. Recent studies have suggested that 5 to 10 percent of patients diagnosed with MS don't actually have the disease, a trend that experts blame on an overreliance on MRI testing. A component of the diagnosis since the nineties, an MRI is supposed to be interpreted in the context of other clinical signs and symptoms raising suspicion. But too many doctors seem to give out an MS diagnosis whenever they see white matter abnormalities on the MRI image, instead of doing the harder work of figuring out what all the clues—including the patient's report of her symptoms—are collectively pointing toward.

───────

Even once the possibility of autoimmunity was accepted, many autoimmune diseases remained vulnerable to psychological explanations. Between the lingering disbelief that the immune system could mess up so badly and the popularity of psychosomatic theories at the time (particularly for female-predominant conditions), searching for the personality traits or hidden traumas that made people prone to develop autoimmune diseases like RA, lupus, or MS was considered a topic worthy of research into the nineties. According to Virginia Ladd, executive director of the AARDA, the thinking went that it was so "unnatural" for the body to turn against itself that "you must have had something terrible happen in your life that caused you to want to attack yourself." For example, apparently RA patients like me are "self-sacrificing, masochistic, conforming, self-conscious, shy, inhibited, perfectionistic, and interested in sports and games," according to a review of the research on personality factors in RA. "They also tend to overreact to their illness."

Of course, during this time, the subspecialty of psychosomatic medicine was developing cancer and heart disease personality profiles as well. The difference is that in those cases, such research was dwarfed by massive investments in scientific research to uncover the biological mechanisms and risk factors for the diseases. Autoimmune disease, on the other hand, was recognized as a major women's health threat only in the nineties and, despite significant increases in funding for research over the past twenty-five years, is still relatively underfunded. In recent years, the NIH has devoted about $820 million annually to research on autoimmune diseases. By comparison, cancer research gets over six times that much. It's hard to brush off the early efforts to probe women's psyches for the root cause of autoimmune disease when comparatively little scientific progress has been made on that question even today.

Instead, experts lament the fact that, until relatively recently, each individual autoimmune disease has been studied separately; there's been little coordinated effort to uncover the basic mechanisms driving the auto-immune process. That's the kind of research that's needed to develop not just treatments that suppress the symptoms, which is all that's currently available for autoimmune patients, but also a way to cure or prevent them. According to experts, autoimmune disease should be treated as an umbrella category in the same way that cancer has been for decades. Cancer, like autoimmune disease, can affect pretty much any organ or cell in the body, and we started to win the "war on cancer" when we began looking at the common pathology that underlies all cancers (mutated cells that evade the immune system and grow uncontrollably), regardless of their location in the body. "It's just a disaster the way it's all split up," Ladd says. "If cancer research was like that, we would never have made the progress that has been made in cancer."

"CHRONIC COMPLAINERS"

"I wish I could say things have changed significantly from an older generation to a younger generation," Ladd says. "Some things have improved: autoimmune disease is now recognized as a disease category, which it was not twenty-five years ago. But getting a diagnosis is still difficult." According to the most recent survey by the AARDA, it takes an average of three and a half years and nearly five doctors before patients with serious autoimmune diseases get diagnosed. This is a slight improvement from when the organization first began its surveys in the nineties, when it took seven years and six doctors. Because good data on prevalence rates for many autoimmune diseases is lacking, it's unknown how many autoimmune patients remain undiagnosed.

This delay is sometimes blamed on the diseases being "difficult to diagnose." But while diagnosing an autoimmune disease may be less straightforward than diagnosing some other diseases, the larger problem is that doctors just are not well trained in them. According to a 2013 AARDA survey, nearly two-thirds of family physicians feel "uncomfortable" or "stressed" when diagnosing an autoimmune disease. Almost three-quarters said the education they'd received on them had been inadequate, with 60 percent reporting they'd gotten only one or two lectures on the topic in medical school. Even extremely low-hanging fruit that would make diagnosing an autoimmune disease easier has not been pursued: despite the fact that they often run in families, it's not standard practice to inquire about them on health history forms. A change as simple as this, prompting doctors to consider an autoimmune disease, could make a huge difference, Ladd says. "That is the first step in diagnosis: for somebody to think of it."

As it is, many primary care physicians don't even think of the possibility of an autoimmune disease. When they do, they may not know what to test for or how to interpret the results. Usually they'll just refer the patient on to a specialist. But there is no specialist in autoimmune disease—no autoimmunologist—comparable to an oncologist when it comes to cancer. Instead, autoimmune diseases have remained siloed in different organ-specific specialties. Rheumatologists (experts in diseases of the muscles and joints) deal with RA and lupus, neurologists take care of MS patients, gastroenterologists are in charge of inflammatory bowel diseases, autoimmune thyroid diseases are left to endocrinologists, and so on. In the AARDA survey, even specialists reported that they find autoimmune cases difficult. Ladd says that, in their surveys, many specialists admitted, "I'd rather not see these people."

Even if the doctor thinks of the possibility of an autoimmune disease, a quirk of the diseases themselves can pose another barrier to prompt diagnosis: the symptoms of autoimmune diseases often come on months or even years before blood tests reveal objective evidence of an activated immune system and a pattern of autoantibodies that points to a particular disease. In other words, there is often some lag time between when the symptoms begin and when they are "medically explained"—a gap that many patients fall right through.

To some degree, waiting for positive test results is necessary, and a delay in diagnosis in the early stages of an autoimmune disease is sometimes inevitable. Take my experience, for example: When, overnight, I began experiencing pain and stiffness in my knuckles shortly after a bad bout of the flu, I got in to see my primary care physician within a few weeks. At that point, though, blood tests didn't turn up any evidence of inflammation or an elevated rheumatoid factor, an autoantibody that is found in 80 percent of people with RA. My doctor told me that was a good sign but that if the pain didn't go away or started to spread to other joints, I should come back in. Within a few months, the pain having spread to nearly every major joint in my body, my blood tests were decidedly positive for RA.

My RA simply couldn't be diagnosed three weeks after my immune system started going haywire. Joint pain is a symptom of many conditions, including multiple autoimmune diseases. Thankfully, my doctor knew that the fact that my symptoms weren't yet "medically explained" didn't mean they wouldn't be eventually—and didn't doubt my report of joint pain just because there was no objective evidence to support it yet. Too often, in the early stages, Ladd says, "The patient will say, 'My knees hurt.' And the doctor will think, 'Well, your knees aren't swollen and aren't red; do I believe your knees are hurting?'" And many doctors don't do what mine did: keep an eye on the patient to see what happens. "Doctors don't like to follow those patients," Ladd says. "They'd rather have them go to somebody else; they'd rather tell them there's nothing wrong."

Complicating matters further is the fact that some patients never fit cleanly into a particular autoimmune diagnosis. If you have a textbook case of a relatively common autoimmune disease (as I did), it's not actually very difficult to diagnose. But many patients have atypical presentations. Their test results may be borderline or conflicting. Here's where the lack of an autoimmunologist—someone who is looking at the big picture, an expert comfortable dealing with the many cases that aren't clear cut—really hurts patients. Most specialists are "boxologists," autoimmune expert Dr. Abid Khan has explained to *Self*. "As a patient, you have to meet their narrow criteria to be taken seriously, or you're dismissed." And organ-specific specialists are especially ill prepared to deal with patients suffering from multiple autoimmune diseases, even though it is common for someone with one autoimmune disease to develop others. As Ladd says, "You live long enough, it seems like you get to collect them."

Advocates say what would really help would be the establishment of autoimmune centers, like heart and cancer centers, where patients with a suspected autoimmune disease could be diagnosed by an expert. Currently, there is only one such center in the United States, the Autoimmune Center at MidMichigan Health, which was started by Khan after he witnessed the difficulty his wife had getting a diagnosis for her lupus, which nearly killed her. "In my own practice, I started seeing a lot of patients, especially women, who have seen other specialists and who were dismissed as having fibromyalgia, chronic pain syndrome, depression, anxiety. A subset of those patients, in fact, did have those diagnoses, as well as an autoimmune disease, but were dismissed as being complainers," he explained. "No workup was done. Their leads were not followed up on. There were never any biopsies done or blood tests done. And when they were done, the right kind of test may not have been ordered, or the test may have been appropriately ordered but testing methods at the lab may not have been optimal."

"THE LONGER THIS WENT ON, THE MORE I FELT LIKE NO ONE BELIEVED ME"

While doctors' lack of training can explain some of the delay in getting a diagnosis, it cannot account for the dismissal that Khan describes and that so many patients say they experienced during their search. According to the AARDA survey, 45 percent of autoimmune patients report being labeled "chronic complainers" or hypochondriacs in the earliest stages of their illnesses. "Many were told that their symptoms were 'in their heads' or that they were under too much stress." Ladd tosses out some of the common responses patients get during their search for a diagnosis: "'You're too concerned with your health,' or 'You should be tired, because you are working when you have a family,' or 'Do you have any marital problems?'"

Since autoimmune diseases can affect pretty much every tissue of the body, their symptoms vary widely from rashes to joint pain, but one common to most of them is fatigue—the kind of zapped-of-all-energy exhaustion you feel when you're battling the flu. For many women, it proves difficult to convince doctors that the fatigue they're experiencing is not the fatigue of depression or the drowsiness of sleep deprivation and that their other subjective, often transient symptoms are not just those of a somaticizer. In fact, fatigue—the primary early symptom of most autoimmune diseases and, for that matter, of a great many serious conditions—is so easily dismissed that Khan has advised patients that to improve their chances of an early diagnosis "they should not describe their fatigue as fatigue."

Katie was in college the first time (of what would be many) that her symptoms were blamed on depression. She was experiencing pain in her joints, her hair was falling out in clumps, and she had a rash, symptoms that in retrospect were probably caused by lupus—which she was eventually diagnosed with years later—though they could also have been side effects of the new birth control pill she'd recently started taking. Her doctor, though, thought depression was the culprit. The fact that she didn't feel depressed, as she repeatedly explained to him, did not seem to be a barrier to the diagnosis. Neither did the fact that none of the symptoms she was experiencing are found in the diagnostic criteria for depression. She remembers being incredulous. "I said, 'How does depression cause pain in my knees, my hair falling out, and a rash?' And he said, 'Well, when you're depressed, any ache and pain can feel like agony—that explains the joint pain.' And I was like, 'Okay, what about my hair falling out?' And he was like, 'Well, when you're really stressed out, your hair can fall out.'" And the rash? "'Well, that I can't explain, but people just get rashes.'"

"If you went to a psychiatrist or a psychologist and they diagnosed you with depression on the basis of those symptoms, that would be malpractice," Katie says. Indeed, many general physicians seem to have more extreme ideas about the limitless range of physical symptoms that they can pass off as psychogenic—even in the absence of any psychological symptoms—than those held by trained mental health professionals. Here's striking evidence of that: according to Stanley Finger, vice chairperson of the board of the AARDA, "even as late as 2000, mental health professionals were often the first to make a correct diagnosis" of an autoimmune disease.

Between the ambiguity of the diseases themselves in their early stages, the lack of training among doctors, and the ease with which doctors reach for psychogenic explanations when stumped by women's symptoms, it is no wonder that so many women with autoimmune diseases at some point fall into the snare of a psychogenic label as they navigate this fragmented system in search of a diagnosis. "I started collecting all of my medical records, taking them everywhere with me, and keeping this detailed list of every single hospitalization and doctor's appointment," Jackie says, "because the longer this went on, the more I felt like no one believed me."

While the lack of knowledge about autoimmune disease certainly affects all patients, regardless of gender, studies from around the world have found that men tend to be diagnosed faster than their female counterparts. A 2010 Chinese study found a longer diagnostic delay in female lupus patients. A 2014 Finnish study found that over a third of women, versus less than a quarter of men, experienced symptoms for more than ten years before being diagnosed with celiac disease. A 2013 survey of myasthenia gravis patients in Australia found that the average delay in diagnosis was 3.7 years for women and 1.9 years for men. According to a 2010 German study, less than 30 percent of women, compared to half of men, are diagnosed with adrenal insufficiency (most commonly caused by the autoimmune condition Addison's disease) within six months.

Diagnostic delays can, of course, stem from delays in seeking care on the part of the patient in addition to delays in reaching the correct diagnosis on the part of the medical system. And as I've already discussed, it's a myth that women always seek medical attention more quickly than men. Still, studies that have teased apart what part of the delay happens on the patients' end versus the physicians' end suggest that women often experience a longer delay than men once they enter the medical system.

For example, a 2001 study from the Netherlands found no difference in how quickly men and women with RA saw a general practitioner once their symptoms began. However, men were referred to a specialty arthritis clinic in an average of fifty-eight days, compared to ninety-three days for women. A 2005 study of RA patients in Norway found the same pattern. The lag time between when symptoms began and the patient's first encounter with a doctor was about a month for both men and women. The gender gap emerged during the "physician's delay" period of the diagnostic journey: men were referred to a rheumatologist three weeks after that first doctor's visit; for women, it took ten weeks. This extra delay can be of great consequence: not only can untreated RA eventually lead to permanent joint damage, but if the disease is treated within twelve weeks, the odds of successfully inducing remission increase dramatically.

Given that men make up the minority of patients with most autoimmune diseases, findings like these are quite remarkable. Many diseases more common in men—including heart disease, the nation's number one killer of women—are so thoroughly stereotyped as "men's diseases" that doctors often act as if they're impossible in women. Yet the fact that most autoimmune diseases are, statistically speaking, "women's diseases" has somehow not translated to a knowledge-mediated bias that leads to faster diagnoses for women than for men. In some cases, Ladd suggests, men may be more rapidly recognized because they tend to get more severe forms of some diseases. But that's not always the case: RA, for one, is not only two times more common in women than in men but tends to be significantly *more* severe in women.

Instead, it seems that the typical autoimmune patient is not viewed as a typical autoimmune patient because she's already stereotyped in another way: A young or middle-aged woman complaining of fatigue and other "vague" subjective symptoms? She's profiled as being a stressed-out so-maticizer with "medically unexplained symptoms." Indeed, the diagnosis of autoimmune diseases would likely improve significantly, even without new cutting-edge diagnostic triage centers or an overhaul of medical training, if doctors would simply suspect them in every woman they're about to send home with an antidepressant prescription and some advice about reducing stress. Given how common autoimmune diseases are among women and how often they are missed, that would be a pretty safe guess.

That this shift hasn't happened organically—despite the fact that as many as a quarter of American women suffer from an autoimmune disease—is a stark consequence of the woeful lack of feedback doctors receive about their missed diagnoses. If doctors had any idea how many of the women they'd initially determined were "just stressed" turned out to have an autoimmune disease, Katie suggests, they'd surely start to think, "Maybe I should start looking for autoimmune diseases." Instead, "If a woman goes to a doctor and the doctor says this is 'all in her head,' she'll go to another doctor, and then another doctor." Three and a half years later, on average, she'll go to a fifth doctor who makes the correct diagnosis of an autoimmune disease. "But the first four doctors who said it's all in her head never learned that they were wrong."

This leaves doctors without an accurate sense of their diagnostic errors, and the assumption that she really was the "chronic complainer" they viewed her as, in turn, affects how they view the next woman with similar symptoms who comes into their exam room. In this way, the misdiagnosis of autoimmune diseases is self-perpetuating: the longer the diagnostic delay, the more doctors get the impression that their offices are filled with doctor-shopping women with "medically unexplained symptoms"—rather than women with very good odds of having an undiagnosed autoimmune disease.

"I ALWAYS THOUGHT IT WAS JUST ME"

In 2015, inspired by her struggle to get diagnosed with lupus and her mother's experience getting a Sjögren's syndrome diagnosis, Katie started a blog,

Miss•Treated, where women can submit their own stories of being misdiagnosed and dismissed by doctors. She quickly realized that many women's experiences had been even worse than her own and that it wasn't just autoimmune patients who had very similar tales. "I haven't met a single woman with a chronic health condition—maybe one—who hasn't, at some point, had their problems attributed to anxiety or depression," Katie says.

Though the problems women with autoimmune disease have getting diagnosed may be exacerbated by factors specific to autoimmune disease, they are hardly unique. With the exception of diseases that can occasionally be caught through regular screening, like breast or cervical cancer, most medical conditions are still diagnosed the old-fashioned way: by a health care provider listening to a patient's symptoms, thinking of possible diagnoses, running some tests, and, hopefully, figuring out what's wrong. If the challenge for a woman suffering a heart attack or another acute life-threatening event is to quickly overcome an initial tendency to underestimate the severity of the problem, for a woman with an autoimmune disease or another chronic illness, the problem is how to hang on to her credibility as a reliable reporter long enough for the mystery to be unraveled.

Take the experience of women with brain tumors. Compared to an autoimmune disease, there's little that's ambiguous about a brain tumor. There aren't borderline tests to interpret. There certainly isn't a lack of awareness. Promptly making the diagnosis of a brain tumor comes down to being concerned enough about the early symptoms—which range from fatigue, headaches, and balance problems to seizures and paralysis to changes in personality, memory, and the ability to communicate—to order a CT scan or an MRI to get an image of the brain. Either the tumor is there or it isn't.

In 2016, the Brain Tumour Charity released a report on the treatment of brain tumor patients in the United Kingdom. It found that almost one in three of them had visited a doctor more than five times before receiving their diagnosis, and nearly a quarter weren't diagnosed for more than a year. Women, as well as low-income patients, experienced longer delays. They were more likely than men to see ten or more months pass between their first visit to a doctor and diagnosis, and to have made more than five visits to a doctor prior to diagnosis.

The initial responses that the female brain tumor patients reported receiving are familiar: one twenty-eight-year-old woman quoted in the report, who was finally diagnosed after three years with a low-grade tumor, explained, "On every hospital admission they accused me of attention-seeking, and on one admission they thought I was on illegal drugs." Another, a thirty-nine-year-old woman, recalled, "One of the GPs I saw actually made fun of me saying what did I think my headaches were, a brain tumour? I had to request a referral to neurology. I went back repeated times to be given antidepressants, sleep charts, analgesia, etc. No one took me seriously."

Similar findings have been found in various cancers in the United Kingdom. A 2015 study revealed a longer lag time from the onset of symptoms to diagnosis in women patients in six out of eleven types of cancer. And, again, at least part of the longer delay experienced by women is due to a gender gap after they seek medical attention. A 2013 study, for example, concluded that more than twice as many women as men had to make more than three visits to a primary care doctor before getting referred to a specialist for suspected bladder cancer, as did nearly twice as many with renal cancer.

There's also a gender disparity in the diagnostic delay when it comes to rare diseases in general. Officially defined as one that affects fewer than 200,000 people in the United States, rare diseases are only individually rare. Collectively, they affect one in ten Americans, or 30 million people. On average, it takes them over seven years to be correctly diagnosed. Along the way, these patients visit four primary care doctors and four specialists and receive two to three misdiagnoses. That it takes longer to be diagnosed with a rare disease than a more common one is not surprising. Doctors are taught that when they hear hoofbeats, they should think of horses, not zebras, and it may take some time to rule out more likely conditions and realize that they may, in fact, be looking at a zebra. But this staggering seven-year delay is decidedly not simply because it takes that long for doctors to crack a challenging case.

According to a survey of 12,000 patients with several rare diseases in Europe, published by Eurordis in 2009, those who were initially misdiagnosed experienced longer diagnostic journeys. And, in an illustration of just how dangerously sticky a psychogenic diagnosis can be, while being misdiagnosed with the wrong physical disease doubled the time it took to get to the right diagnosis, getting a psychological misdiagnosis extended it even more—by 2.5 to 14 times, depending on the disease. Given women's vulnerability to a psychogenic misdiagnosis, it is perhaps not surprising that women reported significantly longer diagnostic delays than men. For example, it took an average of twelve months for men to get diagnosed with Crohn's disease, an autoimmune disease of the gastrointestinal tract, compared to twenty months for women. Men were diagnosed with Ehlers-Danlos syndrome, a group of genetic disorders that affect the connective tissue, in four years. For women: sixteen years.

The authors of the report emphasized that this gender disparity shows that the diagnostic delay cannot be blamed solely on the rarity of the diseases themselves: "Being a woman should have no influence on a physician's clinical ability to diagnose a disease. It is, therefore, difficult to accept that overall women experience much greater delays in diagnosis than men. The more rapid diagnosis of men illustrates that the capacity to do so exists." Indeed, the experience of rare-disease patients seems to be a particularly good illustration of the gender bias women face. After all, when doctors are facing a disease so uncommon they usually haven't encountered it more than a handful of times, if ever—one they may, in fact, have never even heard of before—there are no knowledge-mediated biases at play. A relatively shorter time to the correct diagnosis depends largely on the doctor not prematurely giving up and deciding that the symptoms must be "medically unexplained."

Laurie Edwards, author of *In the Kingdom of the Sick: A Social History of Chronic Illness in America,* has described how gender bias contributed to her decades-long diagnostic search. "I was 23 before I was given a correct diagnosis of a rare genetic lung disease called primary ciliary dyskinesia. I'd been sick since birth, but long diagnostic journeys are occupational hazards of living with conditions doctors don't often see. Still, my journey was unnecessarily protracted by my doctors' dismissal of my symptoms as those of a neurotic young woman." For years, admitted to the hospital unable to breathe and unresponsive to the steroids they gave her, she'd be asked if perhaps she was just a little stressed out. "No matter how many times I explained that being sick and missing school and work was what caused me stress, rather than the stress causing my symptoms, I never felt they listened to that." While some delay may be inevitable, some of it is just sexism.

The extended diagnostic delay if patients are initially given a misdiagnosis, particularly a psychogenic compared to a physical one, surely reflects the fact that once doctors have settled on one answer, they stop looking for another. But, in the worst-case scenario, the *patient* stops looking too. That's one thing Katie has realized from the stories she's collected since starting her blog. She'd found her doctor's suggestion that her symptoms were due to depression to be "annoying," and, unimpressed with his diagnostic skills, she simply went to someone else. But plenty of women, figuring their doctors must know what they're talking about, accept the possibility that they actually do have a psychiatric problem. When Jackie's primary care doctor also decided—since there was nothing else to conclude—that she must be depressed and prescribed antidepressants, Jackie, then a teenager, took them. They didn't help at all, but at that point, she was "still just accepting whatever the doctors said."

Jackie was lucky that the antidepressants at least didn't *hurt*. A psychogenic misdiagnosis can harm patients not just indirectly, by extending the time to get to the right diagnosis, but directly too. Katie has gotten many submissions from women who suffered serious side effects from psychiatric medications that were not appropriate for them. One woman, diagnosed with anxiety when doctors couldn't figure out why she was vomiting as many as a hundred times in a night, became depressed on the antidepressants she was prescribed. When she suggested her deteriorating mental health might be caused by the medication, her doctor told her to try a higher dose. She became so suicidal that she was committed to a psychiatric institution for three days. Finally, another doctor determined that her gallbladder was functioning at just 1 percent capacity. She was told that if she had not gotten surgery to remove the gangrenous organ when she did, the condition would have killed her within a week.

Another side effect of internalizing doctors' dismissal is that it contributes to a collective silence about a problem that is quite widespread. "I think a lot of women are very nervous to ever tell anyone that doctors are saying that they're either making up their symptoms or that they're depressed or whatever," Katie says. The experience can leave you doubting your own grasp of reality. "You start wondering if maybe you *are* making up your symptoms"—or at least making too big a deal of them. Perhaps this really is what stress feels like, and everyone else is just able to push through it. Until she started her blog, Katie says, she hadn't talked about her own experiences with even fairly close friends. "Because it's humiliating."

The result is that a lot of women may assume the problem lies with them, that there's just something about how they present themselves or communicate that makes doctors doubt their reports. That is, until they do start talking about their own stories—and suddenly realize how many other women have remarkably similar ones. Katie says, "I keep getting emails from women saying, 'I always thought it was just me.'"

"YOU'RE SEEKING DRUGS"

After a few years, Jackie finally got one correct diagnosis. In college, a friend—a well-off white woman—urged Jackie to go see her doctor at a top-notch practice in a wealthy suburb. From a middle-class black family in Detroit, where medical care is still informally very racially segregated, she had never gotten such quality health care. "This man listened to every word I said and looked at every document I gave him and just sat there with me for an hour. And I had never experienced that before. I mean, this guy was thorough. He had me doing every test in the book." He quickly diagnosed her with endometriosis, and a surgery alleviated a good deal of her pelvic pain.

But the other problems that had been plaguing her for years persisted and eventually worsened. After moving to a new city for graduate school, it took another few years to find another set of doctors who would take her symptoms seriously. "In the meantime, I had a lot of, 'You're just hysterical,'" she remembers. "One of the more common things, especially in emergency rooms, was 'You're just drug seeking.' More than 'you're depressed or crazy,' I got 'you're seeking drugs.'"

Like that of most women in the United States, Jackie's experience was impacted not solely by gender bias. A growing body of research explores how "implicit" bias—unconscious biases that are usually not linked to consciously held prejudiced attitudes—contributes to disparities in medical treatment based on many different factors, including gender, race/ethnicity, class, and weight. "We want to think that physicians just view us as a patient, and they'll treat everyone the same, but they don't," says Linda Blount, president of the Black Women's Health Imperative. "Their bias absolutely makes its way into the exam room."

The evidence showing that patients of color, black patients especially, are undertreated for pain in the United States is particularly robust. A 2012 meta-analysis of twenty years of published research found that, across all the studies, black patients were 22 percent less likely than whites to get any pain medication and 29 percent less likely to be treated with opioids. Latino patients were also 22 percent less likely to receive opioids. As is the case with gender disparities, racial/ethnic disparities were most pronounced "when a cause of pain could not be readily verified." But black patients were less likely to get opioids after traumatic injuries or surgery too. And the authors warned that the gap "does not appear to be closing with time or existing policy initiatives."

In explaining this disparity, experts point to a stereotype—one widely held by health care providers—that black patients are more likely to abuse prescription painkillers. That clearly seemed to be part of the problem in Jackie's case; she was often accused directly of seeking drugs. Not that it would justify the treatment gap if that stereotype were based in truth, but it is, in fact, entirely false. White Americans have the highest rates of prescription drug abuse, are most likely to die from drug overdoses, and, for that matter, use illegal drugs in general at the same or higher rates as people of color do. The fact that the racial pain-treatment gap extends to children suggests that it's not just the assumption of drug seeking at work, though. A 2015 study found that white children with appendicitis were almost three times as likely as black children to receive opioids in the emergency room.

A 2016 study published in *Proceedings of the National Academy of Sciences of the United States of America* suggested that health care providers may underestimate black patients' pain in part due to a belief that they simply don't actually feel as much pain—a myth that dates all the way back to the days of slavery. For centuries, the claim that black people were biologically different from whites was "championed by scientists, physicians, and slave owners alike to justify slavery and the inhumane treatment of black men and women in medical research," the authors write. Black people were thought to have "thicker skulls, less sensitive nervous systems," and a superhuman ability to "tolerate surgical operations with little, if any, pain at all."

In the first phase of the study, over two hundred white medical students and residents were asked whether a series of statements about differences between black and white patients were true or false. Some of the statements were true, while others—for example, "blacks' skin is thicker than whites" and "blacks' nerve endings are less sensitive than whites"—were false. They found that a full half of the respondents thought that one or more of the false statements—many of which were "fantastical in nature"—were possibly, probably, or definitely true. Also, notably, many of them *didn't* agree with the statements that were actually true; only half of the residents knew that white patients are less likely to have heart disease than black patients are. When asked to read case studies of two patients complaining of pain, one white and one black, the respondents who had endorsed more false beliefs were more likely to believe that the black patient felt less pain, and undertreated them accordingly.

————

Midway through graduate school, Jackie finally caught a break. She had been sick for months, burning up with a fever that the doctors, despite soaking her in antibiotics, could not break. "A primary care doctor—a woman of color—believed me, and she collected all of my medical records and literally took them home with her and started trying to piece them together like it was a puzzle."

She suspected that Jackie might have lupus, and a test confirmed it. Ninety percent of lupus patients are women, and black women are three times more likely than white women to have the disease. They also tend to get it at younger ages and have more life-threatening complications. After ten years, Jackie had a diagnosis that explained everything. She thought her battle to be taken seriously was finally over.

"DISAFFECTED PATIENTS" VERSUS "OBJECTIVE FACTS"

Indeed, the long, frustrating search for a diagnosis is such a common theme running through the stories of women patients that many, like Jackie, feel immense relief to finally get a diagnosis—any diagnosis. Being sick without knowing why is very stressful; being sick without knowing why and being told "nothing's wrong" is more stressful still. But women with chronic illnesses like autoimmune diseases may find that the distrust of their reports of their symptoms just continues. As Meghan O'Rourke wrote in a 2013 *New Yorker* article on her experience with autoimmune thyroid disease, even after diagnosis, "Worrying about being crazy is part of many autoimmune sufferers' lives."

Some patients run into doctors who just aren't educated on their diagnosis. Since people with one autoimmune disease have a higher risk of developing another one, a scenario the siloed medical system is poorly set up to deal with, some autoimmune sufferers have yet more long diagnostic journeys ahead of them, even after getting their initial diagnosis. Others find that, when it comes to managing these diseases that often relapse and remit for a lifetime, an overreliance on objective tests persists postdiagnosis. Ladd, for example, was easily diagnosed with a textbook case of lupus decades ago, when she was twenty-three. "Still, along the way, if my test would come back negative at a particular time, then a rheumatologist would question it."

──────────

The controversy over diagnosing and treating thyroid disease is a good illustration of how rigidly medicine can cling to objective tests—and how reliably medicine resorts to attributing women's symptoms to their minds when their subjective reports conflict with what the objective tests say.

The thyroid, a small, butterfly-shaped gland in the neck, produces hormones that regulate metabolism. The American Thyroid Association estimates that 20 million Americans have some form of thyroid disease, and up to 60 percent of them haven't been diagnosed. Thyroid conditions are five to eight times more common among women than among men. Women have a one in eight chance of developing one in their lifetime. The most common thyroid disorder is hypothyroidism, in which the gland starts underproducing hormones, and in the majority of cases, the underlying cause is the autoimmune disease Hashimoto's thyroiditis. In contrast, in hyperthyroid cases, many of which are due to another autoimmune disorder, Graves' disease, the thyroid is overactive, producing more hormones than the body needs.

The symptoms of hypothyroidism include fatigue, depression, increased sensitivity to cold, weight gain, joint and muscle pain, a slow heart rate, constipation, and dry skin and hair. The symptoms of hyperthyroidism are essentially the opposite: anxiety, irritability, increased sensitivity to heat, weight loss, racing heart, hand tremors, difficulty sleeping, thinning of the skin, and brittle hair. Since symptoms come on gradually, and depression and anxiety are features of Hashimoto's and Graves' disease respectively, many women are misdiagnosed and treated with antidepressants or antianxiety medications for years before someone thinks to look at the thyroid. Meanwhile, a postpartum form of thyroid disease is often mistaken for postpartum depression, and in older patients, thyroid disease may be attributed to menopause or dementia.

Patients have clashed with endocrinologists over mainstream medicine's reliance on a single test to assess thyroid health. Thyroid-stimulating hormone (TSH) is produced by the pituitary gland and tells the thyroid how much thyroid hormone to make. A high TSH level suggests hypothyroidism, while a low TSH level indicates hyperthyroidism. There are other tests, however, that give a more complete picture of how well the thyroid is working, including the hormones that the thyroid itself produces (free T4 and free T3) and autoantibodies that point to Hashimoto's and Graves' disease. But many doctors rely solely on TSH. If TSH is in the "normal" range, even if someone has symptoms of hypo- or hyperthyroidism and autoantibodies that indicate autoimmune disease, they may go undiagnosed.

However, what constitutes a "normal" TSH level has been the subject of much debate. For some time, it was generally accepted that a TSH level between 0.5 and 5.0 milli-international units per liter was normal. Below 0.5 indicated hyperthyroidism, levels of 5 to 10 were evidence of mild hypothyroidism, and levels greater than 10 were evidence of overt thyroid failure. But by the early 2000s, studies had found that most healthy people, rigorously screened to be free from thyroid problems, fall into a smaller range. Some professional organizations, like the American Association of Clinical Endocrinologists, urged doctors to "consider treatment for patients who test outside the boundaries of a narrower margin based on a target TSH level of 0.3 to 3.0." This was in line with what many patients had been saying for years. Once diagnosed, patients with hypothyroidism are treated with supplemental T4 to replace the hormone that their underactive thyroid is no longer producing, and many patients reported that even when their TSH was back in the "normal" range, their symptoms persisted.

But the new recommended range sparked great controversy, which has never really been resolved. Most laboratories have stuck with the old reference range of 0.5 to 5.0. Some doctors have adopted the new recommendations in their practice, while others have refused. The disagreement means that one endocrinologist may diagnose and treat hypothyroidism when TSH is over 3, another may tell patients they're fine until it goes above 5, and still others think that even treating mild hypothyroidism (between 5 and 10) is inappropriate. At the same time, most doctors *have* accepted a lower normal range for women who are pregnant or trying to be. That means that many doctors will tell a woman with subclinical hypothyroidism battling fatigue, depression, weight gain, and joint pain that nothing's wrong, but if she started trying and failing to conceive, she'd qualify for treatment overnight. As Dr. Sara Gottfried has written, "The implicit message is this: if you are not reproductively viable, sit on the sidelines and suffer through your low-thyroid symptoms. Go to spin class and eat less. But if you're making a baby, we will treat you."

Of course, expert disagreement over reference ranges is not unusual in medicine. Judging what is a "normal" and "abnormal" TSH level is fraught, because it involves imposing a binary on something that is, in reality, a spectrum. Whatever reference range is set, there will likely always be out-liers. (Indeed, some experts think people may have their own unique set point for thyroid hormones.) That's why more integrative practitioners have argued that diagnosing thyroid disease should be more a clinical art than a laboratory science, taking into account not just TSH levels but also other thyroid tests (including antibody tests) and, importantly, the patient's symptoms. But, of course, that requires listening to, and trusting, the pa-tient's report of her symptoms.

And that seems to be part of the problem here. In 2006, Dr. Anthony Weetman, a British endocrinologist, angered patients with an editorial en-titled "Whose Thyroid Hormone Replacement Is It Anyway?" in the jour-nal *Clinical Endocrinology*. He lamented that endocrinologists were "under increasing pressure from disaffected patients who believe their symptoms indicate hypothyroidism despite normal thyroid function tests" and con-cluded that "the majority of patients who demand thyroid hormone treat-ment for multiple symptoms, despite normal thyroid function tests, have functional somatoform disorders." Arguing that in "the age of postmodern medicine" there's been a "derogation of objective facts which are the defin-ing characteristic of science and the replacement of scientific certainty with the view that reality can have multiple meanings," he called for the medical community to launch "a robust defence of the biochemical basis for the diagnosis of hypothyroidism."

As prominent thyroid-patient advocate Mary Shomon pointed out, this robust defense of "objective facts" was remarkable considering the complete lack of consensus among experts over what constitutes a "normal" thyroid test to begin with. TSH under 10? Under 5? Under 3? Weetman never said what he considered "normal"; he just knew that the perspective of "disaffected patients" shouldn't play a role in determin-ing it. "If we have obvious thyroid symptoms, and yet fall into one of these mathematical gray areas that are not clearly agreed upon, some of you will willingly diagnose us and treat us, but others of you will equally confidently insist we're suffering from somatoform disorders and refer us to psychiatrists," Shomon wrote in an open letter to endocrinologists. "Recognizing that you don't agree on any of these crucial issues, the san-est thing a thyroid patient can do is ask questions, look for clarification, and yes, sometimes even push for treatment. And all this insisting that 'normal test result' patients are suffering from mental problems, when you can't even agree on 'normal test results?' Well, *that's* what sounds crazy to most patients."

DO EXHAUSTED WOMEN MAKE A SOUND?

The focus on objective measures of disease is especially problematic since the symptom that tends to most greatly impact autoimmune patients' well-being is one that cannot be measured. Nakazawa writes of the "intolerable, life-altering bouts of exhaustion" most patients experience: "If fatigue were a sound made manifest by the 23.5 million people with autoimmune disease in America, the roar across this country would be more deafening than that of the return of the seventeen-year locust."

In a recent survey the AARDA conducted of more than 7,800 autoimmune disease patients, 90 percent said that fatigue was a "major issue" for them, and 60 percent said it is "probably the most debilitating symptom of having" an autoimmune disease. "The biggest reason for having to quit, the biggest reason for having to go on disability, the biggest reason for family problems was the fatigue," Ladd says. "But the fatigue is not taken seriously by the doctors. They hear you saying it but don't really understand the depth of that fatigue, that you are functionally exhausted." While about 90 percent of the respondents said they had discussed their fatigue with their doctor, only 40 percent said their doctor had suggested treatment options for it. As one patient in the survey said, "It's difficult for other people to understand our ongoing fatigue when it can't be seen by them. It's so hard just trying to get others to really, really understand how very tired you are sometimes; even our own doctors don't understand. One wonders if even our doctors may think we are for the most part just mental cases or whiners."

I thought about this survey as I puzzled over why the autoimmune epidemic gets so little attention, despite the enormous toll it takes—and not just on the sufferers. Given their prevalence, the fact that they usually strike when patients are young and middle aged, and that they—usually—don't kill people, autoimmune diseases are incredibly costly to the medical system. A decade ago, the NIH estimated that they exact about $100 billion in direct health care costs. But since many autoimmune diseases don't even have their own medical code yet, Ladd explains, the data to do a rigorous cost analysis isn't even available yet. That, of course, is to say nothing of the human costs to patients themselves, their families, and society at large. Autoimmune diseases typically affect young women—often before they turn thirty—and affect them for the rest of their lives. Many become chronically disabled. "Yet there doesn't seem to be the passion, because you typically don't die with an autoimmune disease," Ladd says. "That's the difference. But you live a long life with it. And it can ruin your quality of life."

But is that the only difference? Certainly, there's no question that the medical system prioritizes life-threatening diseases over chronic conditions. This is reflected in everything from which diseases attract the most research funds to which specialties see the biggest paychecks and prestige. In recent years, there have been some important critiques leveled against medicine's focus on mortality over morbidity, on preventing death over improving health. The surgeon and writer Dr. Atul Gawande, for example, has argued that, when it comes to end-of-life care, a medical system that tends to favor marginally prolonging life, even at the cost of destroying the quality of that life, has "utterly failed" to help "dying patients achieve what's most important to them at the end of their lives." Meanwhile, a system that rewards heroic interventions—the lifesaving surgery or the aggressive chemotherapy—when something goes seriously wrong has neglected to invest in the less glamorous work of effective management of chronic conditions. "Chronic illness has become commonplace," Gawande writes, "and we have been poorly prepared to deal with it."

Even when critiqued, the relative neglect of debilitating but not directly fatal diseases is often portrayed as inevitable. To some degree, it might be; there may be a deep-seated fear of death that makes people more afraid of getting cancer than an autoimmune disease. And, as someone who has lost loved ones too soon to the nation's major killers, I certainly don't begrudge the funding and attention devoted to life-threatening diseases. But it is not self-evident to me that an epidemic of diseases that strike up to 50 million

Americans in the prime of their lives and cause incurable lifelong illness that interferes with their ability to earn an income, raise a family, and live a full and happy life should be *this* invisible.

Would the autoimmune epidemic be treated with more urgency if it were mostly men who were affected? Would there be greater public awareness, politicians pledging to cure autoimmune disease within our lifetimes, and investments in cutting-edge research and treatment centers? There's no way to know, but that's sort of the point: there *is* no counterpart to autoimmune disease that affects mostly men. There is no class of diseases that don't usually kill you but can ruin your quality of life that is just as prevalent and is twice as common among men. Add in the chronic pain conditions and contested diseases that I'll discuss in the remaining chapters—which, hampered by psychosomatic suspicions, are taken even less seriously and receive less research funding than autoimmune disease—and the epidemic of chronic disease that disproportionately affects women swells even larger.

Chronic illness, with its invisible symptoms of fatigue and pain, is largely the burden of women. And it's worth considering to what extent its relative neglect by the medical system is *because* it mostly affects women, whose complaints are so often heard not as a roar but as a whine.

────────────

It had never occurred to Jackie that she might continue to be stereotyped as a drug seeker once she had a legitimate, serious diagnosis. "I genuinely believed that this was a function of my lack of diagnosis and that once I got diagnosed with whatever this mystery thing is, that they would get it and they wouldn't accuse me of that anymore, because I had a real disease." That her gender and race were factors in the dismissive treatment she'd received from health care providers over the years hadn't crossed her mind. And for several years, she had no problems; she had a great rheumatologist who coordinated her care. "I didn't realize it, but I was really in this great little bubble."

But eventually she left her bubble and moved down south. Her joint pain became crippling, and she began having more episodes of chest pain.

Chest pain often occurs in lupus because of pericarditis, inflammation of the sac surrounding the heart, which usually isn't life threatening but should be checked out and treated. Over time, the chronic inflammation caused by the disease can increase the risk of coronary heart disease. Lupus patients are up to fifty times more likely than the rest of the population to have a heart attack. In other words, while nobody should mess around with chest pain, lupus patients definitely shouldn't.

But Jackie found that, as a young black woman, the assumption she was a drug addict was so automatic that the ER staff often simply wouldn't believe she had lupus. "Sometimes I had a hard time even being allowed into the emergency room at all." If an EKG showed she wasn't having a heart attack, she'd be refused treatment and sent away. "I'd say, 'No, I have a diagnosis, call my rheumatologist, call my primary care doctor. Look, here are their cards. I go to this hospital for care. Please believe me.'" It was like talking to a brick wall. That first time, kicked out of one hospital, she finally got into another. "I had pericarditis, and I had to be admitted for three days." This happened again, and again, and again.

Over the last five years, as her deteriorating health has forced her in and out of hospitals in Virginia and New York City, she's had such awful experiences being denied care that, these days, Jackie won't go to the ER at all unless one of her regular doctors has called ahead to ensure that she is admitted and treated properly. Sometimes even if she's admitted, her pain still isn't adequately treated. "Nine times out of ten, I am terrified of doctors. And I know and love many people who are in the profession. But I am terrified." She used to think there was some trick to avoiding being seen through a health care provider's biased lens; she doesn't anymore. "It doesn't matter how well you speak, or how nice you are, or how you dress, or how stoic you are, or how much you cry. If somebody thinks that you are a hysterical woman or a hysterical drug seeker, there is nothing you can do to make that person treat you well."

She says the racist drug-seeking stereotype tends to be her biggest barrier to having her reports trusted, but that doesn't mean that she's not also affected by the double bind all women tend to be caught in. "Anytime I go into a hospital setting, I know that the highest danger to me is an assumption that I'm a drug addict. But then there's this intersectional thing that

I've run into where, if I'm crying or if I'm visibly in pain, they'll ignore you because now you're a hysterical drug seeker." On the other hand, there have also been times when she's successfully remained stoic and been told that she must be lying because if she were really in that much pain, she'd be showing it more.

Only one thing has made any difference. During one of her most recent hospital admissions, with documented inflammation in her stomach, she was supposed to be getting pain management every couple of hours, but the nurse refused to give it to her. Fed up, she angrily demanded care from the doctor and happened to mention that she was a professor. "Suddenly it's like this light goes off." Clearly, up until that point, she had been being treated like a different sort of black woman. "They assumed I was homeless or extremely impoverished and coming off the street just to get a meal and some drugs. I wasn't a human being worth caring for until I said I had a Ph.D. Then suddenly I'm getting pain management, I'm going to radiology, I'm getting my CAT scan." Jackie says that even though it's antithetical to the politics that she believes in to make a distinction between herself and a poor black woman, she has acquiesced to her parents' insistence that she start playing her Ph.D. card whenever she seeks medical care. Now she adds that to the list of things she does before going to the hospital: putting *Dr.* on all her paperwork.

Despite her traumatic experiences, Jackie remains optimistic that change is possible. "All doctors need to be trained around these common assumptions that doctors have around women and minorities in particular. I really believe that if young doctors were trained to think about their assumptions about women being hysterical from day one of medical school, that it would make a difference."

OUT OF THE WASTEBASKET

More than a hundred years after Charcot distinguished MS from hysteria, autoimmune diseases are still being plucked out of the wastebasket of the "medically unexplained." Some of the diseases that have been added to the autoimmune category in recent decades are long-recognized diseases

whose autoimmune basis has finally been realized. But some newly recognized autoimmune diseases are entirely newly identified diseases. And
while it's tempting to assume that only more mild, subtle diseases could
possibly have remained unrecognized and unexplained until the twenty-
first century, the discovery of various forms of autoimmune neurological
disease in just the last decade shows that's not the case at all.

In 2002, Dr. Josep Dalmau, a neurologist at the University of
Pennsylvania, was called to consult on the case of a young woman in the in-
tensive care unit. She'd been hallucinating when she was admitted months
before and was now unable to speak or breathe on her own. Despite doing
"a million dollars' worth of tests," the doctors couldn't find much wrong
with her apart from a small teratoma, a benign tumor, on her ovary and
signs of inflammation in her spinal fluid. As a Hail Mary move, they treated
her with drugs to suppress her immune system, and she miraculously
recovered.

Dalmau and his team began collecting other similar cases: young women
with ovarian teratomas who'd rapidly developed personality changes, para-
noia, hallucinations, abnormal movements, seizures, and memory loss, and,
eventually, descended into an entirely unresponsive state. Their symptoms,
the researchers later wrote, had often led to "an initial diagnosis of acute
psychosis, malingering, or drug abuse." Dalmau's lab searched the patients'
blood and spinal fluid and soon found the culprit: an autoantibody against a
protein in the brain. In a 2007 article, he described a dozen women with the
disease and gave it a name: anti-NMDA receptor encephalitis, caused by an
autoimmune attack against the NMDA receptors, which control communication between neurons, particularly in areas of the brain vital to memory
and behavior.

Anti-NMDA receptor encephalitis typically strikes young adults and
children, and, as is the case in many autoimmune diseases, 80 percent of
them are women or girls. In roughly half of cases in adult women it is linked
to the presence of an ovarian teratoma. Teratomas are a type of tumor made
of cells that can differentiate into any type of tissue, including brain cells.
It is thought that the disease is triggered when the immune system produces antibodies to tumor cells containing NMDA receptors, which then
cross-react with the patient's own brain tissue.

Susannah Cahalan recounted her terrifying experience with the disease in her memoir *Brain on Fire: My Month of Madness*. In 2009, the twenty-four-year-old reporter for *New York Post* began feeling strange. It started with an uncharacteristic obsessive fear about bedbugs. Some forgetfulness at work. A headache, fatigue, and bouts of nausea. Numbness and tingling on her left side convinced her to see a prominent neurologist, but after a normal neurological exam and MRI, he said it was probably just mono. But soon Cahalan was experiencing sleepless nights and titanic mood swings—from inexplicably crying uncontrollably at her desk to a wave of euphoria minutes later. Then, while watching TV with her boyfriend, she had a seizure. "My arms suddenly whipped straight out in front of me, like a mummy, as my eyes rolled back and my body stiffened. I was gasping for air," she writes. "Blood and foam began to spurt out of my mouth through clenched teeth."

Cahalan has no memory of the seizure. After that moment, she has few memories of the events of the next month at all; her memoir is pieced together from her medical records and interviews with her family, friends, and doctors. When she woke in the hospital after the seizure, she believed the doctors were out to get her. Over the next ten days, she became increasingly erratic and paranoid. After a second seizure, she and her family returned to her neurologist for answers. But with a normal neurological exam, MRI, CT scan, and now EEG, he was convinced that Cahalan was suffering from alcohol withdrawal. He told her mother—who insisted that her daughter wasn't a heavy drinker in the slightest—that while it may be difficult for a mother to accept, Cahalan just needed to "knock off the partying."

Her family demanded she be admitted to the epilepsy ward at New York University Langone Medical Center. Over the next couple of weeks Cahalan deteriorated: she slurred her words, struggled to swallow, and held her arms rigidly out in front of her like Frankenstein's monster. Her psychosis eventually gave way to a catatonic state in which she was barely able to speak. But as test after test came back normal, doctors were increasingly considering a diagnosis of schizoaffective disorder, a condition that shares features with both schizophrenia and mood disorders. "At this point," she writes, "my family needed someone who would believe in me no matter what."

Finally, a spinal tap revealed a high white blood cell count, which suggested inflammation in her brain. One of the hospital's top neurologists—nicknamed Dr. House by his colleagues—was brought onto her case. He went through her full history with her parents, taking "note of symptoms—headaches, flu-like symptoms, numbness, and the increased heart rate—that the other doctors had not explored." Convinced that Cahalan's brain was inflamed, he figured that since an infection didn't seem to be the cause, it was likely due to an autoimmune reaction. He recalled reading Dalmau's case studies and sent her blood and spinal fluid to his lab to be tested for the anti-NMDA receptor antibody. Cahalan became the 217th person in the world diagnosed with the newly recognized disease. With the diagnosis, she went from being a "notoriously difficult patient" to "the ward's interesting consult."

Within a week, she was released from the hospital. And though her recovery was slow and painful, after six months of treatment targeting her errant immune system, she was back at work. With treatment, about 80 percent of patients with anti-NMDA receptor encephalitis recover, which is incredible considering how dire their condition is at its worst. Even with proper treatment, about 10 percent of patients die. Cahalan is well aware of how lucky she was. "If I had been struck with this disease just three years earlier, before Dr. Dalmau had identified the antibody, where would I be?" she writes.

In fact, the fate of at least a few patients who developed anti-NMDA receptor encephalitis before 2007 is known. Of the dozen women Dalmau described in his article defining the disease, some had been retrospectively diagnosed. One of them, a twenty-four-year-old woman like Cahalan, was unlucky enough to fall ill in 2005, just two years before rather than after the disease made its first appearance in the medical literature. Three months after her symptoms began, her family, believing that her mysterious condition was irreversible, requested that she be taken off the mechanical ventilator that was breathing for her. She died within hours. Analysis of her spinal fluid later revealed the telltale antibody, and an autopsy found a teratoma on her ovary.

In the last decade, the field of autoimmune neurological disease has exploded. In addition to anti-NMDA receptor encephalitis, fifteen other types of autoimmune encephalitis, marked by antibodies against other proteins in the brain, have been identified. It is unknown how many people are affected and, therefore, how many are still misdiagnosed. Indeed, Cahalan was lucky not only to get the disease after 2007 but also to get an exceptional doctor who'd stayed so on top of the medical literature that he'd heard of it. Her personal Dr. House estimated that 90 percent of those with autoimmune encephalitis in 2009 would not have been properly diagnosed. The fact that the number of cases has rapidly increased since then—Dalmau's team alone identified over five hundred patients in just five years—two experts point out, suggests that it is perhaps "not a rare disease, but rather a rare diagnosis."

This seems to be a fairly consistent consequence of medicine's history of putting all of women's unexplained diseases into a psychogenic catchall category: as the history of MS so clearly illustrates, once a disease is removed from this category, it tends to be initially considered very rare, and then, as awareness of the new disease permeates the medical system, prevalence estimates increase and increase until they finally stabilize. Hopefully, this process is somewhat accelerated in the twenty-first century, but as Dalmau and a colleague write, only time and more research will tell what "subset of what we currently diagnose as primary psychiatric disorders are in fact due to definable, treatable autoimmune syndromes."

The parallels to some of the most dramatic historical descriptions of hysteria, including during its phase as "demonic possession," have not gone unnoted in the medical literature on anti-NMDA receptor encephalitis. "A Case of Hysteria" reads the title of one article. More to the point: "Not Hysteria" reads another. In fact, British psychiatrist Thomas A. Pollak suggested in a 2013 article in *BMJ* that the possibility that some cases of "hysteria" were anti-NMDA receptor encephalitis caused by ovarian teratomas may explain why early gynecologists claimed some success with oophorectomies in the late 1800s; by removing the teratomas too, they would have eliminated the source of the autoimmune reaction. Ironically, in their sexist focus on the reproductive system as the source of all women's illnesses, they may have stumbled upon a cure for one of them.

These accidental successes, of course, do not make up for the larger harms of hysteria's legacy—which persist today. "History should not forgive the chauvinistic prejudices that dogged historical discussion of hysteria; indeed prejudice still characterises current attitudes towards 'functional' and medically unexplained neurological symptoms," Pollak writes. Thanks to this enduring prejudice, unknowable numbers of women suffered unexplained illnesses and even died unexplained deaths until well into the twentieth century. "The weight and influence of centuries of misogynistic theorising by an all-male medical establishment cannot be overestimated." As the next section explores, this influence has shaped what we know—and don't know—about many common women's conditions, from chronic pain to menstrual disorders to Lyme disease.

PART 3

NEGLECTED DISEASES: THE DISORDERS FORMERLY KNOWN AS HYSTERIA

CHAPTER 5

CHRONIC PAIN: "PAIN IS REAL WHEN YOU GET OTHER PEOPLE TO BELIEVE IN IT"

WHEN ALEXIS WAS ELEVEN, her hips began to hurt. The pain felt as if it was deep in her bone and would radiate to her lower back and to the front to her pelvis. Her mother took her to doctor after doctor. She got X-rays and ultrasounds, and saw spine and arthritis specialists. But they could find no cause for her pain.

We've seen how the distrust of women's reports of pain and other subjective symptoms leads to delayed diagnoses and undertreatment for a range of conditions, from heart attacks to lupus to appendicitis. But perhaps the most long-lasting impact of this bias has been on those like Alexis, who suffer from unexplained chronic pain, in which the objective evidence to confirm women's subjective and ever-suspect reports is simply never found.

As her pain became more and more debilitating over the next several years, Alexis eventually gave up on finding a diagnosis and instead searched for a doctor who would at least take her pain seriously and help her figure out how to better manage it. Even that was elusive. "I just felt like no one ever believed me. I never could find anyone to help me—ever. And I saw a lot of doctors, for a long time."

———

In 2011, the IOM released an influential report entitled *Relieving Pain in America* that offered an alarming indictment of the medical system's treatment of pain. "On the one hand, pain is extremely widespread in American society, exacts a huge toll in suffering and disability, and imposes extraordinary costs on the health care system and the nation's economy," the IOM experts wrote. "On the other hand, all too often treatment is delayed, disorganized, inaccessible, or ineffective." While the report found evidence of inadequate treatment of acute pain (for example, from an injury treated in the ER or in postoperative care after a surgery) the IOM was especially concerned about the large burden, on both patients and the health care system, posed by chronic pain. Chronic pain is generally defined as pain that lasts more than three to six months or persists past the point of normal healing.

By the IOM's new estimate, roughly 40 percent of the population live with chronic pain. That's 100 million Americans, which is more than the number affected by diabetes, heart disease, and cancer combined, and their ranks have been growing in recent decades. Chronic pain is, quite simply, "the most prevalent human health problem" and the leading cause of long-term disability. The IOM estimated that chronic pain costs the nation $560 billion to $635 billion in health care costs and lost productivity each year.

Yet in recent years, the NIH has devoted a minuscule $400 million a year—about 1 percent of its annual budget—to studying chronic pain. That's a mere 5 percent of what goes to studying diabetes, heart disease, and cancer combined. According to a recent study of 117 medical schools, only four schools in the United States offer a required separate course on pain. Students received, on average, eleven hours of instruction on the subject. Unsurprisingly, given this minimal training, a national survey found that almost 30 percent of primary care residents, who are on the front lines when it comes to treating pain, said they felt unprepared to help patients with pain management. And the 3,000 to 4,000 pain specialists nationwide aren't nearly enough to meet the huge need for their expertise.

The majority of the 100 million Americans who live with chronic pain are women. In surveys that ask respondents whether they've had pain in different parts of the body over the last several months, greater proportions of women report pain. It's a finding that's fairly consistent across different populations: a 2008 study of tens of thousands of patients in over a dozen countries found that the prevalence of any chronic pain condition was 45 percent among women, compared to 31 percent among men.

Many of the most prevalent chronic pain conditions, such as osteoarthritis (OA), which affects over 30 million Americans, chronic low back pain (nearly 20 million), IBS (44 million), and migraine (36 million), are more common among women. Women are twice as likely to have autoimmune diseases, many of which bring with them persistent pain. Women are up to four times more likely to experience the bladder pain of interstitial cystitis (IC), the jaw pain of temporomandibular disorders (TMD), and the widespread, full-body pain of fibromyalgia. And some common chronic pain conditions almost exclusively affect women: vulvodynia, which causes pain around the vaginal opening, and endometriosis, which causes pelvic pain associated with menstruation.

Over the last few decades, there has been a paradigm shift in our understanding of chronic pain. Historically, and especially since the twentieth century, medicine has considered pain to be a symptom of disease, one to be alleviated as much as possible, to be sure, but clinically relevant primarily as a clue pointing toward the underlying problem. "Cure the disease, and cure the pain" has been the assumption. While this principle may hold true of acute pain, in many cases, according to the International Association for the Study of Pain, "chronic pain is a disease in its own right."

"This profound recasting," the IOM report declared, "means that pain requires direct, appropriate treatment rather than being sidelined while clinicians attempt to identify some underlying condition that may have caused it. Prompt treatment can derail the progression of pain from the acute to the chronic state. This recasting also means that health professions education programs should include a substantial amount of learning about pain and its diversity, and that people with chronic pain should be recognized by family, employers, health insurers, and others as having a serious disease."

WHAT IS PAIN ANYWAY?

To understand what it means to say that chronic pain is a disease in its own right, it's important to realize that pain is usually vitally important. These days, pain experts generally classify pain into four different types. The kind we're most familiar with from our daily lives is nociceptive pain, which we feel in response to any noxious stimulus (something too sharp, hot, cold) that could hurt us. Usually acute, it's considered adaptive—that is, it's actually very helpful. It's supposed to feel terrible when you touch the handle of a hot pan, for example, because it alerts you that you could get burned. To see just how protective this type of pain is, imagine how risky—and short—life is for people who, due to a rare genetic defect, can't feel pain at all: with nothing telling them it is dangerously hot, they don't let go of the pan.

If a noxious stimulus is able to do some real damage to your tissue, inflammatory pain kicks in as your immune system is activated to repair it. After the initial nociceptive pain signaling you've burned yourself on that hot pan, low-grade inflammatory pain lingers, keeping your hand more sensitive than usual until the wound is fully healed. Like nociceptive pain, inflammatory pain is relatively acute and protective; its purpose is to keep you from further injuring yourself while your body is still vulnerable, and, if all goes as it should, it will stop once mending is complete.

Some conditions that cause chronic pain involve nociceptive or inflammatory pain. And in such cases, the pain, though chronic, is still serving its useful purpose as a warning sign of an underlying problem. For example, in RA, pain in the joints is an expected consequence of the immune system mobilizing against the joint lining; though the autoimmune attack is abnormal, the inflammatory pain it causes is normal. In OA, in which the protective cartilage cushion between bones is eroded, the pain is considered nociceptive.

But a great deal of chronic pain is pathological. It does not seem to be a symptom indicating tissue damage or inflammation: there is no apparent reason for the pain, and that is itself the problem. Harvard neurobiologist Dr. Clifford J. Woolf, director of the F. M. Kirby Neurobiology Center at Boston Children's Hospital, offers this analogy to explain the difference: "If pain were a fire alarm, the nociceptive type would be activated appropriately only by the presence of intense heat, inflammatory pain would be activated by warm temperatures, and pathological pain would be a false alarm caused by malfunction of the system itself." Pathological pain comes in two flavors: In neuropathic pain, the malfunction seems to be triggered by damage to the nervous system itself. And then there is dysfunctional pain (also known, confusingly, as functional pain), in which there's pain in the absence of any injury, inflammation, or nerve lesion to explain it at all.

It's only in the last couple of decades that this way of classifying pain has become accepted. Previously, there were really only two types of pain: "organic" pain that was due to some underlying disease and "medically unexplained" pain that was assumed to be psychogenic. Pathological, particularly functional, pain just didn't fit into the early models of what pain is. In the seventeenth century, philosopher René Descartes imagined the pain-perception pathway as a cord running from our nerve endings to our brain; the pain of a hammer striking your hand, in his example, would pull on the cord and cause a bell located in the brain to ring: the message of pain received. This basic idea stuck around for centuries.

Still, in the 1800s, as the discovery of opiates and anesthesia revolutionized the treatment of acute and surgical pain, doctors regularly encountered patients with chronic pain who didn't fit into this model, who had pain in the absence of anything that seemed to be ringing the bell. For the most part, nineteenth-century physicians believed the reports of patients with this kind of "pain without lesion." With their Cartesian bent, they considered pain without lesion to be an impossibility, but, with a healthy sense of humility, they generally assumed that the lesions that explained their patients' mysterious suffering simply hadn't been uncovered yet.

Post-Freud, however, psychiatry was offering alternative theories for what ailed such patients, and physiological evidence was emerging that seemed to support the theory that there was a straightforward, proportional relationship between a noxious stimulus and the pain it caused. Once this idea—the specificity theory of pain—took firm hold in American medical schools in the early twentieth century, pain that wasn't explained by an organic pathology came to be seen as hysterical—if the patient's complaint was believed at all. "Those who suffered from unexplained chronic pain syndromes were often regarded as deluded or were condemned as malingerers or drug abusers," writes historian Marcia L. Meldrum.

In the 1960s, the gate control theory of pain complicated the simple, cause-and-effect Cartesian model somewhat by positing that not all pain signals sent from the peripheral nerves make it to the brain; they encounter "nerve gates" in the spine that either allow them through or block them. An important step forward, it better accounted for the fact that the relationship between injury and pain isn't very consistent at all; a minor injury can cause great pain in one person, while a major one is barely felt by another. And it helped explain how the perception of pain is influenced by thoughts and emotions—for example, why it seems to hurt worse when you stub your toe just after receiving some bad news. Although this new model recognized that the central nervous system (the spine and brain) played a role in modulating pain, it still held that there had to be something causing the peripheral nerves to fire off their pain signals.

That continued to leave only two options for explaining the mystery of "pain without lesion": either there was pathology affecting the peripheral nerves that had thus far eluded medicine's current tools of perception, or there wasn't, in which case such pain could be labeled "medically unexplained" and, by default, "psychogenic." Lacking the humility of their nineteenth-century predecessors, most in the profession went with the latter option. Chronic pain that wasn't a symptom of an observable organic problem was generally assumed to be caused by psychological factors—though the exact mechanism by which this happened was always left hazy—and categorized as a pain disorder in the somatoform section of the *DSM*. In fact, any pain that seemed to be in "excess" of what would be expected given the extent of tissue damage was blamed on the patient's "emotional overlay."

As Dr. Daniel Clauw, director of the Chronic Pain and Fatigue Research Center at the University of Michigan, explains, a couple of decades ago, "if you went to a doctor with chronic pain in any particular region of the body and they couldn't find anything wrong in that area of the body, they would have a tendency to then blame the patient: 'there's nothing wrong with you, you're stressed, it's a psychiatric problem.'" They'd offer "any mis-attribution for those symptoms" rather than cop to the basic truth: "that we just don't understand pain well enough yet." It was "very frustrating for the patients because they knew in their heart that that was not the nature of their problem."

This duality between organic and psychogenic pain was reflected in the tests the doctors gave Alexis as she searched for an explanation for her pain as a teen in the late nineties. "They would say, 'We'll do this imaging, and then we'll do this questionnaire.'" The questionnaire was a psychological test to determine whether she was suffering from depression, anxiety, bipolar disorder, or another mental health problem. "Nothing ever came back on imaging or on the psychological stuff."

Of course, the convenient thing about psychogenic symptoms is that the patient doesn't actually have to demonstrate any psychological disorder at all to have them. So, faced with pain they didn't understand, doctors would frequently suggest that Alexis's condition was psychogenic despite her normal psychological scores. Sometimes, since it was in the general vicinity of her uterus, her pain would be vaguely attributed to "female problems"—menstrual cramps or a "hormonal imbalance." Often doctors would simply say, "Well, we don't see anything wrong: you're fine," she recalls. "Well, I'm *not* fine; I'm in a lot of pain."

THE EVOLUTION OF INTERSTITIAL CYSTITIS

Since medicine tended to treat pain it couldn't explain as if it didn't really exist, dismissing patients to see a psychiatrist when they couldn't find a cause, just a few decades ago chronic pain was largely invisible to the medical system. Back in the early nineties, when women's health advocates called for more research on health concerns that disproportionately impact women, chronic pain wasn't even really on the agenda. Many functional pain conditions that largely affect women, like fibromyalgia, IBS, TMD, vulvodynia, and interstitial cystitis, were not being studied at all; some had only just been named and defined. It's in large part thanks to the efforts of patient-advocacy groups that organized in the eighties and nineties that "unexplained" chronic pain conditions have been pulled out of the psychogenic wastebasket and put on the radar of the public and the medical community.

In 1983, Vicki Ratner, a thirty-two-year-old third-year medical student, came down with what she assumed was a really bad urinary tract infection. But the doctor found no sign of infection, and a course of antibiotics didn't help. As the constant pain—which felt like a lit match in her bladder—and the need to urinate urgently and frequently continued, she went from doctor to doctor in search of an answer. With negative test results, she was told there was nothing to be done. "I was dismissed to live with debilitating symptoms, told that the problem was due to stress and that I should seek psychiatric care," she writes. "It was further suggested that I had brought the disease on myself, that it was all in my head, that the solution was to quit medical school and settle down to a traditional lifestyle." All told, she saw fourteen physicians (ten of them urologists), but none offered a diagnosis or even relief for her agonizing pain.

"Ultimately, I had to make the diagnosis myself," Ratner says. She marched off to her medical school's library to search the literature. In those wild pre-Internet days, that meant paging through volume after volume of the *Index Medicus*, a large index book published annually that listed the medical journal articles from that year. Finally, as the library was about to close and Ratner was about to throw in the towel after two full days and nights of searching, she came across a footnote, which led her to a 1978 article by Stanford researchers about a condition called interstitial cystitis that seemed to match her case exactly. She brought the article to her original urologist and asked him to perform the diagnostic procedure, a cystoscopy to check her bladder for the tiny pinpoint bleeding called glomerulations that the authors described. After nearly a year of insisting, she got her cystoscopy and a diagnosis.

When Ratner was diagnosed in the mideighties, IC, which was first named in 1887, was described in the medical literature as very rare—estimated to affect no more than 45,000 people in the country—and occurring mostly in postmenopausal women. Predictably, given its unknown cause and largely invisible symptoms, it was also thought to be a psychosomatic condition. The leading urology textbook, *Campbell's Urology*, described IC in the chapter entitled "Psychosomatic Conditions in Urology": "Interstitial Cystitis may present the end stage in a bladder that has been made irritable by emotional disturbance . . . a pathway for the discharge of unconscious hatreds." It could be thought of as "an irritable bladder in an irritable patient." After her diagnosis, Ratner wrote a letter to the authors, and that claim was removed in the next edition.

Though getting a diagnosis was a relief, Ratner was still facing "a disease about which very little was known, on which little research was being done, the diagnosis and treatment of which were surrounded by controversy." Above all, she was desperate to find others in the same boat. "I spent the last two years of medical school in intense, unremitting pain and in isolation, imagining that I was the only one in the world with this disease." Her attempts to get information from the NIH, the CDC, and the American Urological Association were futile.

In 1985, Ratner, by then an orthopedic surgery resident in New York City, "turned to the media as a last resort." Through a serendipitous personal connection, she got an early break: an appearance alongside a urologist on *Good Morning America*. After the five-minute segment aired, the newly formed Interstitial Cystitis Association (ICA), which at that point consisted of Ratner, a few volunteers, and a PO Box, received a flood of letters (10,000 of them in just the first week) that didn't let up for months.

"They were such distressing letters," Ratner recalls. "It was the same story as mine": women, many of them—contrary to the patient profile—young and middle aged, with the same symptoms and same experiences being dismissed by doctors. "Patients had often seen five to ten physicians, had had complete workups that were negative, and had received no diagnosis. They were told that either nothing was wrong or the symptoms were 'all in their head.' These IC patients were suffering from terrible pain and urinary frequency as often as every ten minutes. They were trapped in their own home, cut off from their friends, family and society in general, due to their severe disability. On occasion, even family and friends began to believe that the symptoms were not real since the doctor had said so."

There were women who couldn't work but couldn't get disability compensation, because IC wasn't yet listed as a qualifying disease. There were women, unable to have sex because it was so painful, whose husbands had left them. There were women in their seventies who wrote to say, "I've had this since I was in my twenties and no one believed me." Ratner says, "No one had ever validated them—for their entire lives." Then there were the letters, often accompanied by donations, from family members of sufferers who'd committed suicide to end the agony. "Enclosed are three donations made in memory of my wife, Joanna," wrote the husband of a forty-four-year-old woman with a teenage son. "The extreme pain and despair over chances for a cure caused her to end her life on April 8th. We hope that these donations help in some small way to find a cure and save others from this fate."

The letters were typical of the experiences of many IC patients. According to a 1993 study, 43 percent of IC patients had been told they had an emotional disorder before being properly diagnosed an average of four years later. They reported being informed that their symptoms were "just nerves" and that they should "find a lover," "get married," "have a baby," or "get a life."

From the start, the ICA was supported by a few leading urologists committed to researching IC. But "there appeared to be a complete lack of interest" in the field more broadly, according to Ratner. Urology, which deals with problems of the male reproductive system and the urinary tracts of both sexes, is, to this day, the most male-dominated medical specialty. Back then, 99 percent of urologists were men; in 2015, according to a WebMD poll, 92 percent were. And in the early days, the most common response the ICA received from them was laughter. "They didn't believe it existed," Ratner says.

Only gradually did they begin to come around—especially, she recalls, "once they found out that we were working with Congress and had some say over the funding and where it went." In the early nineties, the

ICA successfully lobbied to get the NIH to put some federal funding, for the first time ever, toward studying the condition. The media coverage that Ratner worked tirelessly to secure also helped. She was amazed to discover how much legitimizing power a piece in a reputable outlet could have in the doctor's office. "When patients come in, they have no credibility. But if you bring in an article by [New York Times health reporter] Jane Brody, the doctors believe you!" Still, it wasn't until 1999 that IC was included in the standard review course for residents planning to take their urology boards.

When Ratner diagnosed herself, she'd thought, "Well, either I'm alone—one in a million—or the lady down the block has the same problem." The avalanche of letters to the ICA confirmed her suspicion that this disease was perhaps not as rare as the medical literature claimed. But they needed research to prove that. In 1987, the ICA teamed up with a urologist on the first epidemiological study of IC in the United States. It concluded that it took an average of 4.5 years and five doctors for someone to get diagnosed with IC, and that for every one patient diagnosed, five more went undiagnosed, which put the prevalence estimate at nearly half a million. The patients in the study rated their quality of life as worse than do patients on kidney dialysis and had four times the rate of suicide as the general population.

Since then, the prevalence estimates have increased even more, in part because the criteria for identifying the condition have changed to be symptom based, rather than dependent on objective signs. Historically, to be diagnosed with IC, a cystoscopy (the procedure Ratner had to push so hard for) needed to show a Hunner's ulcer, an area of inflammation, on the bladder. "As it turns out, very few people have that—the majority of them do not," Ratner explains. "So the diagnosis was never made. Once misinformation is printed, once it gets into *Campbell's Urology,* nobody questions it." In 1987, encouraged by the ICA, the National Institute of Diabetes and Digestive and Kidney Diseases drew up a first consensus definition of IC to standardize research efforts. The term *painful bladder syndrome* (PBS) was adopted in the 2000s as an umbrella term to cover all cases of chronic bladder pain in the absence of observable pathology.

Today, according to the most common terminology, IC/PBS is defined by symptoms (discomfort, pressure, or pain in the bladder area, usually accompanied by frequency and/or urgency of urination) that aren't explained by infection or another condition. About 10 percent of patients have the kind of IC marked by Hunner's ulcers, and a major focus of research efforts is to further pull out different subtypes of IC/PBS patients, who may have different underlying causes for their similar symptoms and respond to different treatments.

In 2011, researchers from the RAND Corporation came up with the first prevalence estimate based on a nationally representative population-based survey. It suggested that 3.3 to 7.9 million women in the United States have symptoms consistent with IC/PBS. On average, they'd had the condition for fourteen years. Most had consulted multiple doctors, but less than half had been given any diagnosis at all and just 10 percent of them had received an IC/PBS diagnosis. Strikingly, a follow-up study found that the many millions suffering without a diagnosis reported symptoms that were just as debilitating as women being seen for the condition in a specialty clinic. In other words, while IC/PBS pain can vary in severity, those who go undiagnosed do not necessarily have milder cases that only minimally impact their lives. The women who'd been diagnosed were just more likely to be white and have health insurance. And while it was originally thought that IC affected nine times more women than men, a 2007 study estimated between 1 and 4 million men have IC in the United States.

Today, thirty years after Ratner's diagnosis, this once-rare psychosomatic condition of postmenopausal women is thought to affect 8 to 10 million Americans.

"IT IS HARD WORK BEHAVING AS A CREDIBLE PATIENT"

By the early eighties, as Ratner was being told that this apparently unending UTI from hell was all in her head, scientific research was starting to challenge the notion that any pain not attributable to organic pathology in the body was "unexplained" and psychogenic by default. Growing knowledge of the central nervous system began to point toward a third option. Studies demonstrated an intriguing phenomenon that came to be called central sensitization: in experiments, when volunteers were exposed to a relatively short spurt of nociceptive pain, for a while afterward their entire central nervous system became hypersensitive to pain signals, not just from the nerves at the site of the injury but also from those in the rest of the body. Apparently, the central nervous system played a role not only in tamping down pain signals but also in amplifying them.

This suggested that perhaps pain could, in fact, be "all in your head"—not because of some theoretical psychological process like conversion but due to changes at the level of the neuron. After all, *all* pain is literally all in your head. Though it certainly feels as though it's your hand that hurts when you burn it on a hot pan, your hand is not capable of hurting; pain becomes pain only in the brain. As Woolf, who conducted some of the early studies demonstrating central sensitization in the eighties, explained, the phenomenon suggested that pain could be an "illusory perception" that was identical to pain caused by tissue damage but occurred due to abnormalities in the pain-processing system itself.

You might assume that medicine eagerly welcomed this transformation in our understanding of pain. After all, labeling unexplained pain "psychogenic" was not actually an explanation for it—at least not in the flesh-and-blood (or, rather, cellular-and-neurochemical) terms most physicians preferred. On the contrary, many doctors seemed pretty satisfied with their existing "explanations" for unexplained pain.

According to Woolf, the implications of central sensitization were not embraced at first. "These notions were generally not very well received initially, particularly by physicians who believed that pain in the absence of pathology was simply due to individuals seeking work or insurance-related compensation, opioid drug seekers, and patients with psychiatric disturbances; i.e., malingerers, liars and hysterics," he writes. "That a central amplification of pain might be a 'real' neurobiological phenomenon, one that contributes to diverse clinical pain conditions, seemed to them to be unlikely, and most clinicians preferred to use loose diagnostic labels like psychosomatic or somatoform disorder to define pain conditions they did not understand."

It's surely not just a coincidence that most of these supposed "malingerers, liars, and hysterics" were women. To be sure, the lack of knowledge about chronic pain has affected all pain patients, male or female, over the years. And certainly many men with chronic "unexplained" pain have encountered their fair share of doctors who disbelieved them or dismissed their symptoms. Still, there's evidence of a gendered difference in how likely doctors are to settle on psychological explanations for chronic pain. Cynthia Toussaint, founder of the organization For Grace, has seen this play out among the patients she's spoken with as an advocate for women in pain for the last two decades.

Toussaint developed complex regional pain syndrome (CRPS) after she pulled her hamstring as a promising young ballet dancer in the eighties. CRPS, which affects over three times more women than men, is a poorly understood neuropathic pain condition in which an injury—which can be as minor as a small cut—triggers wildly disproportionate pain, often accompanied by swelling, skin discoloration, excessive sweating, and changes in skin temperature. The pain spreads beyond the original injury to the whole limb and sometimes moves to the rest of the body too. The condition was first classified as a type of hysteria minor by Charcot and was long dogged by psychosomatic suspicions. These days, approximately 50,000 new cases of CRPS are diagnosed annually, and experts think that the true number is likely higher since patients, particularly those with the type of CRPS that isn't linked to an observable nerve injury, continue to be accused of inventing or exaggerating their pain.

Toussaint's hamstring pain just never went away. A year and a half later, a similar burning pain developed in her opposite leg. After another six years, the pain had jumped to both of her arms. For five years, it ravaged her vocal cords, leaving her unable to speak. But for over a decade, she went undiagnosed. "Women have to prove that we're really in pain," she says. "I spent thirteen years being disbelieved." One doctor suggested she take a truth serum to prove she was making it up. Another thought the pain was a manifestation of "stage fright." Eventually reliant on a wheelchair and at times suicidal, she was accused by one doctor of "enjoying the secondary gain" she was receiving from her "attentive partner."

Toussaint tells me that when other women with chronic pain share their stories with her, typically one of the first things out of their mouths is "I'm not crazy like the doctors tell me." While For Grace is focused on women's pain, Toussaint will occasionally hear from men with chronic pain too, and she's always eager to learn about their experiences. In many ways, the men's stories are just like the women's: the same frustration with doctors offering few answers and even fewer effective treatments, the same isolation from friends and family who can't truly understand, the same mourning the life they once had. But there is often one glaring difference: the men usually don't offer a preemptive defense of their mental health or the reality of their pain. "I would sometimes cut in and ask them, 'So at any point in this long, horrible, frustrating journey, did the doctors disbelieve you or say that you were crazy?' And I would generally get something like, 'No, I can't really relate to that,'" she says. "It was the same story: 'I've lost my life, my career, my dreams.' But with the men they were believed, and that respect was something that we women were not given."

Women with chronic pain face the same challenge as women with acute pain: How do you demonstrate how much pain you're in without being seen as either hysterical or else not in that much pain at all? But for those with "unexplained" chronic pain, threading this needle is a never-ending and often all-but-impossible feat. With no observable cause of the pain, the patient's expression of pain is the only evidence for it. But women's expressions of pain—whether through words, grimaces, or tears—are so often viewed as emotional that many women with chronic pain feel as though they need to be ultrastoic to be taken seriously. In a 2002 New York Times article, a pain specialist at Northwestern University described how, acutely aware of how her fellow health care providers interpreted women's tears as a sign of "emotional issues," rather than physical pain, she'd "coach" her female patients on how to use "every resource [they] can muster to not cry" before referring them to other doctors.

But, of course, if the goal is to better demonstrate the severity of your pain, there are obvious risks to a strategy that amounts to downplaying it. Women with chronic pain often report trying to be "antihysterical" to the point of actually being dishonest about how much pain they're in. As the authors of a 2007 study of doctor-patient interactions in chronic pain management note, "Female patients must strike a balance between conveying their pain experiences accurately without inadvertently undermining their authenticity by being perceived according to negative gender stereotypes." Plus, as Lauron's case of the missed appendicitis illustrated, while a stoic response to pain may be expected in men, it's not expected in women; a woman who is rating her pain as a ten yet is not falling to pieces may be met with suspicion as well, assumed to be a malingerer who is inventing her pain entirely.

As the title of a 2003 qualitative study concluded, "it is hard work behaving as a credible patient." Based on interviews with ten female patients with chronic muscular pain in Norway, it explored the "work" these women had to do in order be "believed, understood, and taken seriously when consulting the doctor." "Their efforts reflect a subtle balance not to appear too strong or too weak, too healthy or too sick, or too smart or too disarranged," the authors write. The women described walking a tightrope between being assertive and not too assertive. They had to fight persistently for their care, yet one patient explained, "You have to tread rather softly; because once you antagonise them it's not certain that you are any better off."

The exhausting balancing act extended not just to how they spoke and acted but also to how they looked: too "put together" and they'd have a harder time being perceived as seriously ill. Many of the women reported feeling as if they needed to adjust how they dressed to avoid comments like "You always look so healthy!" from their doctors. Toussaint recalls her mother telling her to stop wearing makeup to the doctor's office when she was a young woman searching for a doctor who would take her pain seriously. And this perception is right: studies have found that health care providers have a strong "beautiful is healthy" bias, especially when it comes to women. A 1996 study found that patients judged "attractive" were perceived by their doctors to be experiencing less pain, a finding that held only for the female patients.

While those with functional pain conditions face an especially uphill battle in attempting to be a credible patient, women with many kinds of chronic pain complain that health care providers don't trust their reports. In 2014, For Grace teamed up with the online news site *National Pain*

Report to conduct a survey of 2,400 women with a range of chronic pain conditions, including fibromyalgia, back pain, OA, migraine, and neuropathic pain. Over 90 percent of them felt the health care system discriminates against female patients. Over 80 percent felt they had been treated differently by doctors than a man would have been, and two-thirds said they thought their doctors took their pain less seriously because they were women. Forty-five percent said a doctor had told them that their pain was "all in their heads." Nearly 60 percent said a doctor had admitted to not knowing what was wrong with them, and three-quarters had been told they'd just have to "learn to live" with their pain. Almost a fifth had been told that their pain was a result of childhood trauma. Over half had been told, "You look good, so you must be feeling better."

Physicians turned pain patients also attest to the bias that female pain patients face. In journalist Judy Foreman's book *A Nation in Pain: Healing Our Biggest Health Problem,* some of the most striking perspectives come from doctors who, once they found themselves on the other side of the equation, were shocked to realize just how poorly the medical system understands pain. A few male doctors felt it was only their gender and medical expertise that prevented them from being completely disbelieved. Dr. Karen Binkley, an allergist and associate professor of medicine, had to diagnose herself when a broken toe turned into CRPS. The four doctors she saw, as well as the many doctor friends whose brains she picked, didn't have any ideas. "It was only because I was a physician that I had the knowledge and resources to help research my care myself," she said. If she'd just been your average female patient with CRPS? Binkley had no doubt: "I would be institutionalized if I had not been a physician and been so persistent."

———

In For Grace's survey nearly half the respondents thought doctors were more reluctant to prescribe opioid pain medication to them because of their gender. The opioid epidemic has been hovering in the background of a few of the stories in this book so far. With about 33,000 Americans now dying each year from heroin, fentanyl, and prescription opioid overdoses, there's no doubt that the opioid epidemic is a public health crisis. It's also clear that as doctors have become increasingly fearful of prescribing opioids, it has led to a heightened atmosphere of distrust surrounding patients' reports of pain—both chronic and acute—that especially affects certain patients: women, people of color, people with low incomes. As Maggie and Jackie learned, simply seeking care at an ER for pain without an immediately evident cause can be enough to provoke suspicions that you're "narco-savvy."

Pain experts caution that concern about the real risks of addiction must be balanced with the recognition that, while opioids are not recommended as a first-line option for chronic pain, they are a lifesaving last resort for some patients. They also point out that, while the roots of the opioid epidemic are complicated, some of the blame lies in medicine's failure to effectively respond to the chronic pain epidemic. As Dr. Sean Mackey, chief of the Stanford Division of Pain Medicine, recently explained to *Vox*, in the nineties there was growing awareness that pain should be treated, but doctors didn't have much training on how to do so. The result: physicians "who've got little education around pain, who are aware that there's an increased awareness to treating pain, who've got very few tools that they can use to treat pain, who now are hearing a message that, 'You know what? It's okay to use opioids to treat pain,'" Mackey says. "It was easier to prescribe an opioid than do anything else."

Take Alexis's experience. She was never denied pain medication, but that isn't to say that she ever felt as though her pain was being taken seriously. When doctors concluded that there was "nothing wrong," Alexis would insist that obviously *something* was wrong since she was in a great deal of pain. "And then it was like, 'Well, if you're in pain, we can prescribe you something,' and then that was it." She says that it often seemed as though painkillers were offered as the fastest way "to get me off their back."

Pain medication was not what Alexis was looking for. "I was eleven, twelve, thirteen, fourteen, fifteen, sixteen; I didn't want to be on drugs for the rest of my life." She particularly had no interest in opioids that left her unable to function at school. (Eventually, she found a nonnarcotic painkiller that helped somewhat.) "I wanted someone to find a diagnosis and then to really work on the issue and help me find a way to manage my pain."

Instead, the medical system seemed to have only two unappealing options to offer: take pain pills for the rest of her life or "just deal with it."

Alexis eventually gave up. "When I was about seventeen, I decided I was done." She'd sought help from a primary care doctor, who gave her yet another psychological test. "I was like, 'I've taken this a hundred times. I'm not suffering from depression. I just need help with the pain.'" She acquiesced to filling out the questionnaire. Even though her results were normal, the doctor suggested the pain was psychogenic. Alexis walked out of the doctor's office and announced to her mom through tears that she'd had enough. "I said, 'I can't do it anymore. I can't go to any more doctors who tell me that I'm crazy.' It was too much of a battle to try and get the help I needed."

So for the next ten years she didn't try. She saw doctors for birth control refills, but she dealt with her pain herself. Besides, newly married and putting herself through college, she didn't have co-pays to waste to see doctors who didn't listen and likely had no help to offer anyway. During this decade, she developed "a pretty good pain management routine" of painkillers, heat pads, and natural creams, though she "couldn't really just have a normal life." The pain was always there—"a constant ache" that was "sometimes dull and sometimes severe." There were a couple of semesters that she had to drop her college classes, but for the most part, Alexis says, she "could kind of get through."

EXPLAINING THE INEXPLICABLE

The most frustrating thing is that, until recently, women's efforts at being the perfect female pain patients—not too hysterical, but not too stoic; not too put together, but not too disarranged—were pretty much destined to fail for those with functional pain conditions. At best, they may have found a doctor who believed the pain was real but had no explanation for it or understanding of how to treat it. At worst, their pain would be deemed psychogenic or fabricated by default. What chronic pain patients needed was not advice on how to better communicate their symptoms, nor even individual doctors more willing to trust their accounts. Ultimately, they needed scientific research to explain the inexplicable.

Instead, the most notable thing about research on chronic pain dis-orders, especially functional and poorly understood pain disorders that largely affect women, is how little of it there's been. Even today, chronic pain conditions are grossly underfunded, relative to how many people are affected by them, how disabling they can be, and how much knowledge we lack about how to treat them. According to an estimate by the Chronic Pain Research Alliance (CPRA), vulvodynia, TMDs, IC, fibromyalgia, endome-triosis, IBS, chronic tension-type headache, chronic migraine, chronic low back pain, and chronic fatigue syndrome research received $110 million total from the NIH in 2014, an average investment of just $1.06 per affected patient. By comparison, it spends about $35 on each person with diabetes.

Meanwhile, as with any "medically unexplained symptoms," much of the research that has been done on chronic pain has been focused on uncovering the psychological factors and personality traits that were as-sumed to cause it. Higher rates of depression and anxiety among chronic pain patients have been pointed to in order to suggest that mood disorders somehow cause the pain—which, given the nature of pain, is an especially ridiculous case of mistaking the consequences of illness for the cause. Pain is not just a sensation but also an emotion. What makes pain pain is that it makes us feel bad. By evolutionary design, it is deeply unpleasant in order to compel us to avoid what is causing it. That many people who live with chronic pain are psychologically distressed would seem to be an entirely unsurprising finding, one that's notable only if you're starting from the assumption that chronic pain is psychogenic and looking for evidence to support that belief.

In fact, almost every perfectly understandable way that someone might react to the nightmare of living with unending pain for which medicine has no explanation has just been reframed as evidence that the pain is due to psychological factors. By the nineties, pain experts were starting to critique the concept of psychogenic pain that was enshrined in the *DSM*. One of their concerns was that patients with allegedly psychogenic pain were often described as having a tendency to "visit physicians frequently, use analge-sics excessively, ask too often for surgery and assume an invalid role"—a position, pain expert Dr. Harold Merskey pointed out, that tended "to treat as psychological problems, behavioural activities which were quite likely to be consequences of protracted illness rather than evidence of some peculiar personality problem causing the disorder."

Perhaps most unfairly, "unresponsiveness" to treatment has been seen as a red flag that pain was not organic but instead maintained by some unconscious hidden motive on the patient's part. As Paula Kamen, a feminist writer and chronic headache patient, writes in her 2006 memoir *All in My Head: An Epic Quest to Cure an Unrelenting, Totally Unreasonable, and Only Slightly Enlightening Headache,* "Doctors in each era, including our own, tend to consider their diagnostic tools definitive, and they are likely to include drug responsiveness as an important measure of validation." In the ultimate victim-blaming reversal, doctors managed to turn the very fact that, with no real understanding of chronic pain, they very often failed to successfully alleviate it, into a reason to let themselves off the hook.

To add insult to injury, patients' understandable frustration with this inadequate treatment has *also* fed into psychogenic theories. Studies have found high levels of "hostility" among chronic pain patients, another fairly unsurprising finding that was just added to the pile of evidence against them. In a 2000 volume published by the American Psychological Association entitled *Personality Characteristics of Patients with Pain,* Merskey suggested that the resentment long observed among chronic pain patients could, just maybe, "be attributed to experiences of unsatisfactory treatment. It is not surprising that people with chronic pain become irritable and perhaps resentful and difficult. A new, deeper explanation may not be necessary."

"When medical 'proof' of the legitimacy of one's illness is missing, often it is just a matter of waiting for technology to catch up," Kamen writes. And in the 1990s and 2000s, thanks to new advanced imaging technologies, chronic pain patients finally got some corroborating evidence of their reports. Functional MRIs and PET scans allowed researchers to observe, via measurements of blood flow, which particular structures of the brain are activated when a person is experiencing pain. Though pain may still be subjective in the exam room, in the lab, it's increasingly something that can be seen, if indirectly.

By 2001, influential pain researcher Ronald Melzack, one of the authors of the gate control theory, pulled together the emerging evidence in support of a new model of pain, the one widely accepted by pain experts today: far from the cord that Descartes had imagined, the experience of pain is "the output of a widely distributed neural network" across multiple parts of the central nervous system, including the spinal cord, brain stem and thalamus, insular cortex, limbic system, and prefrontal cortex, that together create its sensory, emotional, and cognitive aspects. According to this neuromatrix theory, though pain is often triggered by tissue injury or inflammation in the peripheral nerves, it doesn't have to be.

This pain neuromatrix, though in part genetically determined, is, like our nervous system as a whole, changeable. The same neuroplasticity that's helpful when it allows us to learn to play an instrument or master a new language seems to work against us when it comes to chronic pain. As those early studies of central sensitization suggested, pain itself can alter the neuromatrix profoundly in a case of "practice makes perfect" gone terribly awry. During prolonged pain, nerve cells can become more and more responsive to weaker and weaker pain signals. Eventually the central nervous system's ways of inhibiting these pain signals received from the periphery can malfunction as well, ramping them up instead. And the whole system can become so revved up that it may no longer need even low levels of noxious stimuli to keep it in a hypersensitive state: the pain response has essentially become self-perpetuating.

Over the last few decades, research has suggested that abnormalities that lead to an amplification of pain within the central nervous system may contribute to many "unexplained" functional pain conditions. Clauw offers this analogy to explain this kind of "centralized" pain: Imagine your body is an electric guitar and its strings are your sensory nerves. The guitar is constantly getting played, but if the amp is set at the optimal level, you have to strum a string really hard to create a sound (sensation) that's unpleasantly loud (painful). In centralized pain, however, it's as if the amp is turned all the way up: the strings are getting played as normal, but suddenly everything sounds too loud. In this state, sensations that would normally just feel like a touch—a gentle brush of the skin—now provoke pain (this is called allodynia), while those that would usually only be mildly painful now feel excruciating (hyperalgesia).

In studies in which patients are poked and prodded to measure pain sensitivity, patients with functional pain conditions, including IBS, TMD, chronic tension-type headache, idiopathic low back pain, vulvodynia, IC, and fibromyalgia, show widespread hyperalgesia and allodynia compared to healthy controls. And functional imaging studies confirm that the pain-processing areas of the brain light up in these patients in response to stimuli that would typically not be experienced as painful. They also seem to share other abnormalities in common: dysregulation of the hypothalamic-pituitary-adrenal (HPA) axis, autonomic nervous system and immune system abnormalities, and even changes in the volume of gray and white matter in various parts of the brain.

The progress made in explaining unexplained pain is shifting our understanding of all chronic pain. Even chronic pain conditions in which there is nociceptive and inflammatory pain can involve centralized pain, which helps explain why the degree of tissue damage in these conditions does not correlate very well with patients' reports of their pain. For example, 30 to 40 percent of people who, according to their X-rays, have severe knee OA don't have any pain, while 10 to 15 percent of people without evidence of OA have painful joints. Approximately 20 to 30 percent of people with autoimmune diseases like RA or lupus also meet the criteria for fibromyalgia; it's as if centralized pain is overlaid on top of their nociceptive and inflammatory pain.

The long shadow of hysteria has also hindered scientific progress on understanding why many people develop multiple pain conditions. As far back as the eighties and nineties, small studies were showing a large degree of overlap between functional pain disorders; patients with one were more likely than the rest of the population to go on to develop another or several others. But at that time, since each individual disorder was suspected of being psychogenic, these comorbidities were just further cause for dismissal. After all, the more "medically unexplained symptoms" someone had, the more likely she'd be seen as having somatization disorder—or Briquet's syndrome or hysteria in earlier generations. According to the *DSM-IV* criteria for somatization disorder, pain in four areas of the body, plus two gastrointestinal complaints, one sexual/reproductive symptom, and one pseudoneurological one could get you the diagnosis.

The thing is, exactly such a history may well be the rule rather than the exception. In the last decade, larger studies have suggested that "there actually are more people that go on to have multiple conditions than there are that just end up with one primary disorder," says Chris Veasley, director of the CPRA. And the more conditions, the worse the outcome. "As the number of conditions you have increases, the less likely you are to benefit from treatment, the higher the likelihood of disability, increased costs, mood disorders," Veasley says. And even today, with "multiple conditions that have long been thought of as psychological, the level of stigma that's attached to these patients is even greater."

Studying why this overlap occurs has become a major area of research focus. One of the key open questions: to what extent the development of such "chronic overlapping pain conditions"—as the NIH has dubbed them—reflects a progression that could be derailed. Since about half of the risk for developing centralized pain disorders appears to be due to genetic susceptibility, it's possible that some people would eventually develop multiple pain disorders no matter what, their central nervous systems being destined to tip into dysfunction. But for some, Veasley says, if the first pain condition had been treated better—"if we were able to intervene early and stop the cascade of centralizing"—perhaps the development of additional disorders could have been avoided. In other words, how many cases of so-called hysteria, Briquet's syndrome, or somatization disorder could have been prevented if women's unexplained pain was taken seriously from the start?

FIBROMYALGIA AND "A MEDICAL SEXISM THAT'S HARD TO MISS"

Alexis's pain remained manageable until a few years ago, when her husband was in a serious motorcycle accident. Alexis quit her three jobs to become his 24/7 caregiver, as he spent six months in a wheelchair and another six learning to walk again. She lifted him to the toilet, to the bathtub, in and out of bed. She wasn't sleeping enough. She was, to put it mildly, under a lot of stress. "I wasn't able to take good care of myself, and so my symptoms started to get really, really bad."

Alexis's most severe, persistent pain had always been localized to her back and hips, though she'd had more transient pains in her shoulders, elbows, neck, and jaw before. But during this difficult time, she started to get episodes "where the pain would be everywhere" in her body, down to the tiny joints in her hands. She became so fatigued that she couldn't function. By the time her husband had recovered enough to go back to work, Alexis sometimes couldn't even get out of bed to feed herself. She eventually managed to go back part-time to her job as a receptionist, but "it was a battle every time."

Though she was anxious about consulting a doctor about her pain again, she eventually felt she had no other option. "It just got to the point that I couldn't ignore it or handle it on my own anymore," she says. "I wasn't really able to live life." Still, she put off making an appointment for weeks, because she "didn't want to go have someone not listen again." The first couple of doctors she saw did exactly that: "It was just the same story, so I quickly gave up." She was prescribed antianxiety medications and an antidepressant. "I didn't stay on them for long; they didn't improve any of my symptoms."

Among chronic pain experts, fibromyalgia is something of a poster child: the prototypical condition in which the problem seems to be largely a malfunction of the pain-processing system itself.

Fibromyalgia's history follows a familiar trajectory. In 1592, the French physician Guillaume de Baillou first introduced the term "rheumatism" to describe muscular pain, and since the nineteenth century, the medical literature has described various types of muscular rheumatism and theories for its cause. In his 1859 *Clinical and Therapeutic Treatise on Hysteria*, physician Pierre Briquet (whose name would eventually be given to Briquet's syndrome) observed that "pain in the muscles is so common that there is not a single woman with this neurosis who does not have some muscle pain during the course of the illness." Widespread pain was also a symptom included in George Beard's description of neurasthenia in 1880. In the early twentieth century, the British neurologist Sir William Gowers suggested that it should be called "fibrositis" on the assumption that it was caused by inflammation of the fibrous tissues of the muscles. The term stuck around for over seventy years, used loosely to describe any pain in the muscles, chronic or acute, widespread or localized, that couldn't be explained by something else.

But as the decades passed, no evidence of inflammation was found. And as the specificity theory of pain was increasingly accepted, that left fibrositis, like all chronic pain not explained by organic pathology, ripe for psychogenic explanations. In the 1930s, a Scottish doctor argued that chronic rheumatism was simply a manifestation of "anxiety states or hysteria": a "complaint of pain . . . is, in the absence of structural change or inferiority, not infrequently a symbol." The prevalence of fibrositis among soldiers during and after World War II drew attention and reinforced the psychological suspicion. In 1943, two U.S. military physicians suggested that it be renamed "psychogenic rheumatism." For the next few decades, as psychosomatic medicine's influence peaked and then fell, the term fibrositis was often used interchangeably with psychogenic rheumatism. And as with other unexplained symptoms, outside the context of war it was increasingly seen as a particularly female ailment. In 1968, one American physician described most of the features of fibromyalgia as occurring mostly in women who tended to be "worry warts."

In the early seventies, Dr. Hugh Smythe, considered the grandfather of modern fibromyalgia, made the case that there was a distinct syndrome of fibrositis that was distinguishable from the catchall category of psychogenic pain. He suggested that fibrositis could be identified by widespread pain, along with fatigue, poor sleep, morning stiffness, and the presence of multiple "tender points." During the eighties, a small cadre of rheumatologists worked on developing standardized criteria for the ill-defined condition (which was renamed fibromyalgia) so that it could be researched and consistently diagnosed. In 1990, the American College of Rheumatology released the first official fibromyalgia criteria: a combination of widespread pain and pain in at least eleven of eighteen specified tender points. When these criteria were revised in 2010, the tender points were dropped; the diagnosis is now based on widespread pain, fatigue, unrefreshing sleep, and cognitive problems ("fibro fog," as patients often call it).

While initial research on fibromyalgia focused on trying to uncover some pathology in the muscles, fairly quickly the focus turned to looking at abnormalities in the central nervous system. Many pain experts now see fibromyalgia as a kind of end-stage centralized pain state, in which the pain volume control has been turned up system-wide so that basically everything that can hurt does hurt. Why exactly the pain-processing system becomes so hypersensitive is still poorly understood. Those with fibromyalgia seem to have an imbalance of neurochemicals: too much of those that tend to ramp up pain signals and too little of those that inhibit them. These same neurotransmitters are involved in sleep, alertness, mood, and memory, which likely explains the other symptoms of the condition. Some fibromyalgia patients have evidence of small fiber neuropathy. Another intriguing emerging line of research is exploring whether the central sensitization seen in fibromyalgia, and perhaps other chronic pain conditions as well, is due to the inappropriate activation of immune cells in the brain.

Though fibromyalgia may not yet be fully "medically explained," to pain experts, it is clearly not psychogenic. As pain expert Joel Katz pointed out in an article opposing the new category of SSD in the *DSM-V,* as our understanding of the neurophysiology of pain has become progressively more sophisticated, many mysterious characteristics of pain that were once considered inexplicable and therefore, by default, attributed to the mind have been explained: "The complexity of the pain transmission circuitry," he wrote, "means that many pains that are currently poorly understood will ultimately be explained without resorting to a psychopathological etiology."

Yet as recently as 2008, skeptics questioned whether fibromyalgia exists at all in a *New York Times* article entitled "Drug Approved. Is Disease Real?" As brain-imaging advances have helped erase any doubt that fibromyalgia patients are certainly experiencing the pain they claim to be, some have tried to make the mounting evidence of neurobiological abnormalities fit into the existing psychogenic framework. Yes, they say, the pain is real, but the hypersensitive state is of the patients' own making.

In a 2000 article in *The New Yorker,* proponents of a psychosocial explanation for the condition repeated tired ideas about somatization. According to one psychiatrist, patients develop fibromyalgia because they become increasingly obsessed with everyday aches and pain: "They become trapped in the belief that their symptoms are due to disease, with future expectations of debility and doom. This enhances their vigilance about their body, and thus the intensity of their symptoms." By giving them a diagnosis of fibromyalgia, another physician claimed, they become "card-carrying members of the fibromyalgia club" and "pain is allowed to dominate their life." Since patients are thought to become more and more sensitive to pain signals only because they're continuing to focus on them, the way to "cure" it is by diagnosing it less. "If we underplay this, it will come down to a more minor level or disappear."

There is little about this explanation that squares with reality. People who develop fibromyalgia are somewhat more likely than others to have had a history of depression or anxiety, but the majority of them have not. For most people with fibromyalgia, the pain begins fairly suddenly after a trigger. In some cases, it's an episode of acute pain, such as an injury or a surgery, that would normally last a few weeks that seems to set the pain-processing system off on this pathological roll. But essentially any stressor (mental or physical, the body doesn't make a distinction) seems to be capable of turning up the volume control in those who are susceptible. Other common triggers include trauma from car accidents, sexual violence, or deployment to war; certain infections, including hepatitis C, the Epstein-Barr virus, parvovirus, and Lyme disease; and prolonged emotional stress. And a significant subset of people with other "explained" pain conditions, like RA or OA, eventually develops fibromyalgia.

And it is difficult to imagine how the medical system could possibly "underplay" fibromyalgia any more than it already has and does. Three-quarters of doctors say they don't feel comfortable diagnosing the condition at all; some outright refuse to see fibromyalgia patients. Unsurprisingly, then, a 2012 population-based study that estimated that about 4 million American adults have symptoms consistent with fibromyalgia found that three-quarters of them have not been officially diagnosed with the condition. And yet, despite not being "card-carrying members of the fibromyalgia club," half of them are so disabled that they are unable to work. Alexis, for one, had never heard of fibromyalgia when pain and fatigue suddenly took over her life.

Fibromyalgia has become somewhat more accepted as a legitimate diagnosis since 2007, when the FDA approved the first of three drugs, which act on the central nervous system, specifically to treat the condition. As it has for many invisible diseases whose exact mechanism is still unknown (from depression to ADHD), a pharmaceutical treatment helped validate the condition as real, and it also provided an opportunity for experts to educate other physicians. But patients continue to encounter dismissive health care providers. And the stress and frustration of having to prove you're really in pain can make it worse: a 2013 study based on a survey of 670 fibromyalgia patients found that those who had more experiences of medical professionals invalidating their symptoms had a worse quality of life, and those who had more trust in their doctors reported less pain.

Perhaps the most generous explanation for the lingering skepticism toward fibromyalgia is that it takes a long time for new knowledge to trickle down throughout the medical system. "The biggest fibromyalgia haters statistically are always the male, and also older, physicians, because they were taught in a different era," Clauw says. "They didn't learn anything about any of this." Even today, what doctors are taught about pain typically does not reflect the current state of the knowledge of chronic pain. "The number of medical schools that give good pain education is extremely low," says Clauw. Generally, schools are still teaching to the tests, which emphasize basic science information about the different nerve fibers: C fibers, A delta fibers, B fibers. "It's very objective," and it's "totally useless and irrelevant" to actually caring for people in chronic pain. But "medical school curricula tend to change at a glacial pace." Clauw urges patients not to waste their time trying to convince the "Neanderthals" who don't "believe" in fibromyalgia or other functional pain conditions. "I can barely win against those people when I have an hour with slides and my reputation."

But, even compared to other functional pain conditions, fibromyalgia has been met with greater skepticism. While most cases of chronic low back pain, for example, similarly aren't accounted for by a structural problem, you don't see articles debating its very existence. Fibromyalgia expert Dr. David Edelberg has suggested that the medical community's response to the condition displays "a medical sexism that's hard to miss even if you're not looking closely."

It's true: in the medical community, as well as the culture at large, there's a particularly virulent disdain toward fibromyalgia patients, 90 percent of whom are women, that can be described only as misogynistic. In her book

Tender Points, writer Amy Berkowitz, who suffers from vulvodynia and fibromyalgia, collects some online comments about fibromyalgia sufferers: "They're just nasty fat women who want to collect disability checks. 'Doing stuff makes me tired, give me some money and/or drugs.' Lazy-ass slugs who sit at home and watch *Judge Judy* while the rest of the world works for a living. 71% of them are fat women who don't ever get off their ass. Sorry if you don't like facts." "Anyone who can read an Internet article and say 'ow' 11 times can have it." "I have to deal with these nutcases at work and I flat out call them fakers to their face. They need to get up off their lard-asses and get a job. They're just whiney people who love to be 'sick.'"

I think the enduring disbelief toward fibromyalgia really only makes sense within the context of how such patients have historically been viewed by the medical system. "Fibromyalgia patients are those that physicians don't want to see. They are 'heartsink' patients," a 2012 article on the condition noted. "'We think they are all crazy,' a distinguished rheumatology division head and Professor of Medicine told us, reflecting a not uncommon view."

At this point, medicine no doubt has a certain investment in this view. It's difficult to avoid the conclusion that there may be some reluctance to accept that chronic pain in the absence of observable peripheral pathology is a real neurobiological condition—a disease in its own right—because, for decades, medicine has been treating it as if it is not. For most of the twentieth century, physicians, by and large, had acted as though much of women's chronic pain was someone else's problem. Functional chronic pain conditions have been relegated to the very bottom of the research agenda. Patients have been treated as if the only thing perpetuating their persistent, disabling pain is the "secondary gain" they received from being ill.

While it takes a long time for the medical system to incorporate any new scientific knowledge, not all new knowledge requires such a drastic revision: from seeing millions of mostly women patients as "malingerers, liars, and hysterics" to seeing them as people with a serious disease—who have been criminally neglected by the medical community. Accepting the paradigm shift in our understanding of chronic pain necessarily means admitting that, for decades, the approach medicine took to our largest health problem was fundamentally incorrect.

MIGRAINE: REAL BUT STILL NOT SERIOUS

There's also the fact that a neurobiological explanation for functional chronic pain still leaves it subjective. While brain imaging advances have offered some objective proof of patients' pain in research settings, in the exam room, pain is still a subjective experience that must be communicated by the patient. Presumably, if and when a biomarker for fibromyalgia is discovered that offers an objective way to confirm the diagnosis, the medical community will accept it as a legitimate disease. But as it stands now, believing in fibromyalgia and other functional pain conditions requires believing individual patients when they say they are in pain. As the damning IOM report on pain concluded, health care providers "must rely on a person's ability to express his or her subjective experience of pain and learn to trust that expression." And the history of migraine suggests that even when pain is well accepted as being a neurobiological disorder, extending that trust to women remains difficult.

Thirty-eight million Americans suffer from migraine, and three-quarters of them are women. That means a whopping 18 percent of adult American women have migraine. Some of them get only a few episodes a month, but roughly a quarter of migraine patients are severely incapacitated by the disease. And it's estimated that 2.4 to 7.1 million Americans have chronic migraine, in which the headaches gradually become more frequent until they are occurring at least fifteen days a month for three months in a row.

That's a lot of people who spend at least half their days often unable to work, sleep, or sometimes even get out of bed. The pain of a migraine, which typically lasts between four and seventy-two hours, can be unimaginably bad. According to writer and migraine sufferer Joan Didion, "That no one dies of migraine seems, to someone deep into an attack, an ambiguous blessing." Cindy McCain famously said she could imagine her husband Senator John McCain's experience of torture in Vietnam because the "unbearable" pain of a migraine "may come close," a comparison the senator didn't dispute. Even those who don't get migraines all that frequently say that the condition shapes their whole lives; the unpredictable nature of the attacks leaves them constantly worried about how to avoid triggers.

In many ways, migraine is a couple of decades ahead of where other chronic pain conditions are today. "For the past 100 years, migraine has been thought of as an imagined disorder and as only a woman's problem," the chief operating officer of the International Headache Society, Valerie South, said at a 1998 conference. "Physicians believed women were stressed out from taking care of children and the lack of ability to cope, but recent research has underscored the fact that migraine is a real biological problem." A European neurologist added, "Ten years ago, if you asked physicians if migraine was a real disease, about 70 percent thought it was not. Now, probably about 40 percent of physicians think it is not a real disease." In a 2000 radio appearance, headache specialist Stephen Silberstein summed up the shift: "We used to believe that migraine was a disorder of neurotic women, whose blood vessels dilated and they couldn't face up to life. We now know that migraine is a disorder of the brain."

As Joanna Kempner, a sociologist with chronic migraine, has explored, the evolution of Western medicine's view of migraine and other types of headache tracks with the broader history of hysteria. Since ancient times, migraine had been largely understood as an organic disease that could be influenced, like all disease, by emotional or mental factors. In the Victorian era, migraine and other types of headache were closely associated with nervous disorders. In the late nineteenth century, two competing theories were offered for the biological mechanism that explained migraine. Some suggested that it was a vascular disorder in which the cranial blood vessels either constricted or dilated inappropriately, while others framed it as a neurological disorder in which the pain was brought on by a "nerve storm." In both cases, those with a "nervous temperament"—whose "brains are very excitable, their senses acute, and their imaginations free," as one nineteenth-century doctor put it—were seen as especially at risk.

Curiously, while today migraine is known to be more common in women, back then, doctors often spoke of the typical migraine patient as male. This may have been because, while nineteenth-century doctors appeared to believe that headache disorders were more prevalent among women—after all, women were thought to be especially prone to nervous disorders—there was an inconsistent terminology of different kinds of headache, and women and men tended to get different labels. Women were more likely to be given a diagnosis of clavus hystericus (hysterical headache), which was seen as a symptom of hysteria and was related to but distinct from "true migraine," though exactly how the two actually differed, apart from the gender of their sufferers, is unclear.

As psychosomatic medicine took off in the thirties, Harold G. Wolff, the "father of modern headache research," popularized the notion of the "migraine personality." Wolff was a proponent of the vascular theory of migraine, but he believed that was just the mechanism; the root cause lay in the patient's emotions. Based on interviews with patients, he decided the "migraine-type" was an ambitious perfectionist preoccupied with achievement and success. Surprisingly, considering that most migraine patients were women, Wolff spoke more about the migraine personality in men. Perhaps not that surprisingly, considering he himself had migraine, he portrayed it in a pretty positive way. Though their perfectionist tendencies may have brought on their migraine attacks, migraine-types were "responsible, conscientious and reliable."

There was no such upside to the migraine personality in women, however. For Wolff, the crux of the problem in a migrainous woman seemed to be her inability to accept her feminine role—particularly in sex. He claimed 80 percent of his female patients were sexually dissatisfied. Other headache specialists at the time were even more clear about what kind of women got migraine: "Whenever a woman is having three attacks of migraine a week," one physician wrote, "it means that she is either psychopathic or else she is overworking or worrying or fretting, or otherwise using her brain wrongly."

The migraine personality and vascular theory dominated the medical thinking from 1930 to the early 1970s. The first crack in the edifice came in the early sixties, when the FDA approved the drug methysergide as a preventive treatment for the condition. Since the drug, which affected serotonin levels, worked without changing the emotional state, let alone the personality, of the patient, it dealt a blow to the notion that migraine was psychogenic. Experts started to question the research upon which Wolff had developed the migraine personality profile to begin with. With the first population-based epidemiological studies came the conclusion that the myth of the migraine personality had emerged simply because upper-middle-class professionals were more likely to seek treatment from doctors than low-income sufferers.

Discussions of the migraine personality could be found well into the eighties, even as a neurobiological explanation of the condition gradually took over. In the nineties, functional MRI and PET scan studies gave some clues into the pathophysiological mechanisms behind the attacks. Studies also began to show that migraine is, in part, inheritable, and identified a number of genes that are associated with the disorder. Perhaps most importantly, in the early nineties, the drug Imitrex (generic name: sumatriptan) hit the market. Able to stop a migraine in process in many patients, the drug and its several copycats became a blockbuster, giving doctors something that actually helped their migraine patients, as well as combating the lingering stigma and suspicion around the condition. As Imitrex's creator explained, "The discovery of sumatriptan confirmed, once and for all, that migraine truly is an organic disease and not just the figment of imagination of 'neurotic' patients."

But, in her 2014 book *Not Tonight: Migraine and the Politics of Gender and Health,* Kempner reaches the depressing conclusion that while medicine has accepted migraine as a neurobiological disorder, this shift has not been powerful enough to erase the specter of the hysterical woman that has long haunted the condition. In the last few decades, she points out, migraine has successfully checked off pretty much all the boxes a disease needs in order to be respected as a real disease in modern medicine: well-established diagnostic criteria, its own subspecialty, brain imaging that makes it visible, pharmaceutical treatments, a genetic link. And yet the condition continues to be undertreated, underfunded, and belittled as a minor affliction of hypersensitive women. In short, she argues, it still suffers from a "legitimacy deficit."

Medical students get little formal training on headache disorders. They're not a required part of the curriculum, and, according to surveys, medical undergraduate students get an average of two to four hours of education on the topic. As headache specialist Peter Goadsby has said, "Headache is the commonest symptom found in neurologic outpatients—and, paradoxically, the least taught to neurology residents. It's like training electricians, but not telling them about light bulbs." The discrepancy tends to leave young doctors with the impression that migraine is a trivial problem, a perception reinforced when they enter residency and find that neurologists don't much like dealing with headache patients.

According to a recent survey by the American Academy of Neurology, nearly half of the respondents said they found headache patients more time consuming and a third found them more emotionally draining than other patients. Half of those surveyed judged headache patients to have more psychiatric problems than other patients, and a quarter felt they have "motivation to maintain their disability." This leaves headache specialists in high demand but not in high prestige. As Kempner explains, it seems that the negative stereotypes about women with migraine rub off on the doctors who treat them too. Headache specialists often joke that "headache is the Rodney Dangerfield of medical maladies: it gets no respect."

It gets no respect in the funding realm either. The NIH has devoted $20–25 million annually to headache disorders in recent years, mostly for migraine, with minuscule amounts for less common types of headache, like chronic daily headache and cluster headache. That's shockingly little considering both the huge number of people affected by them and how disabling headache disorders can be. As a basis for comparison: epilepsy affects 2.1 million people (just 5 percent of the number affected by migraine) and accounts for a third as many years lived with disability as migraine does, but gets four to five times as much funding. In the absence of federal support, most of the research on headache disorders comes from the pharmaceutical industry.

And while the existence of drug treatments for migraine has certainly helped legitimize it as a real biological condition—not to mention, of course, improved many patients' quality of life—the pharmaceutical industry's portrayal hasn't helped much in making it seem serious. Ads for migraine drugs give the impression that the condition is a minor inconvenience for middle-class white women that is easily treated with a pill. In reality, migraine is more common among low-income Americans, is just as common in people of color, and affects 8 million men in the United States too. And effective treatment eludes many patients. Preventive treatments are only about 50 percent effective in 50 percent of those who take them. Drugs like Imitrex don't work for everyone and are very expensive, ranging from twelve to forty-six dollars per pill.

In the public imagination and the medical community, the perception seems to be that while migraine is now unquestionably real, it is still not that serious.

————

Maureen learned that a few years ago, when she had a migraine for eleven days. She'd had the occasional tension headache, and a couple of migraines in college several years prior, but this was like nothing she'd ever experienced before. All of a sudden, there was an "ever-present pounding" in her head. She was oversensitive to light and sound. Her eyes were constantly sore, as was every muscle in her upper body. Five minutes into a meal, she'd become nauseated and often vomit. "It was hell on earth." By day seven of being barely functional, she was starting to get really concerned. Her vision had become so blurry that for part of the day she'd been temporarily blinded. Her speech slurred at times. "Everything that I read online said, if your symptoms last for more than three days and if you experience any changes in your vision, seek care from a health care provider." The nurse at the urgent care center she called for advice agreed: go to the ER to rule out something like a stroke or an aneurism.

In her initial intake assessment, the ER staff seemed concerned that she couldn't put her chin to her chest (a possible sign of meningitis) and assured her she'd be seen within an hour. But hours went by. "It was excruciating waiting in that waiting room" with its bright lights and bustle, but "I was just desperate for answers." After four hours, a nurse practitioner brought her back and told her it would be several more hours before she'd be seen, because it was unlikely that it was anything more than "just a migraine." She told Maureen, "I can offer you Tylenol for your pain, but we need to address the people here who we know are actually sick, and we need to make sure that they are getting the care that they deserve, and we need to make sure that the rooms that we have available are going to the people who are genuinely suffering."

"I was at day seven of this, so having her say that to my face—'Oh, you're not actually sick, you don't actually need to be here, and you don't deserve a room over all of these other people'—I just immediately started crying." Maureen repeated her reasons for being there (the terrifying vision changes) and asked her if she was implying that she wasn't sick. "Well, people will say just about anything to get their hands on strong painkillers," the nurse replied. "My main takeaway was that she just didn't believe me and thought I was just trying to get hysterical and trying to play on her emotions to get her to give me stronger pain meds," Maureen says. "But I couldn't help my reaction."

Maureen got up and left. The next day she booked an appointment with a queer-friendly health clinic. "My partner had to really push me to make an appointment." While she was still in severe pain, she was almost "willing to accept that" rather than return to the medical system and risk being "treated like that again." On day ten of her migraine, she finally got a diagnosis, treatment, and a referral to a neurologist.

Kempner argues that "for a disease to be fully legitimated, the people who have it must be viewed as deserving of care and resources." And migraine patients are mostly women in pain, whose credibility has long been suspect. Consequently, "people with migraine continue to be understood as weak, whiny hypochondriacs who cannot tolerate the aches and pains that come with everyday life, even as they are framed as having a brain disease." As Maureen's experience illustrates, "it hardly matters if migraine is established as a specific disease if individual patients are not believed or, if when they are, they are not thought to have a serious disorder." The same could be said of many chronic pain conditions.

"I FORGOT WHAT IT FELT LIKE TO FEEL LIKE A NORMAL HUMAN BEING"

About a year ago, Alexis finally got the kind of medical care she'd searched for unsuccessfully for years. Her mom, who had long had similar symptoms, had started doing her own online research and had recently found a fibromyalgia expert who'd diagnosed her with the condition. She encouraged Alexis to give her a shot. Finally, at age twenty-nine, Alexis got a diagnosis—and a doctor who validated her pain. "She answered a million questions that I've had since I was eleven years old. All of a sudden I had answers, and I had someone on my side."

Though she still has a great deal of pain and fatigue, she now has someone helping her to get them under control. And she's improved enough that, with the support of her husband and a large extended family nearby to lean on, Alexis can be a mom to her eleven-month-old twins. Though she'd once hoped to become a nurse, for now, taking care of herself and her kids is more than enough. "Unfortunately I don't get to be one of those supermoms who has a career and everything, because I have to take care of myself too. There's only so much I can do in a day before I'm tapped out." By the evening, her body usually hurts too much to do the bedtime routine with her twins. "It's hard to face the fact that this controls my life, but it's reached a point that I can't deny how much it affects."

Now that she has a doctor who takes her symptoms seriously—and who even has some ideas about how to improve them—Alexis's biggest problem may be that she's struggling to afford to be treated. "We have plenty of bills, and my medical care comes last, I guess." She's run out of covered visits to the specialist, so they're now "few and far between" and she's put off getting some recommended tests. "Just for my medications alone, insurance just doesn't help enough for me to be able to afford what I need." For now, her doctor has given her samples of a drug to help with the fatigue, which has been nothing short of life changing.

"I feel human and I can function. I can go grocery shopping and do laundry and do all these things that on a normal basis, I can't. But the prescription is $450 a month, and I can't afford it. Financially it's just more than we can do. I've gotta pay for everything for my kids—bottles and formula and baby food and clothes. And I'm really emotional about it because I forgot what it felt like to feel like a normal human being, and now I know. Every day I beg for a cure or something to help."

CHAPTER 6

THE CURSE OF EVE: WHEN BEING SICK IS "NORMAL"

Ellen got her period at age eleven, and, after a few years, the mild cramps she'd experienced at first began to morph into a different beast entirely. "The pain was shifting from my uterus to my hips, and it got worse and worse and worse. And it was a different kind of pain than I was used to. It felt like a burning, inflammatory pain, like if you had a hot coffee mug and pushed it against your joints." Her back was painful and stiff, all the way up to her neck. "The result was that a lot of times I couldn't really walk or stand or sit. It put too much pressure on that part of my body. I could basically only move back and forth in bed every so often to distribute the pain around."

In high school, she started missing school, usually the one or two days right before her period began, which is when the pain peaked, and became a regular visitor at the nurse's office. "I think they kind of thought that I was making it up a little bit. Because they were like, 'Oh yeah, it's you again.' At least once a month, I'd have to be taken home from school by my mom and carried into the house, or just stay home from school altogether." A couple of times she ended up in the hospital. "They didn't really know what to do.

They didn't really attempt a diagnosis. They just kind of gave me morphine, and the next morning they sent me home."

———

Though the post-Freud shift to attributing unexplained physical symptoms to the mind has been perhaps the most important barrier to increasing knowledge of many women's conditions over the last century, when it comes to disorders that affect women's reproductive and sexual functions, an even older bias has been at play: medicine's tendency to treat women's illness as perfectly normal.

While women's unexplained symptoms were at least treated as real by physicians in the late nineteenth century, they were also largely attributed to the unfortunate but inescapable fate of being a woman. Hysteria was considered an organic disease but one that was innate within all women. "As a general rule, all women are hysterical and . . . every woman carries with her the seeds of hysteria," wrote the French physician Auguste Fabre in 1883. "Hysteria, before being an illness, is a temperament, and what constitutes the temperament of a woman is rudimentary hysteria."

As all symptoms in women tended to be tied back to their reproductive organs, women's routine reproductive cycles and states were considered somehow inherently pathological. In 1900, the president of the American Gynecological Society explained, with great melodrama, that the life of a woman was medically treacherous: "Many a young life is battered and forever crippled on the breakers of puberty; if it crosses these unharmed and is not dashed to pieces on the rock of childbirth, it may still ground on the ever-recurring shallows of menstruation, and lastly upon the final bar of the menopause where protection is found in the unruffled waters of the harbor beyond reach of sexual storms."

As Ehrenreich and English write, "The theories which guided the doctor's practice from the late nineteenth century to the early twentieth century held that women's *normal* state was to be sick." When hysteria underwent its final shift to being seen as psychological, this led to a jarring pendulum swing in some respects. Many symptoms associated with women's routine reproductive states and cycles that medicine had previously taken as evidence that women were physically abnormal and inferior—and touted to justify excluding women as a class from participating in public life—suddenly weren't considered real at all.

Take menstruation: in the late nineteenth century, it was considered a time of ill health when it wasn't safe for any woman to participate in normal activities—let alone pursue higher education or a career. The 1872 book *A Physician's Counsels to Woman in Health and Disease* advised, "Long walks, dancing, shopping, riding and parties should be avoided at this time of month invariably and under all circumstances." But post-Freud, pain and other symptoms associated with menstruation, like other unexplained symptoms, came to be considered largely psychological. One textbook in the 1970s declared that dysmenorrhea "is generally a symptom of a personality disorder, even though hormonal imbalance may be present." Rather quickly, women went from having to resist medicine's pronouncement that their periods were, as a rule, so disabling they disqualified women from being equal participants in the workforce to having to insist that some women did indeed experience debilitating periods.

To some extent there's been a swing back to seeing women's reproductive functions and transitions as pathological. With menopause, this shift was especially extreme. In 1966, Robert A. Wilson argued in his book *Feminine Forever* that menopause was a "curable" state that "no woman need suffer" thanks to treatment with supplemental estrogen. As feminist critics noted, previously medicine had hardly acknowledged that *any* women suffered menopause symptoms at all. "Until menopause became big business, American women were always told their symptoms were all in their heads. With the new business of hormone replacement therapy, there's been a complete flip-flop. Not only have the symptoms become 'real,' but all women are expected to experience all symptoms, and with the same degree of severity," wrote Dr. Susan Love. "The movement is a breathtaking one," Joan Callahan points out, "from 'It's all in your heads' to 'You are all ill and in need of medical intervention.'"

Indeed, these are the two contradictory extremes that medicine has tended to vacillate between: either women's reproductive functions are pathologized as innately abnormal—in which case any symptoms they bring are "normal"—or else it is claimed that they're normal, so if they cause symptoms, it's only because an individual woman's response to them is abnormal—she's just especially sensitive or overreacting. In short, either all women are sick, or some women are crazy. Today, medicine seems to have generally settled into a position that manages to incorporate the worst of both worlds: it's considered "normal" for women's reproductive functions to be a bit abnormal—and if it's really bad, well, maybe it's all in your head.

ENDOMETRIOSIS

Both of these extreme positions obviously serve as a cover for medical ignorance. Clearly, menstruation, pregnancy and childbirth, and menopause are natural biological processes—as normal as respiration or digestion—not states of disease. Yet medicine still doesn't have a good understanding of why some women have painful periods, while others do not, or why some women experience menopause symptoms, while others do not. But, of course, one of the reasons for that knowledge deficit is that for so long "female problems" have been treated as alternately normal or psychogenic; after all, there's little need to study symptoms that are considered the inevitable result of women's innately disordered biology or psychology.

Perhaps no disease has been more hampered by the normalization of women's illness as endometriosis. A common, poorly understood disease that affects at least 6.3 million in the United States, endometriosis occurs when a substance similar to the endometrium (the tissue that lines the uterus in preparation for implantation of a fertilized egg and, if that fails to happen, bleeds and sheds during menstruation) is found in other parts of the body, most often the abdominal cavity, around the ovaries, fallopian tubes, bladder, or bowel. This tissue seems to respond to the hormones that trigger menstruation, also bleeding and attempting to shed each month. The result is pain, inflammation, and the formation of nodules, cysts, and scar tissue. In severe cases, large masses called adhesions can even glue the organs of the pelvis together.

The disease's symptoms include pain before and during periods, fatigue, heavy bleeding, painful bowel movements, painful urination, and diarrhea and constipation during menstruation. About a third of women with endometriosis are infertile, and more than half experience pain during sex. Some women with endometriosis have pain all the time, not just around their period; indeed, the condition is thought to explain up to 90 percent of cases of chronic pelvic pain in women. On the other hand, some don't have any symptoms at all, discovering the disease only once they try to get pregnant.

To get officially diagnosed, you have to undergo a surgical procedure that identifies the endometriosis lesions. Which means that you have to convince your doctor that your symptoms are not just "killer cramps," a task that proves all but impossible for many women. In the United States, on average, it takes ten to twelve years between the time the symptoms begin—which, for 60 percent of patients, is before age twenty—and getting a diagnosis.

THE WANDERING WOMB

There's some disagreement about who deserves credit for "discovering" endometriosis. Descriptions of abdominal growths linked to severe pain and other symptoms during menstruation can be found in Western medical literature as far back as the seventeenth century. In 1921, American gynecologist Dr. John Sampson gave the condition, then known by a confusing array of terms, its modern name *endometriosis*, which is ancient Greek for "abnormal condition of the uterus." He proposed that the disease was caused by a process he called "retrograde menstruation": during menstruation, endometrial tissue flowed back out of the uterus through the fallopian tubes and took root in the abdominal cavity.

If Sampson's explanation for endometriosis (endometrial tissue that wanders back out of its proper place in the uterus) seems to sound an awful lot like the ancient Greeks' "wandering womb" theory of hysteria, that's perhaps no coincidence. In 2012, three leading endometriosis experts published a sixty-two-page historical analysis of the disease. Combing through almost 4,000 years of medical history for descriptions of women's menstrual and pelvic pain, they concluded that there is "substantial, if not irrefutable, evidence that hysteria, the now discredited mystery disorder presumed for centuries to be psychological in origin, was most likely endometriosis in the majority of cases."

Now, I don't know about *that*; it seems to me that hysteria was a tent big enough to cover countless yet-to-be-understood conditions we recognize today, but they make a strong case that endometriosis was one of the diseases labeled as hysteria throughout the centuries. Undoubtedly, during ancient Greek and Roman times, menstrual pain and other irregularities were a central feature of the *hysterikos* family of disorders. And as the authors point out, though these disorders represented "a veritable diagnostic junk drawer," if endometriosis was the cause in some cases, then the ancient recommended remedy (to marry and conceive as soon as possible) may, by suppressing menstruation, have actually appeared to work. Even as hysteria began to be seen as a nervous system disorder, "menstrual difficulties" remained a common symptom of the disease, and some physicians took note that their hysterical patients' complaints recurred cyclically. The French psychiatrist Philippe Pinel, for example, "explained that the 'violent' hysterical outbursts would start when a girl reached puberty; with each monthly menstruation, she would have hysterical outbursts along with 'bowel and urination problems,' with symptoms persisting for '3 or 4 days,' after which the patient would return to normal."

By the nineteenth century, French pathologists were correlating symptoms of heavy bleeding and agonizing menstrual pain with growths in the abdominal cavity revealed by their autopsies. But by and large, endometriosis remained something that the average doctor was not equipped to see. In 1887, one physician lamented that women with small endometriotic nodules were "simply called 'hysterical' because the tumors are still too small to be recognized by palpation, and the uterus may neither be enlarged, displaced, nor otherwise affected." The hints of endometriosis's presence can be found in a nineteenth-century ad for the popular patent medicine Lydia E. Pinkham's Vegetable Compound. Touted as a remedy for "Nervous Breakdown," the patient testimonials describe symptoms of endometriosis and allude to "female trouble."

In the twentieth century, unexplained menstrual pain came to be considered psychogenic—while the myriad other symptoms endometriosis can cause were easily misattributed to somatization. Mary Lou Ballweg, founder of the Endometriosis Association, pointed out in a 1997 article that endometriosis and somatization disorder were clinically indistinguishable, the only thing separating them being surgery to reveal the endometrial lesions. All the main symptoms of endometriosis (pain during menstruation, irregular menstruation, excessive menstrual bleeding, pain during vaginal intercourse, pain in the abdomen, nausea, abdominal bloating, diarrhea, back pain, urinary retention) were also listed as symptoms of somatization disorder. "In all the decades since Freud, women have been told their symptoms are in their heads," Ballweg concluded. "For the majority of the millions of women with endometriosis, the kind of thinking behind somatization disorder is simply a new twist on that old bias about women."

THE CURSE OF EVE

Today, the widespread belief—shared by the medical system and the public alike—that menstrual pain is "normal" poses a barrier to the timely diagnosis of endometriosis even before a patient steps foot in a doctor's office. "It's bigger than just the physicians," Ballweg notes. "It's our society which teaches girls that being female means to suffer. We have to nip that mythology in the bud."

A 2006 study of women who were eventually diagnosed with endometriosis found that one of the reasons for the diagnostic delay was that the women themselves thought their painful periods were normal, so they didn't see a reason to ask a doctor about them. They figured they were just one of those "unlucky" people who got bad cramps. And really, how would they know that their periods weren't normal? There's so much stigma around menstruation that many young women are left without any point of comparison.

Ellen certainly didn't have one. The pain was so bad that she'd become depressed and anxious in anticipation of every period. But she doesn't recall ever talking to her friends about it in high school. "People don't really talk about it—even between women," she says. "I had nothing to refer to when it came to menstrual pain. It seemed like everyone else was handling it and wasn't being bothered by it, so I figured, why wasn't I doing that?"

Her mom's response confirmed that sense. "I'd tell my mom, 'When I feel this pain, I want to die.' And she'd say, 'Well, periods are supposed to hurt.' She'd say, 'When I was your age, I'd have really terrible periods.' She'd have to take painkillers and stay out of work because of her menstrual pain, so she kind of thought it was normal for me to be going through the same thing." This, too, is common. Many women with endometriosis reach out to their mothers or other relatives to gauge their symptoms, only to find that they've had similar experiences, likely because endometriosis runs in families. Someone is seven times more likely to have the disease if one of her close relatives does.

Kate Seear, author of *The Makings of a Modern Epidemic: Endometriosis, Gender and Politics*, has argued that part of the reason menstrual pain is normalized is that there's such a strong "menstrual etiquette" that discourages people from discussing it. In her studies, many women with endometriosis who did tell others about their menstrual pain were criticized for it. Some encountered employers or colleagues who believed they were using it to get out of work, or partners who thought it was an excuse to avoid sex, or other women who implied they were seeking attention for something that everyone else endures without complaint. In the face of such unsympathetic reactions, they decided suffering in silence was the better option. Seear notes that even greater public awareness about what constitutes an abnormal period may not be enough to improve the diagnosis of endometriosis if experiences like these "dissuade women from disclosing menstrual problems in the first place."

"I was raised with the expectation that periods hurt and you just kind of have to grin and bear it. So I felt like I had to be stoic about it," Ellen agrees. "Whenever I had to stay home from school or take a break or cancel an event because of the pain, I felt really, really bad." To this day, Ellen, now twenty, feels like she "can't really talk about" the pain. She struggles to "justify" her absences by offering other excuses. She says, "I'm not feeling well" or "I suddenly came down with something." "Or 'I have a migraine'— migraine is the classic one. I do get migraines too, so it's legit, but not as often as people think I do." She doesn't like copping to this particular kind of pain: "It's embarrassing."

Given this broader atmosphere, it's all the more disturbing that when women do seek guidance from medical professionals, the people who should be equipped to dispel these long-standing cultural myths about what's normal when it comes to menstruation, they're so often met with the same response: that they're just overreacting to "normal" cramps. According to the Endometriosis Association's research registry, 61 percent of women and girls who eventually were diagnosed with endometriosis had been told by health care providers that nothing was wrong with them.

Advocates like Ballweg suggest we should question the entire notion that any degree of menstrual pain is "normal." Menstrual pain is classified as secondary dysmenorrhea if it's caused by an underlying disease, like endometriosis, and other common causes of secondary dysmenorrhea include uterine fibroids and ovarian cysts. Primary dysmenorrhea, on the other hand, refers to menstrual pain not due to any evident pathology. Assumed to be psychogenic for decades—attributed to a woman's inability to accept her feminine role in the seventies—it's now largely considered "normal."

Primary dysmenorrhea is certainly *common*. The majority of menstruating people in the United States have some—usually mild—pain with their periods at some point, typically during adolescence. Fewer but still far too many experience dysmenorrhea that's bad enough to interfere with daily activities, causing them to miss school or work: according to a 2006 estimate by the World Health Organization, severe menstrual pain affects 12 to 14 percent of women. But of course, it's unclear how many women with severe dysmenorrhea are actually suffering from undiagnosed endometriosis. According to a 2016 survey of over 59,000 American women, about 6 percent had been diagnosed with endometriosis. And given how many years most patients go before getting diagnosed, many women with severe menstrual pain likely have the condition. In other words, the normalization of severe menstrual pain—in medicine and the broader culture—is in large part a result of the mass underdiagnosis of endometriosis.

And just because menstrual pain is common doesn't necessarily mean it is normal. While primary dysmenorrhea has been considered "unexplained," over the past few decades, research has suggested that an imbalance in prostaglandins, substances that control the contraction and relaxation of the uterine muscles, is likely to blame. Despite identifying it as an imbalance—one that is clearly not inevitable, since not all women do

experience menstrual pain—medicine still tends to treat primary dysmenorrhea as normal. As does the culture at large. "Women accept that pain
with their period is normal. And I don't accept that," Ballweg says. "There
are many, many reasons in our modern world that periods are painful for
some women, but we need to study that and turn it around. A routine physiological process shouldn't be painful. Whether or not it's endometriosis,
it's a problem."

"THE CAREER WOMEN'S DISEASE"

Sampson's theory that endometriosis was caused by retrograde menstruation led to a corollary one: that the more periods a woman had—say, by
not being pregnant constantly during her reproductive years—the greater
her risk of developing the disease. Doctors started recommending the same
prescription offered for hysteria 4,000 years earlier: pregnancy.

In the 1940s, Dr. Joe Vincent Meigs, an influential expert on the condition, warned that endometriosis was on the rise due to "delayed and in-
frequent child-bearing" and urged that women "be taught how to become
pregnant and not how to avoid pregnancy." By postponing pregnancy,
women were defying "nature's rules," as a comparison between women and
monkeys clearly revealed: "The monkey mates as soon as she becomes of
age, and has offspring until she can no longer have any or until she dies.
Menstruation in this animal must be rare. As women have the same physiology it must be wrong to put off childbearing until 14 to 20 years of menstrual life have passed." Of course, Meigs, writing at the height of eugenicist
thinking in American medicine, wasn't concerned about endometriosis
in all women. He claimed that the disease wasn't as common among "less
well-to-do patients" and advocated "early marriage and early childbearing
among our people"—by which he meant his own "successful" Anglo-Saxon,
well-educated upper class.

By the sixties, as more and more women began to flagrantly break
"nature's rules" and enter the workforce, endometriosis came to be called
"the career women's disease." The typical patient was thought to share a
particular psychological profile. "The patient is said to be mesomorphic

but underweight, overanxious, intelligent, egocentric and a perfectionist. These characteristics represent a personality pattern in which marriage and childbearing are likely to be deferred and therefore predispose to prolonged periods of uninterrupted ovulation." One leading expert in the field wrote in 1971, "It's that type of individual who simply has to clean out the ashtrays all the time." The idea that endometriosis was a disease of middle- to upper-class white women in their early to midthirties who had postponed childbearing in favor of a career persisted officially in the medical literature well into the nineties.

One consequence of this stereotype was that women were effectively blamed for bringing the disease on themselves with their life choices. By the eighties, they were seen as culpable for a veritable epidemic. "Over the last twenty years," two researchers wrote in 1988, "as personal achievement for women in developed countries has become more defined by professional gains than by exacting and rearing a family, the incidence of endometriosis has increased." As Seear writes, the disease came to be imagined as a "product of women's inappropriate and unnatural exercise of agency."

It likely won't surprise you at this point to hear that there's no truth whatsoever to the "career women's disease" stereotype. "The myth came about because it was really only educated, affluent women who forced the doctors to diagnose them," Ballweg explains. They were the ones who had not only the financial ability to get a diagnosis that requires a surgical procedure performed by a specialist but also enough authority to convince their doctors that their symptoms really were abnormal. Endometriosis expert Dr. Marc Laufer put it simply in the documentary *Endo What?*: "When I went to school in the eighties, I was taught that endometriosis was a 'career women's disease.' What did that mean? It meant white women who had insurance—you listened to their pain."

As for other women's pain? Well, racist assumptions effectively kept many women of color from getting diagnosed. "Racial minorities didn't even get endometriosis according to the textbooks even into the 1980s," Ballweg says. "If an African American woman went to the doctor with the very same symptoms as a white woman with endometriosis, she would be told she had pelvic inflammatory disease (PID), i.e., [that she's] sexually promiscuous." One 1993 study suggested that up to 40 percent of black women with endometriosis were misdiagnosed as having sexually transmitted PID. "It was so blatantly racist it just blows my mind," Ballweg says.

Teenagers, meanwhile, were, and continue to be, told they simply haven't yet learned to handle a normal period. Yet studies suggest that about 70 percent of teens who complain of dysmenorrhea are eventually diagnosed with endometriosis. "Eventually" being the key word. On average, women see seven health care professionals before getting a referral to a specialist and starting treatment. "I write this article as a plea to our profession and the health care industry to improve the early diagnosis of endometriosis," Dr. Robert Albee Jr., founder of the Center for Endometriosis Care, wrote in a piece on the psychological impact of undiagnosed endometriosis in young women. "Please believe our young women when they say they are in pain!"

Another reason for the misperception that endometriosis affects only older women is that doctors have historically been most concerned about the threat it can pose to fertility. About half of women with unexplained infertility have endometriosis, and 30 percent of women with endometriosis experience infertility, although half are eventually able to conceive. And many patients report that it was only when they were trying, without success, to get pregnant that their symptoms were finally taken seriously. A 2003 study confirmed that women who complained to doctors of infertility got an endometriosis diagnosis in half the time of those reporting menstrual pain.

Infertility is certainly a concern to many endometriosis patients. But the medical community's focus on infertility reflects a relative indifference to the debilitating pain that many patients, regardless of their ability or desire to conceive, experience. Endometriosis sufferer Lisa Sanmiguel recalls that, when she was finally diagnosed, her surgeon told her, "'The greatest loss associated with endometriosis is the loss of children.' As a young woman who had spent months in bed in my late teens and early twenties enduring excruciating pain, isolated from friends, school, or any other kind of social interaction, I defined the 'greatest loss' of endometriosis as the loss of my own life."

This focus on infertility has been inscribed into the classification system that describes disease severity. When patients undergo laparoscopic surgery, their disease is ranked into one of four stages, based on the location and extent of cysts and lesions. Endometriosis on the ovaries and fallopian tubes gets more points, because it's thought to cause infertility more often. Consequently, a woman with "minimal" endometriosis may have much more pain than someone with "severe" disease, and in fact, that's often the case. The result is that, even though, unlike many chronic pain conditions, endometriosis lesions offer objective proof that something is really wrong, even postdiagnosis, women often continue to find their reports of pain dismissed. If they have only "minimal" disease but report severe pain, they're liable to be told that it's psychogenic, even though the classification system was designed to predict the impact on fertility, not pain—and, in fact, doesn't even do that very well.

Some experts now think that it's how chemically active the tissue is, rather than how much of it has spread in the body, that determines how severe the symptoms are. But for too long doctors have turned to women's psychological traits to explain away the poor correlation between the amount of endometriosis tissue and how much pain the patient is in, suggesting that endometriosis patients are just especially neurotic, anxious, and prone to overreacting to pain. Some have even listed somatization, hypochondriasis, and somatic delusions as *symptoms* of the disease, a rather nonsensical position that suggests that the disease somehow makes people have psychogenic, unexplained symptoms, not that we simply don't fully understand how endometriosis causes all the symptoms it does.

In fact, while pain is most endometriosis patients' primary symptom, for decades, there was an assumption that "gynecology should focus on the treatment of infertility, while pain should be left to psychologists," writes sociologist Emma Whelan. "As one research team put it, 'patients with chronic pain . . . can be arch-manipulators' and psychologists are better trained to deal with such personalities." It's in large part thanks to the patient advocacy efforts that began in the eighties that the agonizing pain of the disease is increasingly being recognized. "From the beginning, we said pain is the really major issue for us, more so than infertility," Ballweg says. "But even with all our work—all around the world—we weren't able to get a medical conference on pain and endometriosis until 2006."

Eventually, Ellen did "a little googling" on her own. "And I found out that pain like this isn't really normal. Most women are able to get through their periods—they're not comfortable, but they're not disabling. That's when I realized that what I was feeling wasn't really normal." She told her mom that she thought she might have endometriosis.

Ellen found a gynecologist, who agreed that it could be but said there wasn't a need to do the surgery to find out for sure. "She just figured that if I could manage the symptoms with birth control, then that would be fine. So I got on the birth control pill and noticed a huge reduction in pain, but then over time, the pain would come back, just as bad as before, and I would have to increase the dose of the birth control pill, which I didn't want, because it had a ton of side effects."

Meanwhile, she became frustrated by her doctor's advice for managing the pain: "'Do yoga. Go get acupuncture. Massage. Exercise. Take Advil.' I'm pretty sure I've already almost OD'ed on Advil. It was getting really tiring not really being listened to. When I was talking about the pain, I was describing it as intensely as I could; it is a really serious pain. I wasn't trying to downplay it." But she gets the sense that other people, her doctor included, underestimate just how bad it is. Ellen's pain hasn't gone away, though getting her period only every three months now has helped her endure it. She's in the process of trying to find a new doctor.

"ENIGMAS WRAPPED IN RIDDLES"

Back in the early eighties, when the NIH set aside a small chunk of funding for research on endometriosis, not a single researcher applied for the funds. "Most doctors assumed women's excruciating pelvic pain was all in their heads," Laurence and Weinhouse explained. "Why should physicians have devoted precious research time to studying a condition that didn't even exist?" Today, there's more interest, but the funds remain scarce. In 2016, endometriosis received just $10 million in NIH funding. That means that for each patient with endometriosis, the NIH spent about $1.50. "Endo is sorely underfunded," says Heather Guidone, surgical program director at the Center for Endometriosis Care. The lack of attention to endometriosis in the research community and in medical education has left the field, as one researcher put it in 2004, in a state of "etiological confusion and therapeutic anarchy."

Despite prevalence rates that make it one of the most common conditions gynecologists are likely to encounter, medical education about the disease remains inadequate. "Physicians are not given the correct information that they need to have," Guidone says. A recent survey of general practitioners found that nearly two-thirds said they weren't comfortable diagnosing endometriosis. The fact that it's a surgically diagnosed disease means that even the average gynecologist doesn't get much training in it. And many doctors, Ballweg adds, "don't even want to deal with endometriosis, because it's really hard to get a happy patient, and they don't know what to do."

Many of the treatments available simply mask the symptoms of the disease by suppressing menstruation. In addition to pain meds, many general gynecologists, like Ellen's doctor, will offer hormonal birth control as a first option. But while it can help minimize symptoms in some patients, it's just a stopgap measure, "a way to buy time," says Guidone. Other hormonal treatments essentially throw the body into menopause, with a host of significant side effects. Incredibly, some doctors still recommend pregnancy as a treatment, even to young patients. A commenter on one endometriosis Facebook group reported, "My doctor told me having a baby would help my pain. I'm only eleven." Others are told that a hysterectomy is the only cure, even though it's not, and some patients who undergo the procedure find that their symptoms continue. Too many patients continue to encounter doctors who are, as Guidone puts it, "just patting them on the back and saying, 'Try this pill and now we'll getcha pregnant and now we'll give you a hysterectomy.'"

Endometriosis experts say women should be referred to a specialist right away in order to get an official diagnosis and surgical treatment instead of relying on these wait-and-see Band-Aids. It is now possible to excise endometriosis tissue with minimally invasive laparoscopic surgery, a vast improvement from a few decades ago when many patients would repeatedly have their whole abdomen sliced open. But these complex surgeries require specialized skills that most general gynecologists don't have.

By the time patients get to a specialist surgeon, many of them have already had multiple failed surgeries, as many as fifteen or more. "So not only do they still have the disease, but now they also have all this surgical destruction and scar tissue," Guidone says. Even if they get to a specialist surgeon, they're not home free; since endometriosis is a systemic disease with many hormonal and immune irregularities, the symptoms frequently return. Patients often end up in "this endless loop of surgery, drugs, medication, surgery, drugs, medication," Guidone says.

Effective treatment remains elusive largely because medicine still has little understanding of how endometriosis works. Over and over again in the medical literature, the disease is referred to as a mystery. As one expert put it, "Endometriosis may be described as enigmas wrapped in riddles." And it's true: the most basic questions about the disease remain unanswered; there's no consensus on the underlying cause nor even exactly how it produces its symptoms. It's not even clear what endometriosis tissue is or where it comes from.

While Sampson's theory of retrograde menstruation has remained the top contender for nearly a century, some experts these days say it's long past time to start thinking way outside the box. A major problem with the theory is that most women (about 85 percent) seem to have retrograde menstruation, but not all of them have endometriosis. To explain this fact, one popular theory suggests that in most women, the immune system mops up these stray endometrial cells before they implant and start to cause problems, while those with endometriosis have an immune dysfunction that allows them to proliferate. There's no doubt that endometriosis patients have immune abnormalities—"just about every immune cell that's been looked at in women with endometriosis is messed up in some way," Ballweg says—but it's not clear whether this is the cause or an effect of the disease.

Others question whether Sampson's theory is salvageable at all and say the field clings to it, despite fatal flaws, simply out of inertia. They point out that endometriosis has been found in prepubescent girls, in fetuses that died in utero, and even, rarely, in cis men. It's not clear how to square these realities with the idea that endometriosis comes from retrograde menstruation. And the cells that make up endometriosis are similar but not actually genetically and chemically identical to those that line the uterus. One theory suggests that hormonal and inflammatory factors trigger normal cells found outside the uterus to transform into endometrial-like cells; another version posits that this transformation happens because of a misstep during embryonic development. Meanwhile, research has linked the disease to environmental toxins, like dioxin; genetic studies suggest that up to half of the risk may be inherited; and some experts have suggested that perhaps endometriosis is not actually one disease but many, with different underlying causes for different subtypes.

An enigma, for sure. But as others have pointed out, this persistent tendency to highlight how mysterious the disease is has a way of sidestepping the obvious question: Why is it that a debilitating disease that is extremely common, that was first named nearly a century ago, and whose symptoms appear in the medical record even further back remains so unbelievably poorly understood? "The conclusion that endometriosis is an 'enigma,' 'conundrum,' 'unknown,' 'perplexing,' 'mystery,' and 'puzzling,' tends to obscure the reality that there's a reason that's so," feminist cultural critic Ella Shohat points out. Echoing a long history of Western scientific thought portraying women and their bodies as vexingly baffling puzzles, medicine acts as though the disease itself is inherently unexplainable—"beyond the powers of mere mortals to solve," as sociologist Cara E. Jones puts it. In truth, there just hasn't been much effort put into explaining it. For hundreds of years, pain in menstruating women has not qualified as a medical mystery worthy of actually *solving*.

VULVODYNIA

"It was the most painful thing. Still, to this day, one of the most painful experiences I can remember," Nicole recalls. At age eighteen, she was getting her first checkup with a gynecologist, and her first pelvic exam. Though she'd never had one, she was pretty sure that this rite of passage, though not known for being exactly pleasant, did not usually cause such burning pain that it brought women to tears. "It hurt bad enough that I was crying as an eighteen-year-old. I didn't think it was supposed to be *that* painful."

No one else seemed to think anything was amiss, though. During the exam, which "felt like an hour" but likely took only a few minutes, Nicole remembers that the nurse reassured her that she would be fine in "the same way a doctor would talk to a kid who's getting a shot." The female gynecologist told her, "Well, you're a virgin, so it's supposed to hurt." At no point, Nicole says, did anyone remotely suggest that the pain she felt was "not a normal way a vagina is supposed to react to a pelvic exam" or suggest that it indicated a health problem that should be checked out.

"I remember leaving the doctor's office crying and ashamed, not just because of the pain, but because of how dismissed I felt. I drove around the neighborhood for a while afterwards just so I could stop crying before I went home," Nicole says. While she knew that her pain wasn't right, and was "stunned" that the doctor had acted as if it were normal, she "didn't know what to do after that." She recalled her unsuccessful attempts at using tampons. "I just was so embarrassed and ashamed, and I was like, 'this is probably why I can't wear tampons—because my vagina is completely fucked up.'" It would be another two years before she got a name for the problem and another seven years before she started to solve it.

———

In calling for the medical system to treat endometriosis with the seriousness it deserves, advocates have often argued its symptoms would be cause for much greater concern if they affected men. Even accepting that menstrual pain has become widely normalized, it's hard to imagine its other symptoms being brushed off so easily in men. As endometriosis advocate Nancy Petersen has said, "if a man had a disease that causes him to be unable to father a child, to have unbearable pain during sex and unbearable pain during bowel movements, [which was] treated by feminizing hormones and surgery, endometriosis would be declared a national emergency in this country."

Pain during sex—dyspareunia, in the medical lingo—especially is highlighted as one symptom that certainly wouldn't be so overlooked in men. The Endometriosis Association created a series of cartoons entitled *Joe with Endo* to illustrate the double standard. In one a woman gynecologist tells the male patient, "Well, Joe, I told you last time . . . this problem is really a mental thing. All men have some tension with sex once in a while . . . you'll adjust." And when Joe argues that he has never had this problem before, suggesting that it may actually be a physical problem rather than a psychological one, she replies, "Look, Joe, let's be honest. We both know you're the high-strung type. Let's try some Valium and see if it helps, o.k.?"

A number of chronic pain conditions common in women can cause pain during intercourse. More than half of patients with endometriosis experience painful penetrative sex, as do almost half of those with IBS. Up to 90 percent of IC patients say their pain has kept them from being sexually intimate. And too many women find their pain during sex is dismissed as normal or, if acknowledged as abnormal, attributed to their own psychological hang-ups. This tendency has especially hindered our understanding of the condition Nicole would eventually be diagnosed with: vulvodynia.

Vulvodynia is defined as chronic pain of the vulva that lasts more than three months and does not have a clear, identifiable cause. The pain, which is most commonly described as "burning," can be generalized (affecting the whole vulva area) or localized to a certain part (for example, vestibulodynia affects the entrance to the vagina). If it's caused only by direct touch—say, by inserting a tampon, penetrative sex, or even wearing tight pants—it's considered provoked, but it can also be unprovoked and cause pain constantly.

Like other unexplained chronic pain conditions mostly affecting women, vulvodynia was, until recently, thought to be relatively rare and more prevalent among white women. That is, until researchers did epidemiological studies, which showed that it is actually disturbingly common and massively underdiagnosed and that it doesn't discriminate by race, ethnicity, or socioeconomic background. In 2003, the first population-based prevalence estimate suggested that at any given time 7 percent of American women report symptoms of vulvodynia. White and black women were equally likely to have the condition, while Hispanic women were 80 percent more likely to have it. Nearly 40 percent of sufferers hadn't sought treatment, and of those who had, 60 percent had seen three or more doctors and usually hadn't received any diagnosis.

Subsequent studies have yielded similar estimates and laid to rest the misperception that vulvodynia is rare among women of color. According to a 2012 study, the largest to date, vulvodynia affects more than a quarter of American women at some point in their lives. It impacts women of all ages, from six to seventy, with thirty being the average age that the symptoms begin. Less than half of the respondents had sought medical help, and under 2 percent had received a diagnosis of vulvodynia. Instead, those who'd seen a doctor had most often been told they had estrogen deficiency or a yeast infection, conditions that should have improved with treatment but obviously hadn't: they reported experiencing symptoms for twelve years on average.

MARITAL PROBLEMS AND FRIGID WOMEN

Though the term *vulvodynia* was coined only in the 1980s, reports of a similar condition appear in ancient texts like the Egyptian papyri and the first-century writings of Soranus of Ephesus. And descriptions of chronic pain or hyperaesthesia (extreme sensitivity) of the vulva can be found in the medical literature in the nineteenth and early twentieth centuries. In 1874, T. Gaillard Thomas wrote in his *Practical Treatise on the Diseases of Women* that unexplained vulvar pain, "although fortunately not very frequent, is by no means very rare" and noted that it was "a matter of surprise that it has not been more generally and fully described." (I, for one, am somewhat less surprised that women's genital pain wasn't a top priority for male doctors in the Victorian era.)

After that, with the exception of one mention in the 1920s, vulvar pain mostly disappeared from the medical view for many decades. That's because, from the fifties to the eighties, it was considered more of a marital problem than a medical one. Early sex researchers like Alfred Kinsey and William H. Masters and Virginia E. Johnson framed vaginal intercourse as an important part of a healthy, happy heterosexual marriage, and medicine defined vulvar pain as a problem only insofar as it interfered with penetrative sex. Thus, as sociologist Amy Kaler has shown in her analysis of how the medical literature on vulvar pain changed over the course of the twentieth century, vulvar pain was subsumed during this time by two sexual disorders: dyspareunia (pain associated with penetrative intercourse) and vaginismus (involuntary spasms of the pelvic muscles that interfere with intercourse).

Doctors focused on helping to fix couples' relationship problems, which were thought to be somatized as the woman's pain. "The dyspareunic patient must be helped to see for herself that the hyperesthesia is a fiction and that the pain is of her own making," one physician advised in 1954. Treatments ranged from hypnosis—repeat after me: "Sexual intercourse is a wonderful act that results in a great deal of satisfaction"—to couples therapy to numbing ointments and, Kaler points out, their success was "generally measured in terms of whether they enabled intercourse to take place, rather than whether they alleviated pain per se."

During the seventies, as the feminist movement brought increased recognition of women's sexual agency independent from their husbands, the root of the problem gradually shifted from the straight couple to the woman alone. No longer were the only mentions of vulvar pain found in medical articles with titles like "Wives Who Refuse Their Husbands." By the eighties, vulvodynia had emerged as a label in and of itself, with dyspareunia considered a symptom of the condition. In some ways, this was a sign of progress; women's chronic genital pain wasn't considered a medical problem only when it interfered with *men's* sex lives anymore. On the other hand, while the condition had previously been seen as "a two party problem," as one researcher put it, in which "the inept and angry husband and his frightened, tense wife produce a sexual disaster," now the blame was squarely on the woman alone. Since liberated women were now supposed to enjoy sex, when one couldn't due to excruciating pain with no organic cause, it was assumed to be an expression of her individual psychiatric problems.

Of course, unexplained pain in *any* part of the body was likely to be labeled psychogenic during this era. But for fairly obvious reasons, psychoanalytic explanations have been especially popular when it comes to vulvodynia. Inexplicable pain in a woman's genital area that often interfered with sex? The symbolism proved too tempting to resist, and pseudo-Freudian theories ran rampant. According to one influential 1978 article, "Psychosomatic vulvovaginitis is a real clinical entity that should be suspected in any patient whose vaginal complaints do not correlate with the physical findings." The patients, the researchers wrote, manifest "signs of neurosis, dependent personality, guilt feelings, emotional lability, while denying psychologic difficulties" and "receive secondary gain from their symptom complex, i.e., a reason not to engage in sexual activity." Another article claimed that "vaginismus is a conversion disorder which is a neurotic symptom symbolically representing a distorted unconscious wish. It is the active, involuntary somatic expression of the wish to prevent intercourse, plus in some cases the additional wish to capture or break off the penis."

There's no doubt that this persistent sexualizing and psychologizing of vulvar pain has hurt sufferers. In interviews Kaler conducted in the mid-aughts with over a hundred women with vulvodynia, when asked if they'd received unhelpful medical advice or treatment, over a third said being told that their problems were "psychological" or "all in their heads" was the single most unhelpful piece of advice they had received. "They reported being told that they were frigid, sexually dysfunctional, repressed, or otherwise sexually abnormal because they experienced pain; in other words, in these women's encounters with medical practitioners, their accounts of pain were generalized into diagnoses that their entire sexual being was somehow sick," Kaler writes. A third of the respondents said that after receiving a name for their condition, their dominant feeling was "relief that [they weren't] crazy."

One woman's doctor gave her some photocopied pamphlets geared toward preteens about anxieties a young woman might have before having sex for the first time. "She implied that I must not have been ready for sex, have since been traumatized by it, and am therefore projecting pain onto myself. Here I am, an adult, being treated like a little girl who's 'not ready.'" Another woman, who sought medical advice after a month and a half of sobbing in the bathroom after sex because it was so painful, recalled what the first doctor she saw told her: "He said, 'We have a name for it. It's frigid. Go home and take care of your man.' I'll never forget the quote."

———

Shortly after her traumatic pelvic exam, Nicole went off to college and quickly began dating someone. "In between getting that first exam at the gynecologist's and trying to have sex for the first time, I had looked at stuff on the Internet and kind of self-diagnosed myself." Her problem sounded like vaginismus or vestibulitis, which is now known as vestibulodynia. She warned the guy she was starting to see that having penetrative sex might be difficult and they'd need to take it slow. By easing into it, she was able to have intercourse at nineteen, "but it still really, really hurt." And then one particularly painful time left her unable to do it at all. "I really wanted to, and I tried, but I just couldn't."

Now in a long-term relationship, Nicole was determined to solve the problem. She found a new gynecologist and described her condition. "She was just like, 'Relax more, or do more foreplay, or use lube,' and I'm like, 'I'm doing all of these things.'" Just as she'd felt after seeing the first gynecologist, Nicole felt certain that the doctor was wrong. She remembers thinking, "'This should not be impossible. The fact that it's impossible to have sex is not normal. It's not just because I didn't use lube.' And I knew that, but I didn't know what to do."

Except go to yet another doctor. This physician diagnosed her with vaginismus and vestibulitis and gave her various treatments to try, including tricyclic antidepressants, anticonvulsant meds (both often used for chronic pain), and topical creams. But nothing really worked. "It felt like I was hopeless."

A CHRONIC PAIN DISORDER

The notion of vulvodynia as a psychological sexual disorder began to fade in the late eighties. In 1986, the president of the International Society for the Study of Vulvovaginal Disease warned that a psychological cause of vulvodynia shouldn't simply be assumed by default, since "in this imperfect world it is never possible to be absolutely certain that all organic causes of disease have been ruled out." While the condition "was long thought to be an unusual psychosomatic gynecologic problem," one article noted in 1989, "initial physician insistence on a major role for psychological factors has gradually given way to sophisticated searches for evidence" of other possible organic causes. Still, in the early nineties there was a flurry of studies attempting—and failing—to show a causal link between psychiatric problems and vulvodynia.

As with so many diseases, it was really only after vulvodynia patients organized that the old psychogenic model started to crumble. In 1994, five patients formed the National Vulvodynia Association (NVA), and one of the first items on their agenda was to get the NIH to begin funding research on the condition. "The only reason NIH started looking at vulvodynia is that we went over there in 1996 and said we need a conference," says NVA founder and former executive director Phyllis Mate. At that first symposium, sponsored by the NIH in 1997, experts started to call for a reconceptualization of vulvodynia as a chronic pain condition, rather than a sexual disorder. By the next NIH workshop on the condition, in 2003, most of the papers presented focused on the biological mechanisms of the pain.

In the mid-aughts, this trend was reflected in calls for a wholesale restructuring of the classification of pain during sexual intercourse in the *DSM*. Many vulvodynia experts argued that it didn't make sense to list dyspareunia and vaginismus as "sexual pain disorders" and include them in the section on female sexual dysfunction. As a group of Canadian researchers wrote, "Although interference with vaginal penetration and sexual intercourse is often the problem that brings vulvodynia sufferers to clinical attention, it is the pain that typically causes the sexual problem rather than the reverse." They made an analogy to low back pain, which is also often "unexplained," to illustrate the problem with viewing vulvodynia as a sexual disorder: "Although the inability to function at work is what brings many low back pain sufferers to clinical attention, it is not appropriate to conceptualize this problem as a work disorder."

Of course, this final shift in medical opinion just represents an alignment with what vulvodynia patients have long insisted: that they were not anxious, depressed, or fearful of sex before the pain began and that they very much *wanted* to have intercourse, or would, if it didn't feel like getting stabbed in the vagina. Of course, the beauty of psychogenic theories was that it didn't really matter what the patient claimed; she could genuinely want to have sex, but her "unconscious mind" may be more interested in breaking off penises. Some researchers even argued that vulvodynia patients consciously hid their psychological problems. One 1992 study gave patients a series of quantitative tests of psychological distress, depression, and anxiety. Faced with the (unexpected and unwanted) result that the patients scored in the normal range, the researchers decided to do follow-up interviews with some of them and concluded, simply based on their impressions from talking to them, that they actually *were* psychologically disturbed and had just deliberately downplayed it on the tests because they didn't want a psychosomatic label.

Indeed, as we've seen with other "unexplained" disorders, proponents of the psychogenic explanations of vulvodynia tended to simply incorporate patients' adamant rejection of their theory into the psychopathological profile of the disorder. The medical literature frequently described women with vulvodynia as noncompliant, aggressive, and difficult to deal with. According to the authors of that article on "psychosomatic vulvovaginitis," the typical patient "often pleads for help but is absolutely resistant to any suggestion that her symptoms might be psychologic in origin." The stereotypes were so prevalent that in a 1994 article, one researcher warned her colleagues to keep in mind that "a clinical impression that many women with VVS [vulvar vestibulitis syndrome, a subtype of vulvodynia] show certain personality traits including being particularly conscientious, intense and assertive has not been conclusively borne out by any formal study to date."

The transformation in the medical thinking about vulvodynia has mirrored the evolution that other unexplained chronic pain conditions have undergone since the eighties. But in comparison to other disorders, it's taken even longer. The fact that the pain affects women's genitals and impacts their sex lives proved a potent barrier to seeing it as anything other than a psychosexual disorder, even as knowledge about the neurobiology of chronic pain grew. Indeed, as late as 2007 dissenters tried to resurrect old-school psychoanalytic theories of the condition. Claiming that "the vulva has naturally evolved as a sexual communication organ," one group of researchers argued that "vulvodynia may represent the best way that a woman found to hide the conflict she does not want to face. A basic concept in psychosomatic medicine reveals that when it is not possible to show a conflict or a distress condition by psychologic symptoms, it is possible to use the body as a stage. Thus, the vulva can be the theater on which some issues are played out."

———

"No one directly said to me, 'Oh, it's all in your head,'" Nicole says. "But being told, 'You just need to relax more' made me feel like this is my burden, or this is something that I'm bringing on myself." She remembers thinking, "I feel like I *am* relaxed—I want to have sex, I want it to feel good, I'm doing everything I can." And when doctors' advice to "use more lube" or "just relax more" didn't alleviate the pain, she'd end up feeling even worse. "It caused this cycle of me feeling bad that I couldn't fix myself. And then just never getting better."

Of course, while vulvodynia is not caused by relationship problems or psychological distress, it can certainly *lead* to both. Biologically, chronic pain affecting the vulva may be no different than pain in another part of the body, but emotionally, it can be especially difficult to cope with. Some vulvodynia patients struggle with partners who don't believe their pain is real or who become frustrated about being unable to have penetrative sex. Nicole's college boyfriend, thankfully, was always 100 percent supportive. "He never ever said anything that made me feel bad about it. Not once." But she felt trapped in the relationship, dreading the prospect of having to tell a new partner about her problem. "Had I been able to have sex 'normally,' I probably wouldn't have stayed in it."

More generally, the stress of not being able to have penetrative sex took a toll on her psyche. "We're made to think that penis-in-vagina sex is what sex is, and that that's the ultimate representation of a relationship, or that sex is this great normal thing, which it is, but what comes along with that is this feeling that if you're not having sex, then there's something wrong with you," Nicole says. In addition to the pain, she was weighed down by a sense that she was abnormal—and that she couldn't discuss it with anyone. "It just felt really shameful. If I had a broken arm, or some other part of my body was malfunctioning, it would not be as big of a deal, but for some reason having sexual problems was really, really embarrassing. And I think part of it was I was made to feel like if you're not having full penetrative sex, then you're not in a normal relationship or you're not normal."

"'JUST USE MORE LUBE' IS NOT SUFFICIENT MEDICAL ADVICE"

Nicole's experience of seeing two doctors before she found one who seemed to know anything at all about her condition represents significant improvement since the early nineties, when Mate developed vulvodynia. Back then, Mate estimates, there were maybe two hundred health care providers in the United States who were familiar with vulvodynia; today there are tens of thousands. Patient advocacy has played a key role in raising awareness within the medical community. "The doctors don't get two minutes on vulvodynia in medical school, and most of them don't learn about it in their internship or their residency, so if they don't self-educate, they haven't got a clue," Mate says. "The NVA decided that to crack this nut, we had to go ahead and educate the doctors ourselves." In 2007, they used a large donation to develop an online Medscape tutorial for which health care providers can get continuing medical education (CME) credits. Somewhat to Medscape's surprise, there were lots of takers. They quickly had 22,000 learners signed up, and it is currently the third most popular CME program on Medscape. "That has educated more gynecologists than anything else," Mate says.

Thanks to the increased awareness, Mate estimates that more than half of vulvodynia patients don't have to see more than two doctors before they're diagnosed these days, while prior to 1996, five to seven doctors would have been the rule. "And more doctors believe it to be a legitimate disorder. On the other hand, there are still women who go to doctors who say, 'Drink a glass of wine before sex.' And in rural states, you're lucky to find someone who can treat this," she says. A 2013 survey of eighty-five patients eventually diagnosed with provoked vestibulodynia confirmed that women who began experiencing symptoms after 2005 were diagnosed in less time than those who began experiencing symptoms before. Still, 35 percent of them reported that it took over fifteen doctor's appointments to get a correct diagnosis, and 37 percent said it took over thirty-six months. And of course, studies like that capture only the experiences of those women who do ultimately get diagnosed, not those who gave up after one dismissal or who couldn't afford to get a second opinion or who never sought help to begin with.

And, as Nicole found, a diagnosis, while it usually comes as a relief, doesn't automatically bring treatment that works. Like other unexplained conditions, vulvodynia likely describes a number of conditions with different underlying pathologies united only by the fact that they cause chronic pain in the vulva and have yet to be understood by medicine. "They've figured out that there is no one single cause of vulvodynia," Mate says. Experts suspect a variety of causes, from an overgrowth of nerve fibers to pelvic floor muscle dysfunction to hormonal abnormalities to an uptick in inflammatory substances to a hypersensitivity to vaginal microorganisms. Unsurprisingly, then, a therapy that works for one patient may not be helpful at all for another, and treatment remains largely a matter of trial and error. There have been very few randomized controlled clinical studies on treatments for the condition. One of the only ones that has been done, funded by the NIH in 2010, found that a tricyclic antidepressant, which has long been used to treat chronic pain and has been the first-line option for vulvodynia for over thirty years, was no better than a placebo.

In general, research on the condition is woefully inadequate. In 2000, the NIH began funding studies on the condition for the first time, promising $5 million over the next five years. In the last few years, they've devoted $2 million annually to the condition, but that amounts to only a minuscule thirty-three cents for every patient thought to be affected—making it underfunded even in comparison to other chronic pain conditions. Over the past two decades, only about thirty-six research articles on vulvodynia have been published each year, and most studies have been done by just a couple dozen dedicated researchers. According to the *NIH Research Plan on Vulvodynia*, published in 2012, "many more investigators will be needed to establish a body of research sufficient to address diagnosis, etiology, prevention, and treatment of vulvodynia."

It wasn't until Nicole found her way to a specialty vulvar pain clinic during graduate school, after five years of being unable to have penetrative sex, that she found a combination of therapies that led to some improvement in her condition. Today the twenty-nine-year-old neuroscientist still has pain, but it's not as severe as it used to be, and she feels better equipped to manage it.

She remains frustrated that there's so little research on the condition. "I feel like if this was something that affected guys, it would be a major priority of the National Institutes of Health to figure out what's the problem." And she's angry that she suffered, physically and emotionally, for so long simply because there's not even basic awareness among doctors. "It was seven years between when I went to the first gynecologist and when I could have a really normal sex life. In between then, I had seen probably five-plus different physicians, and I felt so many times that the ball was just dropped in trying to help me get better," she says. "If that gynecologist when I was eighteen had acted differently, then I could have saved myself seven years of just terrible feelings and traumatic experiences. If that one doctor had done something different, it would have really changed a lot of negative things about my life."

The experience, she says, has made her far more skeptical of medicine, more painfully aware of its limits, than many of her peers. "I am a neuroscientist; I work with physicians in research. But I still have very little trust in the medical community. I've learned to not just trust whatever doctors say. Because they're not always right. 'Just use more lube' is not sufficient medical advice."

IF YOU JUST LOST WEIGHT . . .

When she was seventeen, Rebecca came down with walking pneumonia and bronchitis. Most of the symptoms improved with treatment, but the cough lingered for months. A year later, she still couldn't breathe properly; it was like her pneumonia "just never really went away." Doctors eventually told her that she had bronchospasms—constrictions of the walls of her airway—due to asthma brought on by being overweight. She was told that if she lost some weight, the bronchospasms would likely go away.

At first, Rebecca accepted this explanation. For two years of college, she was dancing a couple of times a week and trudging up the massive hill—nicknamed Cardiac Hill—on campus daily. "I was very active, and I wasn't losing weight and my breathing was just getting worse. Any time I went to see the doctor to figure out why I couldn't shake this cold, or that cold, I was given an antibiotic and told to lose weight." Upon moving home, she remained as active as she could. "I was going to the gym. I was walking quite a lot. I was working three jobs"—that all kept her on her feet—"and going to school full-time."

The first time Rebecca started to think "Maybe it's not just weight" was when she coughed up blood when she was twenty. The doctors at the ER told her it was probably just a broken blood vessel and sent her home with an inhaler. "They said, 'If you lost weight, you wouldn't have this many coughing fits.'" But she didn't know anyone else with asthma who coughed *that* hard. "I felt like I was stuck in a nightmare, and that the cough would never go away." Meanwhile, "it was getting harder to exercise when I was getting out of breath doing things that I had done for much of my life. I was hardly able to climb a flight of stairs without getting winded. I was tired all the time."

By age twenty-three, Rebecca began to have trouble controlling her bladder during coughing spasms and finally had to rely on adult diapers. The fits sometimes made her throw up. She spent many nights curled around a bucket in a hot shower, coughing and vomiting, hoping the steam would make it easier to breathe. She'd been walking a couple of miles to and from work, but eventually she had to stop because it now left her too exhausted. She was taking so many medications that they couldn't fit in a gallon-sized ziplock bag: cough syrups, antacids, steroids. "Nothing was working." Rebecca began to wonder whether she was a hypochondriac; desperate for help of any kind, she researched inpatient mental health facilities. "I thought I was losing it."

But when blood tests kept coming back normal, her doctors would say, "We don't know what to tell you—it's clearly just weight related."

————————

Women aren't the only group of patients who frequently find their symptoms dismissed as "normal" by health care providers. The tendency to normalize symptoms associated with women's reproductive functions finds echoes in the way elderly patients, trans patients, and overweight patients are often treated. In all these cases, doctors too often can't see past some aspect of the patient's identity that's considered somehow inherently abnormal—the patient's symptoms are at risk of being dismissed as the "normal" result of their "abnormal" age, gender identity, or body type.

It's fairly ironic that elderly patients also find their symptoms brushed off as normal, given that the risks of many serious diseases increase with age. But experts warn that treatable conditions, from Alzheimer's to depression, are frequently overlooked in older patients, dismissed as just part of the normal aging process. Doctors—and even patients themselves—often view chronic pain conditions as an inevitable result of old age. As one older patient with severe OA reported being told, "What do you expect? You're just getting older."

A similar dynamic happens with trans patients. Many trans patients face enormous barriers to accessing the unique transition-related medical care they need. Some insurers deny coverage for gender-affirming surgeries and hormone therapy. A 2011 study found that, on average, American medical students get just five hours of education on LGBT-related topics during medical school. And while most schools reported teaching doctors-to-be to ask patients if they have sex with men, women, or both when inquiring about their sexual history, only about a third included information on gender transitioning. Consequently, finding doctors who are knowledgeable about transition-related care is a challenge.

But trans people, like all people, also have general health care needs. And the biases and ignorance of medical professionals can often prevent them from seeing a doctor when they need to. In a 2011 survey, a quarter of trans people in the United States said they'd delayed seeking medical care because they feared they'd face discrimination, and 19 percent had been refused medical care altogether. When they do seek care, trans patients often find all their symptoms attributed to their trans status—whether blamed on hormone therapy or simply on the fact of being trans. This phenomenon is so common that a 2015 article on the British LGBT site *PinkNews* coined the term "trans broken arm syndrome" to describe it: "Healthcare providers assume that all medical issues are a result of a person being trans. Everything—from mental health problems to, yes, broken arms."

Just as the trust gap leaves women with conditions stereotyped as "men's diseases"—from heart disease to cluster headaches—at a particular disadvantage in trying to get doctors to see past their knowledge-mediated bias, women may have an especially hard time overcoming this tendency to normalize their symptoms. When you're stereotyped as an overly emotional hypochondriac, it is all the more difficult to convince doctors that something is not right for your body when some aspect of your identity tempts them to view your symptoms as normal.

When it comes to the dismissal of fat patients' symptoms, the combined effects of sexism and weight bias are especially clear. All overweight patients, regardless of gender, face enormous bias in the medical system. Rebecca Puhl, an expert in weight stigma and deputy director of the University of Connecticut's Rudd Center for Food Policy and Obesity, has pointed out that doctors quite openly admit to their bias against fat patients. "If I was trying to study gender or racial bias, I couldn't use the assessment tools I'm using, because people wouldn't be truthful," she said. "They'd want to be more politically correct."

But women bear the brunt of this bias. According to patient surveys, women are more likely than men to have been advised to lose weight by a health care provider. Studies of physician behavior confirm that. A 2001 study found that doctors were more likely to encourage a woman with a body mass index (BMI) of 25—a hair outside the "normal" range—to lose weight. When the patient was a man, they were more likely to discourage dieting and encourage the patient to accept their appearance. In one 2014 study, 53 percent of women reported being shamed by a physician, compared to 38 percent of the men, and their weight and their sexual activity were the top two reasons for such experiences.

"Smaller amounts of 'overweight' are taken much more seriously in women than in men," says journalist Harriet Brown, author of *Body of Truth: How Science, History, and Culture Drive Our Obsession with Weight—and What We Can Do About It*. Given the more narrow beauty standards imposed on women, that is perhaps not surprising. Indeed, women are more likely than men to be discriminated against due to their weight in a variety of realms. According to a 2008 study from the Rudd Center, men are not at serious risk for discrimination until they reach a BMI of 35—or sixty-eight pounds "overweight"—while women experienced a notable increase in discrimination at a BMI of 27—an "excess" of just thirteen pounds. The disproportionate concern over women's weight is, however, particularly unjustified; if doctors were actually basing their concern about weight on science, not sexist biases, the opposite would be true.

Studies consistently confirm that women are more likely than men to be fatter and healthy. To be clear, judging *anyone's* health based on weight is unwise. According to a 2016 analysis, relying on BMI as a crude measure of metabolic health leads to the mislabeling of 74.9 million adults in the United States. But it is women especially that are mislabeled. A 2008 study found that 57 percent of overweight women, compared to 48.8 percent of overweight men, were metabolically healthy, as were 35.4 percent of obese women, versus 29.2 percent of obese men.

Being constantly lectured about their weight only makes women reluctant to see a doctor for preventive care—and even sometimes for acute problems. According to a 2016 nationally representative survey of over a thousand women, over a third had been advised by a doctor to lose weight, and 45 percent said they'd somewhat commonly canceled or postponed a doctor's appointment because they wanted to drop a few pounds first. Studies have found that overweight women are less likely to get pelvic exams, breast exams, and mammograms than average-weight women. In a 2002 study, even many women who fell into the "normal" BMI range reported delaying health care if they perceived themselves to be overweight.

When they do seek medical treatment, fat patients regularly find, like Rebecca did, that many doctors are quick to attribute all their symptoms to their weight. A recent *New York Times* article highlighted the stories of a few patients whose symptoms were immediately brushed off as weight related. One woman complained of hip pain to an orthopedist, who, without even examining her, immediately diagnosed it as "obesity pain." She actually had progressive scoliosis, which is unrelated to weight. Another woman, who'd suddenly began experiencing shortness of breath after walking just a few steps, was told by an urgent care doctor that she just had too much weight pressing on her lungs. "Have you ever considered going on a diet?" he asked. It turned out she had several potentially life-threatening blood clots in her lungs.

While this bias certainly affects overweight men too, it seems to be worse for women, whose reports of their symptoms are so often distrusted. "Anecdotally, many, many, many more women than men talk to me about experiencing that at the doctor's," Brown says. "When it comes to stories like, 'I went to the doctor's for a wrenched knee and was told to lose weight,' the vast majority of those come from women."

───────────

Finally, Rebecca went to a new primary care physician, the first doctor yet to suggest that she see a pulmonologist to do some tests of how her lungs were functioning. "That was the first time in a while that any physician had taken my concerns seriously and hadn't just dismissed them on my weight. She listened. She listened when I said, 'Look, I've been working out.' And she listened to my daily activities and the food I was eating. And she said, 'Okay, if you're still having these symptoms and doing all these things, we need to talk to a different person.'"

Before Rebecca made the appointment with a pulmonologist, another coughing fit that produced blood landed her in the ER. This time, the doctors did a more powerful CT scan, rather than an X-ray, and, noticing an abnormality, also told her to follow up with a pulmonologist. When she did, he found a tumor in her bronchial tube. Less than two weeks later, she had surgery to remove her left lung, the bottom half of which was a black, rotting piece of dead tissue.

Rebecca's surgeon told her that a diagnosis five years prior could've saved her lung. "I remembered the five years I spent looking for some kind of reason why I was always coughing, always sick. I remembered being consistently told that the reason I was sick was because I was fat."

"THIS IS NOT NORMAL"

When Natalie was eleven years old, she developed sudden, severe abdominal pain and nausea. Her mom, a physician, quickly took her to the emergency room. After being given a full exam, the doctor concluded her pain was most likely due to menstrual cramps. Just barely into puberty, Natalie hadn't gotten her period yet. Though her mom disagreed with the diagnosis, she also recognized her bias as a mother, so she tried to trust the ER doctors. Natalie returned home mortified. "I was sure I was the first kid in history that had gone to the emergency room for cramps."

That night, the pain kept Natalie awake. "Embarrassed, I tried to hide my discomfort from my parents. The next morning, a full twenty-four hours after my pain began, it was so excruciating that I couldn't move. My dad had to carry me back into the ER, and my mom had to use her doctor voice to demand that I be given an ultrasound." It showed severe appendicitis, and she was rushed to the operating room. "After the procedure, the surgeon told me it was the largest unruptured appendix he'd ever removed. I think it's safe to say that had I been a little boy and not a little girl, I would not have gone those twenty-four hours without proper treatment."

————

The normalization of symptoms associated with women's reproductive cycles and states hasn't just hurt women with endometriosis, vulvodynia, and other conditions that cause chronic pelvic pain. If any pain "down there," no matter how severe, can be blamed on cramps, if any pain during sex is something to be alleviated with a glass of wine, it opens up fertile ground for missed diagnoses of a whole range of conditions. After all, the reproductive tract is pretty close to other vital organs.

Recall what the campus clinic workers asked Maggie after she'd fainted from severe abdominal pain from a perforated ulcer: Are you pregnant or on your period? "It was so striking to me, even in that moment, that those were the two questions they asked me—like, 'What are the female explanations for this pain that you're describing?'" she recalls. Or the woman with colon cancer whose worsening pain was blamed on menstrual cramps for three years. Or Alexis's hip pain: "So often it was just put off on being a 'female issue.' If a man would have had the same pain, I think a lot more tests would have been done," she suggests, "because there's not as much going on there to attribute it to."

In a recent *BuzzFeed* article, women readers shared tales of times their pain was not taken seriously by doctors. Several reported that their medical conditions had been initially misdiagnosed as "normal" menstrual cramps. One of these women was in such terrible pain she had to be carried by her husband into the ER, where doctors eventually discovered a trapped gallstone that required surgery to remove. Another had heavy and painful menstrual bleeding for forty days straight that was due to polycystic ovary syndrome. Another was passing kidney stones for four days. Another was crying and throwing up from pelvic pain and was ultimately found to have massive ruptured cysts on both ovaries. Another had been having abdominal pain, diarrhea, vomiting, and a fever for two days and ultimately spent the night in the hospital, hooked up to an IV, for an *E. coli* infection.

And menstruation is not the only "female issue" that doctors may be tempted to attribute a wide range of symptoms to throughout women's lives. When they're pregnant, women may find their symptoms blamed on pregnancy, and then, after giving birth, on the normal postpartum healing process, and then simply on motherhood itself. I heard from one woman who was chronically sick for a few years after her kids were born, suffering monthly infections and multiple bouts of pneumonia. "The doctor kept telling me I was just a new mom, and this was to be expected, and basically to get over it." After a switch to a new doctor and a thorough workup, she was diagnosed with two autoimmune diseases. "If I had listened to the first doctor who blamed all the illness on being a new mother, I'd still be sick and miserable."

Once women make it out of their childbearing years, they reach the final bar of menopause. A range of conditions are often dismissed as menopause—and not just diseases, like non-Hodgkin lymphoma or hyperthyroidism, that also cause hot flashes or those, like uterine or cervical cancer, that can mimic the irregular periods of perimenopause. Women have reported receiving a diagnosis of menopause for everything from brain tumors to hepatitis C. My aunt's doctor initially attributed her back pain and bloody urine to menopause; within six months, she'd died of kidney cancer that, by the time it was found, had spread too far to cure.

Great swaths of women's lives may no longer be considered periods of ill health, as they were a century or so ago, but great swaths of women's lives are still apparently periods during which it is considered somehow normal for women to be sick. And once it's normal for women to be sick for large chunks of their lives, it tends to bleed into a more generalized sense that women are inherently sick that seems straight out of the nineteenth century: in a 2015 article in *The Telegraph,* a twenty-four-year-old British woman recalled that when she reported having abdominal swelling and pain, her male doctor told her "some women's bodies 'don't run as tight a ship as others' so it's perfectly normal to be out of sync."

Thankfully, young women like Ellen aren't buying that. She still doesn't have a certain diagnosis for her pain. Maybe it's endometriosis; maybe it's something else. But she does have a spot-on diagnosis of what's wrong with how medicine—and the culture more broadly—approaches women's menstrual pain: "You won't label menstrual pain as abnormal but you'll label women's responses to it as abnormal." Guidone says that over the twenty-five years she has worked with endometriosis patients, she has begun to see a shift: women are less willing to accept it when doctors try to send them off with a paternalistic pat on the head and the assurance that debilitating pain is simply "a part of life." "I think it's a result of the patients becoming more empowered, more educated, more informed. Women now are saying, 'This is not normal. If you can't help me, please send me to someone who will.'"

CHAPTER 7
CONTESTED ILLNESSES: WHEN DISEASES ARE "FASHIONABLE"

IN 2011, JEN BREA was traveling with her then boyfriend in Kenya and Tanzania. Both were sick on and off during the trip, and a couple of weeks after she returned home, Brea spiked a high fever that lasted for ten days and was 104.7 degrees at its peak. When it finally broke, the relief was short lived. The next day, she woke up to find a new problem. "I was so dizzy that I couldn't really leave the house for three weeks. I would have to hug the wall to get to the bathroom and would bump into doorframes." That too eventually passed, and Brea returned to her graduate school classes. But throughout that spring and summer, her energy lagged and she kept getting infection after infection: a sore throat, then the worst sinus infection of her life. Each time she'd get profoundly dizzy again for a time and then improve.

"After that fever, I went to see a doctor for the first time, because the dizziness was very strange; I'd never had anything like that in my life. I'm not someone who runs to the doctor for any little thing, but I was going constantly because I was constantly getting sick." Almost from the start, Brea says, the doctors seemed focused on "comforting me and helping me understand that I wasn't really sick, as though it was my anxiety about being sick that was causing the problem. The emphasis was on making me feel as though nothing was wrong, because if there was nothing wrong on the lab tests, it meant nothing was wrong.

"I can't tell you how many times I went into the clinic and was told I had either an inner ear infection or dehydration because I was dizzy." She took to drinking a liter of water before appointments just to preempt the suggestion. "I'm like, 'I've been alive for twenty-eight years—I'm telling you that something is wrong that I've never experienced before; I didn't just forget to drink water.'" Another trick she started doing pretty early on, as she began to get the sense that doctors thought she was exaggerating her symptoms, was to bring her fiancé with her. "I felt like if I had a man in the room with me—and a man who vouched for me to the extent that he was planning to marry me—that somehow I would be treated better. And I was."

A biracial young woman in a Ph.D. program at Harvard, Brea found it jarring to find herself in such a position. "This was the first time in my life that I had ever been like, 'What I really need in this situation is a chaperone.' It was the first time in my life that anyone had ever doubted my account of the world. I felt suddenly like I had gone from being an expert and authority on myself to being in this really helpless position, where I felt like I couldn't be too challenging, because I was afraid people wouldn't help me."

───────

As historian of medicine Charles Rosenberg has written, "In our culture, a disease does not exist as a social phenomenon until we agree that it does." And whenever you hear a condition described as a "contested disease," the odds are good that the "contest" is between, on the one hand, mostly women patients who believe their condition to be an organic one and, on the other hand, a medical establishment that assumes their "medically un-explained symptoms" are all in their heads. Indeed, all "functional" syndromes could be described as "contested," as patients typically consider their symptoms to be physical, while medicine has largely assumed them to be psychogenic by default. We've seen how this assumption, when it comes to unexplained chronic pain conditions—from IC to vulvodynia to fibromyalgia—has been a hindrance to furthering our scientific understanding of pain and addressing the enormous suffering it causes in this country.

Debates over contested diseases have tended to become especially acrimonious when it comes to "medically unexplained" conditions that have attracted widespread media attention, which has been the case with fibromyalgia, as well as the conditions discussed in this chapter: chronic fatigue syndrome, chronic Lyme disease, and multiple chemical sensitivities. That's likely because, as we saw with fibromyalgia, those who insist that these conditions are not poorly understood emerging diseases but actually just new labels for the psychogenic symptoms of somatizing women tend to think that media coverage itself exacerbates the problem.

Indeed, these "contested" diseases have sometimes also gone by the even more revealing moniker "fashionable illnesses." According to a 1997 article by one physician, somatizing patients who "make illness a way of life" have found a "contemporary hiding place" in "fashionable" diagnoses, like fibromyalgia, chronic fatigue syndrome, and multiple chemical sensitivities. "Patients who, in the past, were identified as hysterics or invalids have, with the facilitation of mass communications, adopted current and fashionable means by which to seek solutions to their psychosocial distress. Hysteria has not gone away, it just has a new style."

As the highly gendered language of "fashionable illnesses" suggests, implicit in discussions of these contested diseases—though, as we'll see, sometimes made explicit too—is an assumption that they are unlikely to be real, organic diseases, because women constitute the majority of their sufferers.

MYALGIC ENCEPHALOMYELITIS / CHRONIC FATIGUE SYNDROME

Between 800,000 and 2.5 million Americans, over 80 percent of them women, are estimated to have the disease known as "chronic fatigue syndrome." In much of the rest of the world, it's known as myalgic encephalomyelitis, and now it often goes by both names: ME/CFS.

The condition first came on the radar in the United States in the mid-eighties. A handful of physicians across the country began taking note of patients complaining of unexplained debilitating fatigue accompanied by recurrent sore throats, tender lymph nodes, headaches, muscle pain, and cognitive dysfunction. Initially, the condition was called "chronic Epstein-Barr virus syndrome" because many patients seemed to have high levels of antibodies to the virus that causes mono. Indeed, it looked sort of like a never-ending case of mono on steroids, and it often came on after an acute flu-like illness. An especially large outbreak was reported by two doctors in the wealthy resort town of Incline Village, Nevada, near Lake Tahoe. Investigators from the CDC came to check it out but concluded that the Epstein-Barr virus wasn't the problem. In 1988, a working group convened by the CDC released criteria for diagnosing the condition and proposed it be called "chronic fatigue syndrome" (CFS) until its cause was uncovered.

But after the initial hypothesis that the disease was caused by a chronic Epstein-Barr virus infection failed to pan out, the medical community rapidly shifted to suspecting that there wasn't really any disease there at all, just the usual psychogenic symptoms of neurotic women. By 1988, studies concluding that ME/CFS patients were actually suffering from psychological problems, mostly depression and somatization disorder, were coming out to headlines like "Chronic Fatigue Is Often Mental Illness" and "Fatigue: Fact or Figment?" The next year, the same conclusion was reached by an NIH study that found that twenty-one of twenty-eight ME/CFS patients "had been or were currently affected by a psychiatric illness." The disease has faced an uphill battle for legitimacy—and funding for research—ever since.

Patients have always hated the name chronic fatigue syndrome, which appears to invite responses like, "Yeah, I'm tired all the time too!" Most people know what it feels like to be exhausted from sleep deprivation or temporarily fatigued after a hard workout. But the fatigue of ME/CFS is on a different level and doesn't improve with rest. Patients have compared it to "permanently having the flu, a hangover, and jet lag while being continually electrocuted." Or being too exhausted "to change clothes more than every seven to ten days." Or being so tired that a trip to the bathroom requires going "back to bed struggling for breath and feeling like [they] just climbed a mountain." In the most severe cases, patients can't even sit up in bed, speak, or tolerate light or sound.

It is only in the last several years that major medical institutions have begun to acknowledge that ME/CFS is a severe neurological and immune-related disease. In 2015, the IOM issued a three-hundred-page report, based on nearly 9,000 published articles, on the host of abnormalities that have been documented on the disease. It suggested that the name be changed to systemic exertion intolerance disease and proposed new diagnostic criteria for it. In addition to the prolonged, profound fatigue, patients must experience post-exertional malaise (a worsening of symptoms, or crash, after any kind of physical or mental exertion), unrefreshing sleep, and at least one of two remaining symptoms: cognitive impairments or orthostatic intolerance (symptoms that worsen upon standing).

"ME/CFS," the IOM report concluded, "is a serious, chronic, complex, multisystem disease that frequently and dramatically limits the activities of affected patients." About 50 to 75 percent of patients are unemployed because of their illness, and a quarter have been confined to their homes, or even their beds, for some time because of it. Patients with ME/CFS have been found to be equally or more functionally impaired than those with congestive heart failure, type 2 diabetes, MS, end-stage renal disease, AIDS, breast cancer, and COPD. Symptoms may improve for a time and then relapse, but few patients ever fully recover. The economic burden of ME/CFS in lost productivity and medical costs is estimated at $51 billion annually.

Less than one-third of medical schools include ME/CFS in their curriculum, and only 40 percent of medical textbooks mention the condition. Despite this, surveys show that most health care providers are very aware of the disease, but in the absence of good education, their knowledge appears to be largely based on myths. According to a 2011 study by researchers from the CDC, 85 percent of health care providers believe ME/CFS is fully or partly a psychiatric condition. "Many health care providers are skeptical about the seriousness of ME/CFS, mistake it for a mental health condition, or consider it a figment of the patient's imagination," the IOM report lamented. "Misconceptions or dismissive attitudes on the part of health care providers make the path to diagnosis long and frustrating for many patients." Patient surveys have found that for 78 percent of patients, it took over a year to receive a diagnosis, and about 29 percent reported that it took longer than five years. And those are the ones who got a diagnosis at all. The vast majority (84 to 91 percent) are not diagnosed.

"MILLION-DOLLAR WORKUPS ON NEUROTIC WOMEN"

It was clear to many of the early doctors sounding the alarm about the disease in the mideighties that the gender imbalance among the sufferers was a factor in how quickly the medical community concluded there was nothing to see here. In fact, one wonders whether the disease would have been recognized at all were it not for the minority of male sufferers. Investigative journalist Hillary Johnson's chronicle of the first decade of research on the disease, *Osler's Web: Inside the Labyrinth of the Chronic Fatigue Syndrome Epidemic,* is filled with examples of doctors who learned to showcase their male patients with the condition in order to get half a chance at changing the minds of their skeptical colleagues.

One of them was Dr. Carol Jessop, an internist who saw more than a dozen women in her women's community clinic in San Francisco with a similar constellation of severe and unexplained symptoms throughout 1984. An associate professor of internal medicine at University of California, San Francisco (UCSF), Jessop took advantage of her colleagues' expertise, sending her patients for extensive testing with specialists at the medical school. But finding nothing consistently abnormal, "they told me the patients were depressed," Jessop recalled to Johnson. Several male colleagues chided her for doing "million-dollar workups on neurotic women."

By 1985, with more than a hundred patients with the mysterious ailment under her care, Jessop was increasingly suspicious that a new pathogen may be the cause. She eventually convinced a UCSF microbiologist who was a heavyweight in HIV research to collaborate. Intrigued by Jessop's description of her patients and her hypothesis that an unknown infectious agent, perhaps a new retrovirus like HIV, was affecting their immune systems, he asked her to send over some patients to his lab and said he'd start searching their blood for viruses. But after seeing the first several patients, he started to balk. Suspecting what the problem might be, Jessop sent over one of her male patients with the condition next. "[He] saw ten women, and he thought they were all hysterical," she explained, "then he saw a man, whose complaints he took seriously."

This is not to say that men with ME/CFS haven't been dismissed and labeled as psychiatric cases or malingerers; they certainly have. Insist on being sick for long enough without explanation, and anyone will be at risk of being disbelieved. But, as with chronic pain, doctors seemed to find it far easier to ascribe ME/CFS to the mind in women. A 1996 Australian study of fifty patients eventually diagnosed with ME/CFS, for example, found that 85 percent of the women, compared to 30 percent of the men, had received psychiatric diagnoses during their search for an explanation. "Their expressed emotion or signs of distress appear to have influenced the diagnosis regardless of other symptoms," the authors wrote. "In contrast, men's accounts of their symptoms and their choices about treatment were usually given credence." In fact, trusting in the reality of the men's complaints, doctors had sometimes ignored the "objective" findings when the two didn't match; two of the men received a diagnosis of mono even though they tested negative for it. "Their doctors had chosen to dismiss the test results rather than the men's accounts."

"There was such clear evidence of extraordinary bias," says Johnson, who began reporting on the disease when she fell ill with it herself. "Most of the men I have met with this disease are treated with a great deal more seriousness than any woman I've met. They still get the brush-off a lot of the time, but at least doctors believe them when they say there's something wrong with them. If the doctor doesn't know what to do or what to think about it, he'll refer them to a neurologist or an infectious disease specialist. They get referred all over the place. Whereas a woman is given antidepressants or told to work out her sex-life problems, things like that."

Even before the condition got the CFS moniker in the United States, the predominance of women among its sufferers had been used to dismiss the idea that it was anything more than hysteria. Throughout the first half of the twentieth century, sporadic outbreaks of an illness that many suspect may have been ME/CFS had been reported in the medical literature. In 1955, a mysterious illness affecting over three hundred doctors and nurses forced London's Royal Free Hospital to close for months. At the time, investigators concluded it was caused by an unknown viral infection of the central nervous system, and "benign myalgic encephalomyelitis" was eventually suggested as the name for the condition. By the late fifties, researchers were suggesting that a dozen past outbreaks, from Florida to Australia, may have been ME.

In 1970, however, a couple psychiatrists revisited the case files from the Royal Free Hospital outbreak and argued in an influential article in *British Medical Journal* that it was actually a case of mass hysteria. The primary piece of evidence in support of their hypothesis? That there were more women than men affected. "Characteristically epidemic hysteria occurs in populations of segregated females—in girls' schools, convents, and among female factory hands," they wrote. "At the Royal Free, as at any other hospital, the female population is segregated to a very considerable degree. The attack rate among the females should, according to the hysterical hypothesis, be considerably higher than among the males. There is no dispute that this was so." While they didn't interview any of the patients who had fallen ill, some of whom remained sick, they concluded that there was "a fair case for regarding these symptoms as the subjective complaints of a frightened and hysterical population."

They suggested that many of the other epidemics of ME were also due to hysteria—or else the "altered medical perception of the community" that blew minor symptoms out of proportion—again on the basis that eight of them occurred among hospital nurses, who, as young women in close proximity, were considered inherently susceptible to mass hysteria. They proposed a new name for the condition: "myalgia nervosa."

───────

About a year after Brea's initial fever, she began having terrifying neurological symptoms. Out at a restaurant with friends, she suddenly realized she couldn't sign her name on the check. "My hand wouldn't move, and I didn't know why at first." She realized that she'd lost the ability to draw the right side of a circle. The right side of her body became numb. She struggled to find words. She finally went to the ER, concerned she might be having a stroke. After a series of consultations with neurologists, MS and epilepsy were ruled out. With a normal MRI and an EEG that showed an abnormality in her temporal lobe but one that was "nonspecific"—that is, not associated with a known disease—she was diagnosed with conversion disorder, joining the long lineage of women with ME/CFS labeled as hysterical.

"My neurologist told me that all of my symptoms were being caused by a distant trauma that I couldn't remember," Brea says. "All of a sudden at twenty-eight. After a fever." She thought it sounded "a little bit convenient" for her doctor to blame her symptoms on an alleged cause that he didn't know about and she couldn't recall. She was also skeptical when he attributed *all* the ailments she'd had over the last year to her "mind." That sinus infection? Psychosomatic. The fact that it went away after taking antibiotics? That was psychosomatic too. As were the dizziness, the gastrointestinal problems, and the terrible new headaches that she'd never before had in her life. Plus, as other doctors had begun to suggest that her symptoms were psychogenic, Brea had already been to see a psychiatrist. She figured she should get the opinion of an expert instead of accepting guesses from doctors with no mental health training. He'd told her, "It's clear you're really sick but not with anything psychiatric; I hope they find out what's wrong with you."

"YUPPIE FLU," FEMINIST BURNOUT, AND EDUCATED WHITE WOMEN

While the previous outbreaks of ME could apparently be blamed on mass hysteria merely on the basis that more women than men were affected, the apparently growing number of individual cases of the condition in the mideighties called for some explanation. And as ME/CFS became seen as a psychogenic illness, it was characterized as a condition of a certain kind of woman. The subtitle of a 1987 *Time* piece on the condition had dubbed it "yuppie disease," and the term subsequently spread like wildfire. A CBS segment that same year described the typical patient as "a professional woman in her thirties with a high-pressure job" and the disease as "less a malady than it is a movement."

The same characterization occurred in the United Kingdom, where the name remained myalgic encephalomyelitis. "The one absolutely clear-cut clinical feature in this disease is the personality profile of the people who develop it," one neurologist declared in a 1993 *Frontline* episode on ME. "Many of them have profound psychosexual difficulties with partner relationships and life in general. Something like four-fifths of the people I deal with, if not more, are women in early middle age who have unsatisfactory marriages, who have children who are making life difficult for them." According to two cardiologists featured in a 1988 article in *The Sunday Times* (London), ME patients "have above-average intelligence, high levels of drive, lots of enthusiasm; but they are not quite the superman or superwoman they need to be to achieve their ambition." They are people who "have four-star abilities with five-star ambitions."

Scholars too ran with the "yuppie flu" stereotype popularized in the media and offered psychosocial theories to explain why most of the "yuppies" affected were women. ME/CFS represented a "culturally sanctioned" flight into the sick role during an era in which many were "wrestling with the expanding role of women," two psychiatrists argued in 1991. Many ME/CFS sufferers, they suggested, felt conflicted about balancing their work and family obligations. "The diagnosis of chronic fatigue syndrome provides a legitimate 'medical' reason for their fatigue, emotional distress, and associated psychophysiological symptoms and allows them to withdraw from situations they find intolerable on the basis of illness rather than their own volition."

" 'Liberated' by feminism to enter previously all-male occupations, women in the 1970s found themselves exhorted to 'have it all' by combining a demanding career with a rich and fulfilling family life," another academic article argued. "This meant juggling a number of incompatible identities." By the workaholic eighties, the theory went, many of these women were overextended and subconsciously looking for a way out. The fatigue they felt was a "symbolic resistance" to the culture of hyperproductivity. In fact, as the researchers told it, coming down with ME/CFS was actually a positive transformation for many patients: "The abandonment of expectations of success produced feelings of content and relief."

The influence of the antifeminist backlash occurring at the time is not exactly subtle here. "The false characterization about who gets this disease was so deeply misogynistic," Johnson says. There was this "suggestion that women who get this disease, they almost deserve it, because they stepped out of bounds, they got educations, they got graduate degrees, they were working in professions that men typically work in." Feminism had convinced women they wanted to "have it all"; ME/CFS was imagined to be their excuse when they inevitably realized that they actually didn't.

Such sexist stereotyping by the media and academia was enabled by researchers who were claiming that it was, in fact, female "yuppies" who disproportionately got the disease. In a 1988 article, the NIH's resident ME/CFS researcher wrote, "The demography of this syndrome reflects an excessive risk for educated adult white women. This may reflect either a bias toward the cohort of sufferers who can best afford a sophisticated medical evaluation or some unique constitutional frailty of such individuals." While most patients reported "excellent prior health," he claimed they often had "histories of unachievable ambition, poor coping skills, and somatic complaints." He added, "It is difficult and at times unpleasant to address the demands of such patients or to test hypotheses as to the etiology of their woes."

It's difficult to accept that there could have ever been any question that the overrepresentation of educated white women in early ME/CFS studies probably had something to do with their relative privilege. It was the same reason that migraine was thought to affect professional perfectionists, vulvodynia was initially considered a condition of white women, and endometriosis was the "career women's disease": the only women who were able to get a diagnosis were educated white women—and persistent ones at that. This was a newly defined condition, without objective biomarkers, that the vast majority of doctors dismissed as psychological instead. *Of course* the only patients diagnosed with it were those who had the resources to pay for repeated doctor's visits, enough authority to repeatedly reject those doctors' conclusions that they were just "depressed," and the information and connections needed to find one of the handful of doctors in the country who had taken an interest in the condition. Consider one of the first patients seen by the Incline Village doctors in the mideighties: an upper-middle-class housewife who'd been bedridden for ten years before finding her way to them, she'd spent $400,000 and been to 210 doctors, including some at the prestigious Mayo Clinic, who'd all concluded she was mentally ill.

In fact, as early as the nineties, there were community-based epidemiological studies showing not only that educated white women weren't uniquely vulnerable to the disease but also that other women were: In 1991, researchers knocked on doors in northern Nevada and found that people with less education and with lower incomes were more likely to have the condition. In 1999, researchers surveyed nearly 30,000 people in Chicago and concluded that "the highest levels of CFS were consistently found among women, minority groups, and persons with lower levels of education and occupational status." In 1987, the media even reported on an outbreak of the illness in the Nevada town of Yerington, a poor farming community that was just about as far from the "yuppie" scene at Lake Tahoe as you could get. Yet these facts were overlooked by the media and the medical community in favor of sticking to a story in which the sufferers all shared a certain background and personality—and not a very sympathetic one.

UNHEALTHY SKEPTICISM

The story of how Dr. Lucinda Bateman, founder and medical director of the Bateman Horne Center, became a specialist in the condition offers a good illustration of just now pervasive and automatic the dismissal of ME/CFS patients was in the eighties. In 1987, she graduated from the Johns Hopkins University School of Medicine and started her residency. Her sister, who'd been a healthy young woman when she left for medical school, was now very ill, and no doctor had been able to explain her crushing fatigue. "The last one she saw said, 'You need to take a night class or broaden your life.' He really implied to her that this was all in her head and she was just a busy mother who was overwhelmed with three kids," Bateman says. "And I thought that was just unbelievable, because I knew her, and she was a very talented, highly productive person, who could do more than anybody with her eyes closed."

Desperate to figure out what was wrong with her sister, Bateman followed the discussion of the newly defined CFS closely. "I had no idea that it was going to be anything different than a really interesting new emerging illness." But she quickly realized that she was in a conservative academic environment where her superiors "didn't think these patients really had anything." She became the go-to doctor for the patients that everyone else dismissed. Upon finishing her training in 1990, she opened up a group practice in Salt Lake City. "I was flooded with patients who had chronic fatigue and fibromyalgia, and I couldn't figure out why." She later found out: her former colleagues in the infectious diseases division at the University of Utah had changed their after-hours message to say, "If you're calling about chronic fatigue syndrome, call this number"—and gave out hers. As a hilarious prank.

The fact that so much of the medical community did not share Bateman's open-minded attitude toward ME/CFS, instead greeting the condition with outright derision, is sometimes characterized as an understandable consequence of its mostly subjective symptoms. Except that from the beginning, ME/CFS researchers were documenting plenty of objective physiological abnormalities. By the early nineties, they'd found problems with natural killer cells (a type of immune cell) in patients. MRIs had revealed brain lesions in a pattern distinct from depression and similar to MS. They'd objectively confirmed problems with memory and concentration on neurocognitive tests. They just hadn't—and still haven't—uncovered one smoking gun that explains the disease.

But the doctors sounding the alarm about ME/CFS were convinced that this was a *new* disease, or at least one that, even if it had occurred in sporadic outbreaks or at lower levels in the past, was seemingly becoming much more widespread. If a disease has never been fully described and studied before, then the fact that even a million dollars' worth of tests reveals "nothing wrong" isn't evidence against its existence; it is what you'd expect. As Dr. Thomas English, a doctor diagnosed with ME/CFS, asked in an open letter to his fellow physicians published in *JAMA* in 1991, "Are we to believe that just because symptoms are strange and unfamiliar they cannot be real? Are we to assume that our laboratory tests are capable of screening for new diseases as well as old?" While "healthy skepticism" is a prized quality among doctors, when that skepticism is directed toward patients, English warned, it makes the medical community collectively incapable of unraveling new medical mysteries.

Though medicine has a long history of dismissing women's unexplained symptoms, Bateman suggests that the problem became even worse in the eighties and nineties, with the rise of "evidence-based medicine." This approach, she points out, "can come back to bite you, if you're not careful," because if a disease hasn't been sufficiently studied yet, the evidence base simply isn't there. At the same time, there were increasing financial pressures on doctors to spend less time with patients. "The incentive for doctors to sit and listen to patients has just completely disappeared. It's actually a negative incentive; they are punished if they slow down." ME/CFS, she suggests, "got caught in the change in the way we practice medicine—both scientifically and economically. We've taught people that it's not okay to think outside the box. We've implied that if [something] doesn't fit what we know, it's probably not important, or it's probably psychological. It goes in the garbage can. There's no curiosity. That's a very modern change in medicine."

English concluded his appeal to his colleagues skeptical of ME/CFS with a question: "I would only plant this seed in the mind of skeptics: What if you are wrong? What are the consequences for your patients?"

For Brea, the consequences were immediate and dramatic. Though unimpressed with her doctor's diagnosis of conversion disorder, she was also desperate for any explanation that could help her understand what was happening to her. So she decided to walk the two miles home from the neurologist's office and try to "figure out" how her mind was making the symptoms happen. Once home, she collapsed on the couch in pain and, that night, had another severe fever. "And then I was bedridden for four months, and I have never recovered from that. I've gotten better over the years, but I have never been as well as I was the minute I left his office," Brea says. "When you have this condition, it's not just that doctors are wrong; it's that entertaining their advice can actually make you worse, in ways that you may never recover from."

Like many patients, Brea eventually turned to the Internet, suspected she had ME/CFS, and sought one of the dozen or so specialists in the country, who confirmed the diagnosis. But she was just getting sicker. "A lot of days I wouldn't even be able to lift my head from a pillow. There would be months where I would not even cross the threshold of my house. Maybe every few weeks I would make it to the living room, and that was a big deal." She worried she would have to start using a bedpan soon; she worried she would eventually starve to death because she'd become sensitive to all but a few foods.

The downward spiral was finally turned around when she tried an antiviral drug, one commonly used for HIV-related infections. Suddenly able to walk more than twenty steps a day, she built on that, finding advice from other patients online and better learning how to pace herself to avoid a crash. Finding a treatment that helped made her even more frustrated with the initial psychogenic misdiagnosis she, and so many others, had received. "When you get a label like that, it prevents doctors from looking for things that could actually help you," she says. "I think that's the hardest thing—that I don't know how well I could have been if I had been treated properly. But almost no one is."

————

The skepticism in the broader medical community has often harmed individual patients. But it was the skepticism of a handful of midlevel male scientists whose decisions set the course of research on the disease for the next three decades that had the most long-lasting and devastating impact on ME/CFS patients. The individual doctors who, going against the grain, believed their ME/CFS patients, could only do so much. To have anything more to offer those patients beyond that belief, they needed scientific research.

But for at least the first few years that the CDC was investigating the disease, it was treated as an object of open ridicule by most of the staff of the Viral Exanthems and Herpesvirus Branch that had been charged by Congress with investigating the disease. "There was a pervasive feeling that this just could not be real, this had to be a joke, these people were just whiny, unhappy women," says Johnson, who haunted the CDC cafeteria during the late eighties while she was writing her book. The lead investigator assigned to the disease then told her, "I get constant jokes about this, you know—'Oh, I'm so tired, maybe I've got chronic fatigue.' Nobody wants to fool with this."

The staff even displayed on a bulletin board in the branch's hallway a satirical letter mocking the hypochondriacs who thought they had the disease. According to Johnson, it read, "I am SICK . . . I am so tired it took me 6 days to dictate this letter to my secretary." It continued, "I would also like a list of recommended treatments for the above conditions, in descending order of trendiness, including acyclovir, gamma globulin, WXYZ-2, 3DPG, Vitamins A, B-1 thru 12, C, D, E, F, G, H, I, J, K, L, M, N, O, P, and Q, Zinc, Cadmium, Cobalt, Neodymium, Ytterbium, lecithin, morithin, lessismorithin, sensory deprivations walking on hot coals, alternating sensory deprivation and walking on hot coals, purified fruit-bat guano injections, and bedrest. I have already tried Valium, Lithium, Haldol, and thorazine, but they only work when I take them. Please, also inform me about how to get social security and workmen's compensation benefits for the above diseases. I have had them for over 40 years now, and I am only 29 years old."

And the agency backed up this dismissive attitude in deed. One of the revelations Johnson reported in *Osler's Web* was that the CDC had routinely reallocated funding that Congress had directed to their ME/CFS program to other projects. A couple of years later, the head of the Viral Exanthems and Herpesvirus Branch, claiming whistle-blower status for himself, publicly leveled that charge against his superiors. In 1999, an audit by the U.S. Department of Health and Human Services' (HHS) inspector general confirmed that at least 39 percent of the $23 million that Congress had given the CDC to work on ME/CFS between 1995 and 1998 was spent on other programs, and that CDC officials had lied to Congress about where the money went. In 2000, the GAO reported that progress on understanding the disease had been hindered by the theft, as well as by poor coordination between the CDC's and NIH's programs.

In the mideighties, Congress had charged the NIH with offering funding for ME/CFS research to outside researchers. Yet by 1990, the NIH had provided only two grants. This wasn't because of a lack of interest. On the contrary, despite the general dismissiveness in the medical community, in the eighties, there were plenty of scientists hoping to uncover the cause of a mysterious new disease. But the NIH had already settled on the probable cause and was only looking to fund research that confirmed it. "Many, many premiere scientists of their day who could get funding for anything else, when they got interested in this disease and tried to get funding to pursue it, they were not funded," Johnson says. Their proposals would be rejected with comments like, "'Your proposal to look for a causative pathogen in chronic fatigue syndrome cannot be funded because, as you know, chronic fatigue syndrome is a psychiatric disease.' That was really it."

"All that stereotyping—boy, it was heavy at the federal level," says Bateman, who was on HHS's Chronic Fatigue Syndrome Advisory Committee for years. "I've had occasion to work in some way in almost every federal agency, and they were just like academics; they didn't want to hear about it. They put up roadblocks for years and years. It was amazing." Eventually, the stonewalling drove many prominent researchers away from the field. The result has been that patients have been forced to bankroll much ME/CFS research themselves.

By 2000, in fact, the NIH had largely abdicated all responsibility for ME/CFS. The National Institute of Allergy and Infectious Diseases, which had housed ME/CFS since the mideighties, had booted it from its portfolio. At that point, the disease would have been homeless within the NIH if Vivian Pinn hadn't stepped in and offered to bring it under the ORWH. However, the ORWH, with its minuscule budget, was given no money to fund it. From 2001 to 2008 NIH funding for ME/CFS dropped by 45 percent.

"OLD WINE IN NEW BOTTLES"

The NIH's only in-house investigator on ME/CFS had quickly come to believe it was psychogenic. In 1985, he had helped put the condition on the radar by suggesting that it might be caused by chronic Epstein-Barr viral infection or some new kind of immune dysfunction. But three years later, unable to find consistent abnormalities, he'd decided that it might actually represent a "psychoneurotic condition." As one patient put it to Johnson, "[He] couldn't find out what was causing this illness, and instead of admitting that, he called us psychoneurotic." He began opening his lectures at medical schools on the disease with a slide showing a Victorian-era young lady swooning on a fainting couch and reading from an eighteenth-century text on "The Nervous or Hysteric Fever; the Fever of the Spirits; Vapours, Hypo, or Spleen."

More commonly, proponents of a psychogenic theory of ME/CFS have compared the condition not to hysteria but to its sister nervous disorder that was popular in the late nineteenth century: neurasthenia. One article in the early nineties, noting the "striking resemblance" between the two conditions, predicted, "Chronic fatigue syndrome will meet the same fate as neurasthenia—a decline in social value as it is demonstrated that the majority of its sufferers are experiencing primary psychiatric disorders or psychophysiological reactions and that the disorder is often a culturally sanctioned form of illness behavior." Another influential article that compared the two in 1990 described ME/CFS as "old wine in new bottles."

An identical argument has been made about fibromyalgia, which shares with ME/CFS the symptoms of fatigue, unrefreshing sleep, and cognitive problems. (Though it's difficult to draw neat boundaries around conditions with overlapping symptoms whose underlying mechanisms are unknown, experts generally consider the two conditions distinguishable, with pain hypersensitivity the hallmark of fibromyalgia and post-exertional malaise the hallmark of ME/CFS, though many patients develop both.) A 2013 article arguing that fibromyalgia is "indistinguishable in most respects" from neurasthenia claimed, "Time brings clarity to confusing illnesses of the past, and we now recognize that hysteria [and] neurasthenia . . . were almost always psychogenic disorders."

This conclusion is a testament to medicine's case of collective amnesia about the many organic diseases that would have been labeled as hysteria, neurasthenia, or another "nervous" disorder in the nineteenth century— and continue to be misdiagnosed as such well into the twenty-first century. Never mind that diseases as diverse as MS, temporal lobe epilepsy, endometriosis, and a whole range of autoimmune diseases are also "indistinguishable in most respects" from some descriptions of these historical disorders; it is only conditions that are still currently "medically unexplained" whose similarity to the ever-shifting plethora of loose diagnostic labels of centuries past is somehow considered evidence of their psychogenic origin.

The weakness of this argument is underscored by the fact that one can just as easily look at the very same medical history and reach the reverse conclusion: That the resemblance ME/CFS bears to some nineteenth-century descriptions of neurasthenia suggests that perhaps the disease has been around for a long time. That as the neurasthenia label, like hysteria, splintered into various newly recognized diseases that cause fatigue, there remained one—or, more likely, multiple—conditions that remained "unexplained." And that the only reason the condition "disappeared" for much of the twentieth century was that medicine began to *mis*label its symptoms as psychogenic. As ME/CFS patient Dorothy Wall writes in her 2005 memoir, *Encounters with the Invisible*, "To claim [ME/CFS] as an incarnation of neurasthenia is to demean and dismiss. I think, though, that our view of neurasthenia is ripe for revision."

From this perspective, ME/CFS's reemergence in the mideighties may have been the product of feminist progress above all else. It's certainly possible that ME/CFS—or perhaps some subtypes of it—was new or becoming more prevalent in the eighties. But it's also possible that it simply wasn't until then that a critical mass of women patients had enough social authority to reject medicine's conclusion that their unexplained illness was all in their heads—and there were enough enlightened doctors who believed them. After all, it does seem to be an interesting coincidence that it was just as the large baby boomer generation, the first to have come of age during the women's movement of the sixties and seventies, began reaching middle adulthood that so many unexplained conditions that predominantly affect women and that, it turns out, are quite common—from ME/CFS to fibromyalgia to vulvodynia to IC—rather suddenly appeared on the radar.

The irony is that while the stereotype that ME/CFS patients were feminist "superwomen" trying to "have it all" was quickly used to discredit them, it's perhaps only because some of them *were* such women that the condition was defined at all. A generation earlier, the most privileged ME/CFS patients would have been not conflicted career women plagued by "yuppie flu" but housewives suffering "hysterical housewife syndrome"—a condition even less likely to be taken seriously by medicine.

REVERSING COURSE

Perhaps one of the most far-ranging effects of the early mockery of ME/ CFS was that the longer it went on, the harder it became to walk it back. "I really believe that at a certain point they were so cemented into that early posture," Johnson says. After a decade of dismissing sufferers as over- whelmed working mothers, sexually dissatisfied wives, and middle-aged women with empty nest syndrome, "you can imagine how difficult it would be for either the CDC or the NIH to come out in mainstream media and say, 'You know the disease we've been calling chronic fatigue syndrome or yuppie flu that you all think is a joke? Well, guess what . . .'"

Only in the last few years have the NIH and the CDC finally started to reverse course. In 2015, the NIH announced that it would "ramp up" its efforts on ME/CFS, launching a comprehensive in-house study and in- creasing funding for research on the disease by 15 percent to about $6.5 million, which bumped it above hay fever for the first time in years. NIH director Francis Collins told *The Atlantic*—in a bit of an understatement— that "given the seriousness of the condition, I don't think we have focused enough of our attention on this." In 2017, funding was expected to nearly double from the previous year to $15 million, though it will likely fall short of that thanks to across-the-board cuts to the NIH budget. Still, that's far below the $250 million that experts argue would be commensurate with the burden of the disease, and a strong case can be made that the disease deserves reparations for decades of neglect.

Recently the tide has also begun to turn against some of the bad sci- ence that has been done on the disease. While most American experts on ME/CFS consider it to be a physical disease, a psychogenic model has flourished across the pond. The theory goes that ME/CFS patients hold "unhelpful illness beliefs" that they have an organic disease that is wors- ened by exertion and, as a result, have become deconditioned from too much rest. For years, prominent British mental health professionals have recommended a treatment program composed of cognitive behavioral therapy (CBT) and a steady increase in exercise that's designed to help patients overcome the fear of activity that's allegedly perpetuating their illness. In other words, it's not just misdiagnosed ME/CFS patients like Brea who may be encouraged to push themselves to do the very thing that makes their illness worse.

Several years ago, British government agencies funded a much-hyped study, nicknamed the PACE study, to test the effectiveness of this approach. With a price tag of $8 million, it was the largest clinical study on ME/CFS ever. Its conclusions, first published in *The Lancet* in 2011, were trumpeted in the media to headlines like "Got ME? Just Get Out and Exercise, Say Scientists." The researchers characterized the treatment as "moderately effective," claiming that 60 percent of the patients in the study had "improved" and 22 percent had actually "recovered." Largely on the basis of the PACE results, major American medical organizations, including the CDC and the Mayo Clinic, have listed CBT and graded exercise therapy as recommended treatments in their public information about the condition.

ME/CFS patients were obviously skeptical of these results, given that even mild exertion could cause a dramatic worsening of their symptoms, and they quickly pointed out a number of serious problems with the study. The evidence that the patients had gotten any benefit from the treatment came entirely from their self-reports, which may have been biased by their expectations in an unblinded study. On all of the objective measures of physical functioning—such as a six-minute walking test or whether patients had returned to work—the treatment had resulted in no improvement whatsoever. What's more, the researchers had significantly loosened their definition of "improvement" midway through the study—which is very frowned upon in clinical research—so much so that a patient could actually get *worse* during the study and yet meet the criteria for being "recovered."

For years, patients' criticisms of the PACE study largely fell on deaf ears. Then in 2015, after a detailed exposé was published on the science site *Virology Blog*, scientists outside the ME/CFS field started to take notice; an open letter declared that "such flaws have no place in published research" and called for an independent review of the study. Patients fought a legal battle to get the PACE researchers to publicly release their raw data.

After a court order finally compelled them to do so in 2016, a reanalysis by independent researchers concluded that if the PACE researchers had stuck to their original standards, only 20 percent of the patients would have "improved"—half of whom would have improved just as much with specialist medical care alone and no treatment—and less than 7 percent would have "recovered," a rate that was statistically no different from that of the control group.

As Julie Rehmeyer, a science writer and ME/CFS patient, points out in her 2017 book *Through the Shadowlands: A Science Writer's Odyssey into an Illness Science Doesn't Understand*, the researchers' characterization of their results was so misleading that it was pretty much the exact opposite of the reality. "The researchers' modest results in fact offered compelling evidence *against* the theory that it was psychological problems and deconditioning that kept ME/CFS patients sick. After all, the researchers had given patients the best treatments they could to address those problems, and it had barely helped. CBT and exercise did no more for ME/CFS than for illnesses like lupus, MS, and fatigue from cancer treatment, all of which are known to be primarily biological in origin." In 2017, the CDC removed any mention of CBT and exercise from its online information on the disease. Scientists and patient groups have continued to call for a full retraction of the original study results to "protect patients from ineffective and possibly harmful treatments."

Meanwhile, among practicing doctors, a younger generation that does not feel locked into belittling the disease simply because the medical community has spent three decades doing so will hopefully bring fresh perspectives. Bateman teaches a class on ME/CFS and fibromyalgia at a local medical school. "Before I start the lecture I always have a show of hands from the group: 'How many of you have heard these diseases spoken of disparagingly by your attending physician?' And 80 percent of the hands go up. And then I say, 'How many of you know someone with these illnesses?' And about half the hands will go up."

But even today Bateman says that she still tends to talk more about the men she treats with the disease in her lectures. "I don't think I really examined my biases on that before, but I'm sure that is it: to help the audience take it more seriously because it's a male patient."

POSTURAL ORTHOSTATIC TACHYCARDIA SYNDROME

When Brea started searching online for information about what she might have, there was another condition besides ME/CFS that caught her attention: postural orthostatic tachycardia syndrome, or POTS.

POTS is the most common form of dysautonomia, a dysfunction of the autonomic nervous system. Normally, when we stand up, the autonomic nervous system immediately and automatically responds by constricting the blood vessels and slightly bumping up the heart rate so that our blood doesn't pool downward due to gravity. Orthostatic intolerance is the umbrella term for conditions in which this vital mechanism fails. In people with POTS, the heart rate jumps up in an attempt to make up for this failure. The symptoms they experience are mostly due either to the fact that they're not getting enough blood flow to their heart and brain (light-headedness, diminished concentration, fainting or almost fainting) or to the overactivation of the autonomic nervous symptom to compensate (a rapid, pounding heartbeat; shortness of breath; shaking; chest pain). Patients also often report fatigue, exercise intolerance, nausea, headaches, and sleep problems.

POTS can be caused by other underlying diseases, including diabetes, some genetic disorders, and many autoimmune diseases. But in primary, or idiopathic, POTS, it's not clear why the blood vessels aren't getting the message to constrict as they should. What is clear is that being unable to properly adapt to being upright is a debilitating problem. While some cases of POTS can be mild, other POTS patients are confined to their beds or have to use wheelchairs. Researchers have found POTS patients to be as impaired as those with COPD or congestive heart failure, with a quality of life comparable to patients on dialysis for kidney failure. Approximately 25 percent of them are unable to work or go to school.

Among patients diagnosed with ME/CFS, a significant minority (studies suggest about a third of them) have POTS or another form of orthostatic intolerance. Conversely, if you take a group of POTS patients, a large proportion of them will have severe enough fatigue that they meet the criteria for ME/CFS. In our siloed medical system, which diagnostic label a patient gets often depends on the specialist they happen to see: Autonomic nervous system specialists would say that diagnosing a patient with POTS as having ME/CFS is a misdiagnosis; they consider all the symptoms explained by the patient's POTS. ME/CFS experts, meanwhile, sometimes describe POTS as a subtype of ME/CFS. Since at this point both conditions are syndromes whose underlying mechanism is yet to be determined, the exact relationship between them remains unclear, but at the very least POTS contributes to the problem in some ME/CFS cases.

While both conditions may be poorly understood syndromes, unlike ME/CFS with its subjective symptoms, which skeptics often complain are too "vague" and "nonspecific," POTS has highly specific, objective criteria for diagnosis: adults are diagnosed with POTS if their heart rate increases by 30 beats per minute or is greater than 120 beats per minute within ten minutes of standing up, without a fall in blood pressure. And, to autonomic nervous system specialists at least, POTS is also not really "unexplained." Though it's unknown at this point what causes the autonomic nervous system to fail to adapt to standing in idiopathic POTS, the symptoms seen in patients are those you'd expect if it did.

It is likely for these reasons that POTS is not contested in the way ME/CFS is. There is just remarkably little awareness of it within the medical community at all. Most medical students don't get any training on POTS. It's not part of the board exams. Even many neurologists and cardiologists aren't familiar with it. Lauren Stiles, cofounder of Dysautonomia International, a patient advocacy group for autonomic nervous system disorders, says, "We think part of the reason it's neglected is because it is a young woman's health condition." About 80 percent of POTS patients are young or middle-aged women. About half of POTS patients in Dysautonomia International's surveys first developed the condition in their teens.

Even when doctors are vaguely aware of the condition, there's a tendency to minimize its seriousness, Stiles says. When Dysautonomia International does educational lectures at medical schools, she finds physicians are receptive once they learn about it. "But until they get those facts, there is a lot of eye rolling." There's a sense that this is "just some teenage condition; they grow out of it." In fact, there isn't much research on how POTS patients fare long term. With the underlying cause unknown, treatment is limited to managing the symptoms. In a 2016 study from the Mayo Clinic, less than a fifth of adolescent patients had fully improved with treatment, while just over half reported improved but persistent symptoms two to ten years later.

After reading about how common POTS is among ME/CFS patients, Brea did a home version of the test used to diagnose the condition and found that her heart rate would shoot from about 70 beats per minute when she was lying down to 140 beats per minute when she stood up. In the year she'd spent returning to the Harvard clinic, complaining of being so dizzy she couldn't get out of bed, not one of the doctors she'd seen, including neurologists and cardiologists, the specialists most likely to know about POTS, had tested her for the condition. "They wondered why I couldn't stand up, but they didn't catch that at all."

FROM "IRRITABLE HEART" TO "ANXIETY NEUROSIS"

In a perfect illustration of how the same medical history can look radically different depending on your perspective, Stiles invokes the same images that the NIH researcher who'd become convinced that ME/CFS was a "psychoneurotic condition" used in his lectures in the nineties. "You know those Victorian images of women clutching their pearls and putting their hand on their head and laying on a fainting couch? Pretty sure they had POTS."

Indeed, while arguing that ME/CFS is neurasthenia reincarnated on the basis that both have fatigue as a main symptom seems a little silly, POTS, with its fairly unique collection of symptoms linked to the specific sign of a rapid heartbeat when upright, can much more convincingly be traced back through the historical record—all the way back to the American Civil War. In 1871, Dr. Jacob M. Da Costa published the first major article on the condition he called "irritable heart." The symptoms of the disorder, which he noted often began after an acute infectious illness, included heart palpitations and a rapid pulse that worsened upon standing, chest pain, shortness of breath, dizziness, fatigue after exertion, and sometimes digestive problems.

During World War I, the condition was observed again, going by various names, including "Da Costa's syndrome," "general exhaustion," "effort syndrome," "soldier's heart," and "neurocirculatory asthenia." Most experts continued to view it as an organic condition of unknown origin, but some started to turn to psychogenic explanations. In 1941, American physician Dr. Paul Wood argued that Da Costa's syndrome was caused by "misinterpretation of emotional symptoms, certain vicious circular patterns, the growth of a conviction that the heart is to blame, consequent fear of sudden death on exertion, conditioning and hysteria."

After World War I, a group of American researchers wrote the first medical paper on the condition's prevalence among civilians. They estimated that it affected 2 to 5 percent of the population, with an average age of onset of twenty-five, and that it was twice as common among women. Of course, in women—who could hardly be diagnosed with "soldier's heart"— it had probably simply been called hysteria, neurasthenia, or nerves. Wood suggested that the gender difference probably explained why no one had really paid attention to the condition during peacetime: "It is possible that the curious lack of recognition of Da Costa's syndrome in civilian life is due to the fact that it is commoner in women: the change of sex, plus the lack of khaki uniform, seems to have proved an effective disguise. 'Effort syndrome' in the male soldier becomes cardiac, respiratory, or other neurosis in the female civilian."

By the sixties, the psychological theory of the condition was firmly in place. And as the proposed etiology shifted from organic to psychogenic, there was an accompanying "diminished interest in Da Costa's syndrome as a medical entity," Harvard physician Oglesby Paul noted in a 1987 review of its history. It wasn't considered a rare problem, though. In 1968, Wood estimated that it accounted for 10 to 15 percent of all cases referred to cardiovascular clinics. But by the late eighties, it had been so subsumed by psychiatric diagnoses that it was "infrequently mentioned" at all, according to Paul. "It is unlikely to have disappeared; it probably exists much as before but is more often identified and labelled in psychiatric terms such as 'anxiety state' or 'anxiety neurosis.'"

Paul wrote that "there is no harm in this shift in diagnostic labels as long as the essential importance of the syndrome, its prognosis, and treatment are properly appreciated." That was an odd take, given that the prognosis was considered "life long with remissions and exacerbations" and the treatment offered to patients was nothing more than "reassurance" that they did not have organic heart disease. No doubt to the women debilitated by a condition for which there was no cure—and zero effort being made to find one—it made a great deal of difference whether this shift in diagnostic labels reflected an accurate understanding of the nature of the problem.

To some extent, it's understandable that POTS was undifferentiated from anxiety disorders for so many decades. The autonomic nervous system exists right at the entangled crossroads of mind and body. Panic disorder shares many symptoms with POTS (heart palpitations, dizziness, shortness of breath) for a reason: both involve an overactivation of the autonomic nervous system's sympathetic branch, which is responsible for the fight-or-flight response. That neurocirculatory asthenia was studied mostly among soldiers during wartime for decades perhaps compounded the difficulty; surely some cases of "soldier's heart" would today be diagnosed as PTSD or overlapped with it.

On the other hand, POTS is difficult to mistake for anxiety disorders if you listen to the patients' description of their symptoms. Panic attacks occur sporadically, not almost constantly, and are accompanied by an intense, overwhelming sense of fear; POTS patients are typically just worried about passing out. A 2008 study found that a group of POTS patients scored moderately high on an anxiety test that asked about the physiological symptoms of anxiety (like a pounding heart), but, using a test that focused more on the cognitive aspects of anxiety (e.g., if they feel excessively worried), they were actually slightly less anxious than the general population. Above all, anxiety disorders do not occur primarily after prolonged standing, and they're not improved by lying down, a curious fact that surely must have been noted by countless women during the decades that the condition was considered an "anxiety neurosis."

Finally, in the eighties, experts studying the autonomic nervous system began experimenting with a new technology: the tilt table test. The patient is strapped to a bed that's tilted up to a seventy-degree angle, while their blood pressure and heart rate are monitored to assess any problems with their autonomic nervous system's ability to counteract the force of gravity. In the early nineties, researchers from Mayo Clinic coined the term *postural orthostatic tachycardia syndrome* and suggested that the condition that had been called Da Costa's syndrome, soldier's heart, and neurocirculatory asthenia over the decades was not a form of anxiety but a form of orthostatic intolerance.

"MAYBE YOU WEREN'T CUT OUT TO BE A LAWYER"

By the late nineties, autonomic nervous system experts were noting an "epidemic" of orthostatic intolerance, which they acknowledged probably reflected "an epidemic of disease *recognition*," not an actual increase in prevalence rates. In contrast to just a few years before, one physician wrote, "a 20-year-old woman who appears to be healthy yet has dizziness, palpitations, and fatigue is certainly no longer passed over as having a psychosomatic illness!" Of course, contrary to that doctor's naive optimism, that hypothetical woman most certainly still *is* passed over—even two decades later. While the condition itself may no longer be dismissed as a form of anxiety, individual POTS patients like Brea continue to be dismissed during the many years it often takes to get diagnosed.

Dysautonomia International recently teamed up with researchers from Vanderbilt to conduct an online survey of over 3,000 POTS patients in fifteen countries. The patients reported having seen an average of seven doctors over four years and two months before getting properly diagnosed. A quarter had seen more than ten doctors. Over 80 percent were given at least one psychological misdiagnosis, most commonly anxiety, stress, or depression, or were told that it was "all in their heads." One study explained the challenge of diagnosing POTS: "Patients may repeatedly present with a multitude of symptoms, often without obvious clinical findings: typical 'heart-sink' patients. Although severely incapacitated, they often appear well."

For Stiles, it took about forty doctors over the course of nine months to get the right diagnosis when she fell suddenly ill after suffering a concussion on a snowboarding vacation in 2010. She was told she had fibromyalgia,

CFS, and IBS, and was even misdiagnosed with a neuroendocrine cancer. One doctor suggested that her symptoms were somehow brought on by her job and perhaps she just wasn't "cut out to be a lawyer." Another said it was stress and prescribed a glass of red wine. In an emergency room right after the concussion, she was accused of being hungover from New Year's Eve. Her all-time favorite: An endocrinologist asked her whether she had any children. When she replied that she didn't, he suggested that she was trying to get attention from her husband, because she was thirty-one and didn't have babies yet.

The medical system never accurately diagnosed Stiles at all; like many of the women in this book, she figured it out herself from doing her own research and had a neurologist confirm the diagnosis. Initially told her POTS was idiopathic, after a few years of insisting doctors rule out every possible underlying cause, she discovered it was due to severe damage to her peripheral nerves from the autoimmune disease Sjögren's syndrome.

Stiles formed Dysautonomia International in large part because she was horrified by the thought of the patients who never get properly diagnosed. After all, she'd had a number of advantages going for her: she was white, lived near New York City, had a supportive family, was an attorney with a good salary and great insurance, and went "to the best hospitals money could buy." And it still wasn't enough. "What if I was poor?" she asks. "What if I lived in a rural area? What if my insurance would only cover one doctor? I was bedridden the entire time; what if I didn't have family to drive me to the doctors all the time? Think about all of those women who stopped after the first doctor, or the second doctor, or the third doctor. How many people have the money and time to keep pushing and pushing and pushing?"

The answer is that we have no idea. Because there hasn't been an International Classification of Diseases (ICD) code for the condition, it's hard to know how many people exactly are even *diagnosed* with POTS, let alone estimate how many go undiagnosed. (Stiles recently collaborated with a physician to obtain one in the next ICD edition.) When POTS was first described in the nineties, the number of people affected was initially estimated at 400,000 Americans (which is already not a rare disease, but on a par with MS). The newest estimate is 1 to 3 million.

PATIENTS DOING IT FOR THEMSELVES

One reason that so many doctors still don't know about POTS may be that Dysautonomia International has been around only since 2012. Indeed, one of the key lessons of POTS's history seems to be that, in a medical system that has no formal way of ensuring the dissemination of new knowledge and has long been dismissing women's unexplained symptoms as psychogenic, patient advocacy has become absolutely essential to raising awareness of newly recognized female-predominant conditions. Dysautonomia International's efforts to get coverage of the condition in the media have helped, since "even doctors are susceptible to pop media awareness." They're also empowering patients themselves to educate their doctors, one printed handout at a time. "We're doing a lot of indirect physician education through the patients. They need the professional materials that the doctors will believe, rather than walking in and saying, 'Hey, let me teach you about this medical condition that you've never heard of.'"

The organization is also helping push forward research on the condition. Way back in the early nineties, when Mayo Clinic researchers defined the syndrome, they suggested it might be immune related since many patients developed it after an infection. There's other circumstantial evidence that hints at a possible autoimmune basis: the fact that it's more common among women, that it runs in families, and that patients often develop other autoimmune diseases. (Though, like other unexplained conditions, "POTS likely has many different mechanisms, from inherited genetic traits, to immunological abnormalities, to structural neuropathies," Stiles says.) The autoimmune hypothesis remained unexplored for decades, largely because the condition receives little research funding. "Assuming POTS impacts the more conservative estimate of 1 million patients, it's getting 1 million dollars a year at NIH; MS impacts 400,000 patients and gets over 100 million dollars a year," Stiles says.

In the last few years, though, multiple research teams have come out with small studies showing that many POTS patients have autoantibodies to the adrenergic and muscarinic receptors, which are critical parts of the autonomic nervous system. Dysautonomia International decided to help speed along the scientific process by raising money to fund larger follow-up studies and literally bringing the researchers to the patients. "We went to them and said, 'Hey, we have this annual conference in DC every year; do you want to come to the conference and collect serum from a hundred patients?'" At the last few conferences, several research teams took them up on the offer. In 2018, Dysautonomia International will distribute at least $300,000 in research grants, almost a third of the sum that the NIH, the largest public funder of scientific research in the world, can muster for research on the condition.

Of course, even before a formal advocacy organization like Dysautonomia International was formed, informal online patient communities had radically changed the POTS experience. When a prominent neurologist finally confirmed Stiles's diagnosis, he warned that she likely would never meet another patient with it or find a doctor who knew how to treat it. Instead, to her relief, by the end of the day, she'd found an online support group with 3,000 members ready to share their advice and doctor recommendations. In fact, she credits online patient communities for everything: "I diagnosed myself through the Internet, I found the doctors I needed through the Internet, I found the other patients I needed for support through the Internet. And so, so often we meet patients who were diagnosed first by their friend—their girlfriend from dance class or whatever—and then found a doctor because of a recommendation they got from an online support group. Thank god for the Internet."

Thank god, indeed. But this is not how it should be. We deserve better than a medical system in which an extremely debilitating and common condition remains so unknown more than two decades after it was first described (or 150 years, depending on when you start counting) that patients have to do everything themselves—from diagnosing each other to teaching their own doctors about it to funding the scientific research that's so desperately needed to explain it and cure it.

CHRONIC LYME DISEASE

In the late eighties, Sherrill went to see her family physician. A strange red rash shaped like a bull's-eye had appeared on her thigh, and she had a bad sore throat. He gave her five days' worth of antibiotics for the sore throat and said he had no idea what the rash could be. Both symptoms subsided, but others soon appeared. Her joints ached. Her hands sometimes curled up like claws. She often felt confused by simple things: Did a red stoplight mean stop or go? She was exhausted. As it happened, she'd gotten pregnant a month after the mysterious rash. So for the first nine months, her doctor assured her that the symptoms were "just pregnancy"; once she gave birth, they were "just motherhood."

———

The most common vector-borne disease in the United States, Lyme disease is caused by the spirochete bacteria *Borrelia burgdorferi*, which is transmitted to humans via the bite of a black-legged tick. Between 1992 and 2008, the number of reported cases in the United States (mostly in the Northeast, upper Midwest, and West Coast) more than doubled. The CDC now estimates that there are 300,000 new cases of Lyme disease each year.

There's evidence that Lyme disease has been around for thousands of years, but it has been identified as a distinct disease and linked to *B. burgdorferi* only relatively recently. In the United States, its discovery was thanks, in no small part, to two persistent women who questioned medical authority to bring attention to an outbreak of a mysterious disease in their small town of Lyme, Connecticut, in the midseventies. Polly Murray, an artist, had become sick nearly twenty years prior when she first visited the rural southeastern Connecticut community, suffering headaches, rashes, and swollen joints that eventually abated. By the midsixties, when Murray was living in the area with her young family, her health deteriorated again. She sought a diagnosis for her fatigue, memory problems, nausea, and shooting pains, but when doctors—twenty-four in total over the years—couldn't find an explanation for her symptoms, they dismissed them as psychogenic. "You know, Mrs. Murray, some people subconsciously want to be sick," one physician told her.

Within a few years her young sons and daughter had symptoms too: rashes, headaches, and swollen knees. Eventually, the kids were diagnosed with juvenile RA. But Murray wasn't convinced; juvenile RA is very rare and not known to occur in clusters. Yet she knew that several other children in the neighborhood had the same symptoms. In 1975, she reported this outbreak of alleged arthritis cases to the Connecticut Department of Public Health. Another mother in Lyme did too. Finally, a team of investigators, led by rheumatologists from Yale, came to town to investigate. In 1977, they described the new disease (although most aspects of the condition had actually been described in the medical literature in Europe for centuries) and suggested it was transmitted by a tick bite. Five years later, a medical entomologist identified the previously unknown spirochete, *B. burgdorferi*, that was responsible.

It may seem surprising that an infectious disease with a known cause could be contested. We tend to think of infectious diseases as some of the most straightforward in all of medicine; there is a clear cause and, hopefully, a clear cure. And yet, there's a lot of uncertainty when it comes to Lyme.

Here's what everyone basically agrees on: in its acute phase, early Lyme disease sometimes, but not always, causes flu-like symptoms: fatigue, headache, fever, sweats, and chills. About 70 to 80 percent of people get the hallmark red rash at the site of the bite (called erythema migrans) that in about 20 percent of cases looks like a bull's-eye. If the infection begins to disseminate throughout the body, it may also cause facial paralysis, heart complications, and meningitis. If left untreated, 60 percent of people go on to develop the symptoms of late Lyme disease months or years after the initial infection, most commonly arthritis and sometimes inflammation of the brain and spinal cord. In both early and late phases, patients often have fatigue, cognitive dysfunction, and muscle and joint pain.

When diagnosed early, Lyme is treated with a few weeks of antibiotics, and, in most people, the symptoms resolve for good. But that's far easier in theory than in practice. The main problem is that there isn't an easy way to directly test for infection with *B. burgdorferi*. Even during the acute infection, the organism is difficult to detect, because it doesn't stay long in the blood. Instead, the standard blood tests for the disease are actually tests for its indirect footprint: the antibodies produced by the immune system to fight *B. burgdorferi*. There's a two-tier testing system that is used by the CDC to track cases. If the first test, the ELISA, is positive or indeterminate, a second test, the Western blot, is done that detects specific IgM and IgG antibodies.

Because it takes time for the immune system to churn out antibodies when it encounters a new pathogen, in the first few weeks of infection— that is, when the symptoms would first bring someone to a doctor—the blood test is negative in about half of patients who actually have been infected. Making matters even more complicated, at least four other pathogens are now known to be transmitted by the black-legged tick in addition to *B. burgdorferi*. These infections, which cause somewhat different symptoms, are often not tested for at all and are similarly hard to detect.

Given the limitations of blood tests, Lyme can be diagnosed on the basis of the rash alone in areas where it is endemic. But doctors sometimes aren't aware of that and want to see confirmation with a blood test. Plus, not everyone develops the rash, notices it, and consults a doctor right away. Even when they do, doctors may misdiagnose it. According to one study, over half of patients eventually diagnosed with Lyme who never had the rash had initially been misdiagnosed. Even worse, among those with the rash, Lyme had been initially missed in almost a quarter. And that was in an area in which the disease is endemic.

A missed early diagnosis can be an enormous problem, because as Lyme progresses, it becomes a multisystem disease that is more challenging to diagnose and less responsive to antibiotic treatment. In the late stages of the disease, blood tests are typically more accurate but still not perfect. There's variability from lab to lab and from doctor to doctor about how to interpret them. One key limitation is that exposure to antibiotics during the early stage of infection can blunt the immune response, so that someone never creates enough antibodies to turn up a positive blood test. In a 2015 study, researchers tested over a hundred early Lyme patients both before and after being treated with three weeks of antibiotics. They found that before treatment, just over a third of the patients tested positive. After treatment, 60 percent of them did. This means that someone who wasn't diagnosed in the early stage but took antibiotics for something else—but not enough to eliminate the Lyme infection—may develop late Lyme and never have a positive blood test.

That's what happened in Sherrill's case. After having been sick for a year or so, she happened to watch a PBS show about the newly discovered disease. Recognizing the bull's-eye rash immediately, she called her doctor and was referred to an infectious disease specialist. Despite her description of the rash and her symptoms, he was skeptical she had Lyme, because if she did, he told her, she'd "be really sick." She insisted she *was* really sick and begged for the blood test. But the result was negative. She tracked down the Yale physician featured in the TV program who'd led the team that identified the disease, Dr. Allen Steere, who confirmed that she surely had Lyme and the antibiotics she'd been prescribed for the sore throat had made the test negative. After receiving three weeks of IV antibiotic treatment, Sherrill felt much better, no longer in an exhausted fog, but a migrating pain in her back and neck remained.

MINIMIZE AND PSYCHOLOGIZE

There's also no dispute over the fact that a significant minority of patients (between 10 and 50 percent of them, according to different studies) have persistent symptoms for years after being treated for Lyme. Those who are diagnosed at a later stage, who have an initially severe infection, and who receive inadequate antibiotic treatment are at greater risk for these chronic symptoms, usually of debilitating fatigue, joint and muscle pain, sleep problems, and cognitive dysfunction. Going with the conservative 10 percent estimate, that amounts to about 30,000 Americans who become chronically ill each year due to Lyme infection.

It's the nature of the problem in these patients that has been the subject of the most vicious debates in the Lyme community. On the one hand are the self-described "Lyme-literate" doctors. Mostly family physicians, when some of their Lyme patients failed to get better after the standard antibiotic regimen, they decided to keep treating them until they did—for months or sometimes years—on the hypothesis that they may have a lingering low-grade infection that the first round of antibiotics didn't fully eliminate. Many patients reported they got better eventually after long courses of treatment, while others found they improved while on the antibiotics but relapsed again when they stopped them. On the other side, mainstream Lyme experts insist that there's no evidence of chronic infection, that long-term antibiotic treatment is unjustified, and that the doctors who offer it are quacks flouting the rules of "evidence-based medicine."

As I delved into the Lyme controversy, I was initially—optimistically— curious to hear what alternative hypothesis the mainstream experts offered for chronic symptoms after treatment for Lyme. If not an ongoing infection, then what? But apparently confident that a few weeks of antibiotics *should* have cured the infection, many experts initially viewed post-treatment symptoms the way any "unexplained" symptoms tend to be: they minimized them and dismissed them as psychological. According to one 1993 article in *Science*, "Factors such as the premorbid personality and a tendency to somatization may determine the length of convalescence and the response to postinfection fatigue and joint aches." Another study claimed to find a link between "severe psychological trauma" and ongoing illness after Lyme infection. "In some cases, earlier symptoms may be the result of infection with the invading spirochete, but later chronic symptoms may be partially or entirely conversion phenomenon." In fact, in other cases, they suggested, the symptoms may have actually predated the infection, but afterward, the hysterical patient, in search of an organic cause of her suffering, attributed them to Lyme.

Such doctors were putting an awful lot of faith in antibiotics and their own very limited understanding of a just-discovered disease by turning to psychogenic explanations for post-treatment symptoms. After all, the pathogen that causes Lyme disease had been identified only in 1982, and there were vast unknowns about what it did once it left the bloodstream and entered the tissues. With no routine way to test for active infection, there was also no way to test for a cure. And the symptoms that some patients were reporting after treatment were many of the same symptoms that patients with late Lyme reported; it was hardly an unreasonable leap to suspect that maybe, just maybe, these symptoms had something to do with *B. burgdorferi*.

By the early nineties, skeptics of chronic Lyme were increasingly claiming that patients with ongoing symptoms actually had fibromyalgia or CFS. Certainly, muscle and joint pain, fatigue, and cognitive dysfunction

were symptoms shared among all three just recently defined and "unexplained" conditions. But concluding that patients who developed such
symptoms after being treated for Lyme really had fibromyalgia or ME/
CFS—syndromes for which there was neither a test nor an explanation—
amounted to rejecting one potential explanation for the symptoms, not offering another one. Simply swapping one contested diagnostic label—one
with a proposed underlying cause—with another of completely unknown
origin was saying nothing more than that you didn't believe that Lyme infection had anything to do with the patients' symptoms anymore.

And that was a matter of opinion, not fact, one that seemed to hinge
entirely on confidence in antibiotic treatment. As science journalist
Pamela Weintraub writes in her 2009 book *Cure Unknown: Inside the Lyme
Epidemic*, "Prior to treatment a symptomatic patient testing positive on
a Western blot would be diagnosed with Lyme; if the same patient failed
that treatment," she would be labeled with CFS or fibromyalgia. Sherrill, for
example, was told by a rheumatologist that her chronic back and neck pain
was fibromyalgia and that, despite starting right after her bout with Lyme,
it "had nothing to do with Lyme disease."

And of course, within the broader medical community, fibromyalgia
and ME/CFS were themselves largely seen as psychogenic disorders. No
doubt some Lyme experts who argued that chronic Lyme was just misdiagnosed fibromyalgia and ME/CFS genuinely took the position that the
latter conditions had an underlying pathology that, though unrelated to
Lyme, would ultimately be unraveled. But it's hard not to see the tendency
to shift Lyme patients who failed to get better after antibiotic treatment
into these diagnostic categories as a way of dismissing them as hysterics
and hypochondriacs without coming right out and saying so. In fact, some
mainstream Lyme experts tipped their hand by lumping all three conditions together as made-up diagnoses: one wrote in a 2003 letter to the editor, "We would all be better off without the patient advocacy agencies that
have sprung up for chronic Lyme disease, fibromyalgia, chronic fatigue
syndrome, and other fictitious illnesses."

What Lyme experts really thought about chronic Lyme patients became increasingly clear as patients resisted the new fibromyalgia and ME/
CFS labels. In a 2002 article, one prominent proponent of the mainstream

view of Lyme argued that "chronic Lyme disease is yet another in a long series of 'containers' for ill-defined suffering," one that "holds a certain appeal for patients searching" for explanations for their "medically unexplained symptoms" since it is a real, "curable illness with a well-established treatment." In his view, most patients with post-treatment symptoms had "depression and high levels of stress" before infection, predisposing them to "chronic, nonspecific symptoms and complaints." Encouraged by Lyme-literate physicians to attribute them to Lyme, they "adopt a permanent sick role in light of their firmly entrenched belief that they have an incurable disease" and become angry at doctors who don't agree with the diagnosis, because their illness behavior "has become their only fundamentally acceptable 'language' for expression of their distress."

In its 2006 guidelines, the Infectious Diseases Society of America (the professional group representing the mainstream view of Lyme) put forth a definition of post-treatment Lyme disease syndrome (PTLDS). While granting that ongoing symptoms could be due to "slow resolution of an inflammatory process," they focused on the notion that they may be related to "the emotional state" of the patient before falling ill. In fact, they questioned whether the symptoms were really all that different than the "background complaints" reported by much of the population. "In many patients, posttreatment symptoms appear to be more related to the aches and pains of daily living rather than to either Lyme disease or a tick-borne co-infection. Put simply, there is a relatively high frequency of the same kinds of symptoms in 'healthy' people."

While mainstream Lyme experts have grudgingly started to accept that PTLDS may be real—though absolutely not due to a chronic infection—they argue that many patients who've been diagnosed with "chronic Lyme" have neither PTLDS nor late Lyme—that they have never been infected with *B. burgdorferi* at all. Instead, these patients too really have ME/CFS, fibromyalgia, or "medically unexplained symptoms" not otherwise specified, but push for a Lyme diagnosis because it's considered more respectable. The thinking, as historian of medicine Robert A. Aronowitz has paraphrased, is that "a market for somatic labels exists in the large pool of 'stressed-out' or somaticizing patients who seek to disguise an emotional complaint or to 'upgrade' their diagnosis from a nebulous one to a legitimate disease."

In making this case, mainstream Lyme experts tend to obscure the reality that, given the limitations of the current Lyme tests, the lack of a positive blood test indicating exposure to *B. burgdorferi* is not conclusive evidence that they haven't been exposed. As researchers from the Johns Hopkins Lyme Disease Research Center explain, "Until a gold standard with high sensitivity for exposure to *B. burgdorferi* becomes available the percentage of patients with medically unexplained symptoms that are due to exposure to *B. burgdorferi* infection will remain unknown." In other words, without an accurate biomarker of active infection, cure, or previous exposure to *B. burgdorferi*, it is simply not possible to determine with certainty whether a patient with symptoms of fibromyalgia, ME/CFS, or other "medically unexplained symptoms" has indeed been infected with *B. burgdorferi*—or whether their symptoms were triggered by a Lyme infection that's been cured or are the result of ongoing infection.

An implication of the psychological theory of chronic Lyme was that the condition was perpetuated by those in the medical community and the media who humored its existence. Mainstream experts blamed "sensationalist" media coverage of Lyme for fostering an irrational fear of the disease among "the overanxious 'worried well.'" Never mind that the very first studies on the disease in the early eighties had demonstrated that a minority of patients had persisting symptoms post-treatment. In fact, in a 2005 article, two experts worried that media coverage of a recently published meta-analysis on what percentage of patients have post-treatment symptoms may actually worsen the problem. "We hope that misinterpretation of their report will not exacerbate the anxiety and misattribution that are probably at the root of much of the [PTLDS] predominantly limited to females in the Northeast."

GENDER BIASED AND SEX BLIND

Of course these chronic Lyme patients were stereotyped as women—specifically hypochondriacal, affluent women obsessed with every minor threat in their "suburban splendor," as two skeptics put it. In 1991, a satirical column in *Annals of Internal Medicine* ridiculed them. Adopting the voice of a representative of the "Centers of Fatigue Control," the author wrote of a new disease called "Lime disease": "The growing national epidemic of Lime disease [paralleled] increased public awareness and knowledge of Lyme disease." Rates of so-called Lime were "highest in adults of upper middle to upper socio-economic class, with a female-to-male sex ratio of 3:1 (in contrast to the more balanced age and sex distribution of Lyme disease)," he wrote. "Recent case-control studies of clusters of Lime disease have shown a weak to moderate association with previous attendance at cocktail parties serving lime-garnished mixed drinks, but very strong association with recent exposure to media stories on Lyme disease."

In a 2009 article entitled "Implications of Gender in Chronic Lyme Disease," two prominent mainstream Lyme experts dropped the satire and just made the case straight: that women's overrepresentation among "chronic Lyme" sufferers was evidence against the idea that there is such a thing. In an argument reminiscent of the recasting of the Royal Free Hospital outbreak as a case of mass hysteria on the basis that it mostly affected women, their case went like so: since men and women are about equally likely to be diagnosed with early Lyme (with the slight edge to men), if chronic Lyme were caused by ongoing infection with *B. burgdorferi,* then you'd expect it also would affect both genders equally. "On the other hand, if there is a substantial difference in the gender of patients with chronic Lyme disease, it is additional evidence that this disease is unrelated to infection with *B. burgdorferi.*" Ergo, the fact that more women than men have a diagnosis of chronic Lyme means they probably really have fibromyalgia, CFS (conditions more common among women), or "unexplained symptoms that did not meet criteria for either fibromyalgia or chronic fatigue syndrome," since "there is also usually a female preponderance in patients with unexplained symptoms" in general.

It would seem to be the height of circular logic to argue that Lyme infection couldn't possibly be the explanation for some women's "medically unexplained symptoms" because women are more likely to have "medically unexplained symptoms." But that's not even the biggest flaw in their argument. In fact, they offered a rather selective summary of the known sex/gender differences in the epidemiology of Lyme. On the basis of three studies, they claimed that PTLDS (that is, persistent symptoms in patients who have been treated for objectively confirmed early Lyme) is equally common among men and women. And they used that fact to bolster their argument that most women with a diagnosis of "chronic Lyme" have never actually been infected with Lyme at all. But the majority of studies that have looked at the question over the past few decades suggests that there actually is a difference: women are more likely than men to develop chronic symptoms post-treatment.

They also conspicuously failed to mention another striking gender difference: men are about twice as likely as women to be diagnosed with late Lyme. According to the strict CDC criteria, a late Lyme diagnosis requires objective swelling of the joints or neurological effects and a positive antibody test. Given the relative gender balance in early Lyme diagnoses, this overrepresentation of men in late diagnoses is also begging for an explanation. As Dr. John Aucott, director of the Johns Hopkins Lyme Disease Research Center, has asked, "What happened to all the women?" There are a number of possible explanations: It could be that for some reason women are just less susceptible to aggressive strains of Lyme. It could be that women's more robust immune response more effectively shuts down the infection before it spreads. It could be that women are actually less likely to be infected with Lyme than men but more likely to seek prompt treatment, leading to a gender balance in diagnoses at the early stage, while more men don't get treated early and thus progress to the late stage.

But it could also be that the women with late Lyme are more likely to go undiagnosed, or misdiagnosed—with, say, fibromyalgia or CFS—because they have "atypical" presentations that don't meet the official diagnostic criteria. And if women were both more likely to have chronic symptoms after being treated for early Lyme and more likely to have unrecognized subjective manifestations of late Lyme, then their overrepresentation among chronic Lyme patients wouldn't be a mystery at all—or grounds for concluding that it's simply the result of misdiagnosis. It would be an indictment of diagnostic criteria and a treatment paradigm that appears to be letting many Lyme patients, the majority of them women, fall through the cracks.

But, as in many realms, until recently, potential sex/gender differences in Lyme have been utterly overlooked. Aucott and his Johns Hopkins research team are working to change that. Several years ago, research program coordinator Alison Rebman was inspired after reading new research documenting sex/gender differences in other infectious diseases. Noticing the clues in the Lyme epidemiological research that suggested "that there is something going on there," she started combing through the literature to see what was already known about sex/gender differences in the disease. There was amazingly little. "When we went back and looked at the really foundational work, the patient groups aren't separated out by sex. And in some papers they don't even report the sex in their analyses," she says. Studies directly exploring possible differences in the clinical presentation, response to treatment, and immunology of Lyme infection were virtually nonexistent. A PubMed search of the terms "gender/sex," "immunity," and "Lyme" turned up five papers, only two of which were relevant. "It hasn't been done in general, in a lot of areas, but it *really* hasn't been done in Lyme disease."

The Johns Hopkins team figured that this might be "worth looking into, since in a lot of other areas—including other infectious diseases—there's this new wave of findings that hint at there being some important immunological differences" between men and women, Rebman says. The center is one of the few research groups in the country that's specifically focused on determining the cause of post-treatment symptoms in Lyme. That, in and of itself, is incredible; controversy over chronic Lyme has been rocking the medical community for decades, yet little concerted effort has been made to actually figure out what's going on with such patients.

The center is taking an open-minded approach to the question, looking at the possibility of chronic low-grade infection, as well as some sort of immune dysfunction triggered by the initial infection. The psychological theory, though, is already out: in 2012, they conducted the first prospective study that tracked a group of patients treated for early Lyme to see which of them had persistent symptoms six months later. There were no differences in psychological traits between the group that developed PTLDS (over a third of their sample) and those who didn't. And contrary to mainstream experts' characterization of these chronic symptoms as "mild," comparable to "the aches and pains of daily living," the patients were significantly impacted by them.

In 2010, the center's first study directly looking at sex/gender differences found that the standard antibody test, hardly very sensitive in general, may be even less so in women. Among patients with confirmed early Lyme disease, just a third of the women, compared to half of the men, had a positive result on the two-tier blood test. And a study they did in 2015 suggests that women may be especially unlikely to test positive after antibiotic treatment. If it turns out that, like the standard test for a heart attack, the standard Lyme blood test systematically underdiagnoses women, that of course is just all the more reason to suspect that it's much more likely that women who actually have Lyme get misdiagnosed with fibromyalgia or ME/CFS, or are left totally undiagnosed, than the reverse. "It is an unanswered question because there have really only been a few studies that have started to look at this," Rebman says. Other unanswered questions include the following: Are there any sex/gender differences in the pharmacokinetics of antibiotic treatment on Lyme infection? Are women more likely to have persistent symptoms after Lyme because the infection sets off an autoimmune reaction or some other kind of immune dysfunction?

We don't know yet, but it's remarkable that researchers have just recently started to ask these questions. Weintraub points out that mainstream Lyme experts have continually framed the controversy over the disease as a contest between the unreliable anecdotal experiences of patients versus the rational pursuit of hard science, "as if the antiseptic 'objectivity' of one trumps the sheer desperation of the other, proving they must be right." But, she writes, "if we are rejecting patient anecdote for the 'higher truth' of evidence-based medicine, shouldn't we make sure that the evidence is solid, objective, and sound?" What Weintraub concluded after eight years of investigation is that our knowledge of Lyme is disputed and incomplete at best. "The truth is that the mainstream experts have imposed a rigid template on an entity they don't fully understand." And a complete blindness to the possibility that there may be sex/gender differences—in symptoms, risk of missed diagnoses, accuracy of blood tests, effectiveness of treatment, and long-term complications—is one of the ways our understanding of Lyme has been woefully incomplete.

The story of chronic Lyme is in many ways a perfect illustration of how the knowledge gap and the trust gap create an interlocking circle that allows medicine to maintain the illusion that its knowledge is already complete. On the one hand, medicine has ignored the possibility of biologically based variations in how Lyme affects men and women, operating from an untested assumption that there are no sex/gender differences. On the other hand, it has turned to stereotypes about women's alleged susceptibility to hysteria—the medical "fact" that they are more likely to have "medically unexplained symptoms"—to account for the inconsistencies that don't fit the rigid template it has imposed on the disease. It relies on sexist stereotypes to fill in the gaps in knowledge that it refuses to acknowledge are there.

Thirty-five years after *B. burgdorferi* was identified, after the fight over Lyme disease turned into one of the ugliest doctor-versus-doctor battles in medicine, this pattern is hopefully beginning to change. Some researchers are finally trying to explain Lyme patients' chronic symptoms instead of trying to explain them *away*. And they are finally viewing the predominance of women among chronic Lyme patients not as a reason to dismiss the condition but as a clue that can help solve the puzzle. As Rebman says, "There's a ton to do."

───────

And the work can't happen fast enough, because the controversy over the disease has made the experience of getting a diagnosis and proper treatment perhaps even more difficult for Lyme patients over the last few decades.

In 2008, Sherrill got Lyme again. In a cruel irony, it was after putting tick repellent in the woods on her Pennsylvania property that she found an engorged tick embedded in her hip, and the rash soon followed. All too aware of how important it was to get treated right away, she immediately made an appointment, and a nurse practitioner prescribed ten days of an antibiotic. She assumed she'd be fine. But a few weeks later, she suddenly began having hourly episodes of flushing and sweating. She developed vertigo, ringing in her ears, muscle aches, and fatigue. The whites of her eyes turned red and bloodshot. She rapidly lost thirty pounds. She mixed up words and couldn't think. "Writing a simple email, I'd have to carefully go over every word to ensure it made sense."

Since joint pain wasn't one of the multitude of symptoms she now had, Sherrill at first didn't think it could be Lyme. When she saw her primary care doctor, who'd known her for years, he congratulated her on the weight loss: "Hey, that's a good weight for you!" She burst into tears; she was 118 pounds and terribly ill. He sent her to endocrinologist after endocrinologist, who told her nothing was wrong. Like Brea, Sherrill started bringing her husband to appointments. "That just changes the conversation completely. It's amazing what a difference a guy in the room makes."

Indeed, I spoke to a depressing number of women with a range of conditions who attested to the power of a male relative—whether a partner, a father, or even a son—to help ensure their symptoms were taken seriously. One eighteen-year-old woman went to the ER twice reporting sudden chest pain—once by herself and once with a friend—only to be sent home with the suggestion that it was anxiety once cardiac diagnostic tests came back normal. The third time, she brought her dad. "He was just repeating everything I said," she recalls, but it did the trick. This time, the doctors ran blood tests—and then sent her to emergency surgery to remove her gallbladder. Another woman, who is battling for disability compensation after losing her job due to fibromyalgia and ME/CFS, told me that her "six-foot-seven, deep-voiced 20-year-old son" accompanies her to every medical and legal appointment. "People don't hear me," she says, "but when he opens his mouth, lo and behold, they have ears!"

An ear, nose, and throat doctor finally noticed the tick bite in Sherrill's chart and suggested this was Lyme and she should get IV antibiotic treatment. But many doctors aren't willing to try longer courses of antibiotic treatment on patients who've already been treated, and those who are usually do not accept insurance. Eventually, she found a doctor who would give her three months of IV antibiotic treatment, although when her blood test came back negative, she had to pay for it—all $12,000—out of pocket. She was improved but not completely better afterward. Over the years, additional antibiotics have helped. After one round of tetracycline several years ago, the "fibromyalgia" pain she'd had for twenty-five years disappeared. She found out only years later that she was also infected with two of the tick-borne coinfections that can accompany Lyme: *Babesia microti*, which causes a malaria-like illness, and anaplasmosis, which presents like a severe flu. Eight years later, she says she's about 80 percent better, but episodes of sweating, vertigo, tinnitus, aches, and fatigue still come and go.

As Sherrill searched for an explanation for her mysterious illness, she found that even mentioning the "L word" seemed to make doctors suspicious. The heated controversy over chronic Lyme seems to have created an aura of doubt surrounding the whole disease, as if there are no patients who truly have Lyme disease, only patients convinced they do. When she told one physician that she'd been treated for Lyme, the doctor started to cut her off—as if by reflex: "But you don't live in an endemic area." In fact, Sherrill lives in Chester County, Pennsylvania, which is the *number one* county in the entire United States for Lyme cases. When she saw an infectious disease specialist recently and started to give her medical history— that she'd been bitten by a tick in 2008, had a brief course of antibiotics, and never fully recovered—she got the same knee-jerk response. "He was immediately hostile: 'Who told you you have Lyme disease?'" He interrogated her on every step of her story. Both doctors wrote CFS as the diagnosis in their notes.

CHEMICAL INTOLERANCE

According to surveys, 13 percent of Americans report being hypersensitive to common synthetic chemicals in products like pesticides, formaldehyde, fresh paint, new carpets, diesel exhaust, perfumes, air fresheners, insecticide, cleaning products, nail polish, hair spray, and tobacco smoke. Four percent say they become ill from them every day, which amounts to a whopping 11 million Americans with at least moderately severe chemical intolerance. At least 13.5 percent of people with chemical intolerance are unemployed because of their illness. In the most severe cases, people often become socially isolated and homeless in a desperate bid to do the only thing that improves their symptoms, one that is all but impossible in the modern developed world: avoid chemicals.

Of all the contested conditions that affect mainly women, chemical intolerance—which has also been known as multiple chemical sensitivity

(MCS), environmental illness, chemical injury, and twentieth-century disease—is perhaps the most marginalized. While fibromyalgia, ME/CFS, and PTLDS are at least recognized by mainstream medicine and receive some—far too small—amount of federal research funding, chemical intolerance has been largely ignored for decades. A 2007 survey of physicians found that a little over half of respondents were familiar with chemical intolerance. Under a third had received any medical training on the condition, and only 7 percent were "very satisfied" with their knowledge, although almost all had encountered chemically intolerant patients. And that was of the self-selected group of doctors who'd cared enough to respond to the survey at all. The study's authors noted that, in what may be a telling "indication of the position of MCS in mainstream medicine," one doctor sent a blank survey back with a note that read, "Don't waste my time any more."

Chemical intolerance was first described in the fifties as the "petrochemical problem" by an allergist named Theron Randolph. He observed patients who reported a wide range of symptoms (asthma, headaches, fatigue, depression, joint pain, racing heart, dizziness, nausea, difficulty concentrating) that seemed to be caused by sensitivity to extremely low doses of chemicals but were different from traditional allergies. He isolated his patients in special chemical-free rooms for days, watched their symptoms vanish, then reintroduced chemicals one by one to see which they were reacting to. Randolph's work inspired a movement of "clinical ecologists."

By the eighties, the condition was known as multiple chemical sensitivity, and it provoked fights between clinical ecologists and allergists, who considered the former to be practitioners of a "junk science." Chemical intolerance expert Dr. Claudia Miller, who is an immunologist and environmental health expert at the University of Texas Health Science Center at San Antonio, has suggested that allergists were so resistant to Randolph's heretical ideas because until recently *they* had been the heretics. When the word *allergy* was first coined in 1906, it described a general state of "altered reactivity" of all sorts. But as knowledge of the immune system grew, it was redefined to refer specifically to immune hypersensitivity. Until the discovery of immunoglobulin E (IgE) in the sixties, mainstream medicine was skeptical of the burgeoning allergy specialty. "Allergists had been accused by their colleagues of practicing witchcraft and 'voodoo' medicine when they treated their patients by injecting them with tiny amounts of the same substances to which they reacted. With the discovery of IgE, allergists at last had a scientific basis for their practices," writes Miller. They guarded it defensively.

Then there was the fact that most of the patients were women. "Many of the first cases of [chemical intolerance] described involved individual, upper-middle-class women. Such cases often were viewed as depression or 'hysterical housewife syndrome' and referred accordingly," Miller writes. The patients' many symptoms with no discernible cause were pretty much destined to be read as somatization. "In medical school, young doctors-to-be often are taught that the more symptoms a patient reports, the less likely there is to be anything to them, i.e., the diagnosis is probably a psychological one."

While it was especially easy to dismiss individual cases, even some of the first cases of mass illness from chemical exposures were written off as hysterical women. Many of the early outbreaks of "sick building syndrome" were among female clerical workers, and the initial response was to attribute their symptoms to "mass psychogenic illness." As historian Michelle Murphy writes in her 2006 book, *Sick Building Syndrome and the Problem of Uncertainty: Environmental Politics, Technoscience, and Women Workers*, "In debates between experts over the reality of sick building syndrome, the fact that women made up the majority of complainants opened up the possibility of using the diagnosis of hysteria to explain worker unrest." Experts eventually concluded that new energy-efficient building standards adopted in the seventies had led to poor ventilation and high levels of volatile organic compounds, which were already well known to have negative health effects, in many "sick buildings."

Throughout the nineties, the medical literature described MCS patients as well-off women between the ages of thirty and fifty years old. In 1999, the first population-based survey found that the condition was indeed more common in women but—you guessed it—occurred across all races and income levels. But the stereotype allowed MCS to be dismissed, alongside "yuppie flu" and so-called "Lime disease," as a "fashionable" diagnosis for stressed-out hypochondriacs. One doctor quoted in a 1994 media article on the condition declared, "It's a belief, not a disease. It's a culturally acquired anxiety disorder, without known cause."

Similar to the charge against chronic Lyme patients, women with MCS were portrayed as latching on to chemicals as the cause of their ill-defined suffering because it offered a legitimate explanation. As Murphy writes, MCS was seen as a "version of women's age-old ability to psychosomaticize their distress; in the 1990s, symptoms take the form of chemical phobias instead of hysterical paralysis." Again, as with Lyme, the media and other cultural forces were blamed for fostering an irrational fear, in this case not of an infectious pathogen but of an increasingly toxic world.

A WHOLE NEW THEORY OF DISEASE?

But of course, the reality was that the world *was*—objectively, unquestion-ably—becoming increasingly toxic. (Just as Lyme was, *actually*, a growing epidemic thanks to shifting land-use patterns and suburban development in forested areas.) Medicine managed to blame chemical intolerance on a fear of chemicals, rather than on chemicals themselves, despite the fact that there's been an exponential increase in the use of largely untested synthetic chemicals in everyday products since World War II. In the early nineties, the National Research Council warned that of the 70,000 commercially used chemicals, less than 10 percent had been evaluated for neurotoxicity. Every day about 15,000 new substances are added. Meanwhile, the average American now spends 90 percent of their lives inside, in indoor air that is far more polluted than outdoor air.

And it's not as if anyone denies that many synthetic chemicals can have serious impacts on health. Most people with chemical intolerance re-port that their symptoms began after a particular chemical exposure or a series of them. And it is well accepted that at *large* doses, the chemicals that patients most commonly say triggered their illness are toxicants—man-made poisons—that can make people sick. Many natural exper-iments have demonstrated that when people fall ill from toxic chemical exposures—from oil-spill cleanup crews to Gulf War veterans to workers in remodeled buildings—some of them remain permanently sick. In 1987, for example, 225 employees got sick after 27,000 feet of new carpet was installed in the headquarters of the Environmental Protection Agency. Most recovered, but a couple dozen developed long-term chemical intolerance and sued the building owners.

In 1997, Miller proposed the theory of toxicant-induced loss of tolerance (TILT) to explain chemical intolerance. It's a two-step process: A genetically susceptible person gets sick after a large chemical exposure (say, after spraying a pesticide) or repeated lower-level exposures (say, working every day in a nail salon). That initial exposure damages the neurological and immune systems, and they begin to lose their usual tolerance to the many chemicals we all encounter on a daily basis. Gradually, they start reacting to not just the particular chemical that first made them sick but others as well. That's in line with what most chemically intolerant patients describe: they were fine until one day they weren't, and then it got worse and worse.

While the exact physiological mechanism underlying TILT is unknown, it is hardly unlikely that certain people, due to differing levels of exposure or genetic vulnerabilities, are affected by the known poisons in our environment in ways that medicine does not yet understand. An Australian study that looked at the differences between physicians who "believed" in chemical intolerance and those who didn't found it simply came down to how comprehensive they considered our current knowledge of the effects of toxic chemicals on human health. Those who thought it was at least *possible* we didn't know everything tended to treat the experiences of chemically intolerant patients as a source of knowledge.

Indeed, the loss of knowledge that has resulted from medicine's distrust of women's accounts is staggering to think about. The nineteenth-century physician Sir William Osler, who is often described as "the father of modern medicine," famously said, "Listen to the patient. He is telling you the diagnosis." And there is perhaps no better indication of just how far medicine has drifted from that wisdom than the skepticism toward chemically intolerant patients. Here, after all, are patients who not only are telling medicine that they are sick but also have identified what makes them sick and what makes them better. In the real world, where common sense reigns, the fact that chemically intolerant patients become ill when exposed to chemicals and improve when they avoid them is rather good evidence that the chemicals are causing their symptoms. But in medicine, women's reports count for so little that even their experience of a cause-and-effect relationship is not trusted. A demonstrable fact, it is treated as if it is something that can be "believed in" or not. The specter of the hysterical woman is apparently so powerful that invoking her is enough to cast doubt on an empirical reality.

Researchers have put forth a few different hypotheses about how people become "TILTed." Perhaps the most popular is one that borrows from research on epilepsy and chronic pain. Toxicants travel straight to the limbic system of our brain—bypassing the blood-brain barrier—via the olfactory receptors in our nose. Perhaps one large chemical exposure or many smaller ones permanently sensitize the olfactory neurons; as in chronic pain, in which neurons respond to weaker and weaker pain signals, smaller and smaller exposures become necessary to excite the limbic network. Laboratory studies have implicated both central nervous system sensitization and inflammatory processes in the condition. Brain-imaging studies have shown abnormally reduced blood flow to particular regions of the brain when chemically intolerant patients are exposed to normal levels of common chemicals.

Experts believe chemical intolerance may be behind a large share of today's chronic illness. In a 2012 study published in *Annals of Family Medicine,* Miller and her colleagues measured the prevalence of the condition in four hundred patients visiting medical clinics in San Antonio, Texas, for chronic health problems. Of the mostly low-income and Hispanic patients, one in five reported chemical intolerance. In over 6 percent, the problem was severe. Far from being an affliction of the well off, the condition was more common among patients from lower socio-economic backgrounds: 9 percent versus nearly 25 percent. Compared to those without chemical intolerance, the patients reported seeking medical care more frequently and had higher rates of allergies, depression, panic disorder, and generalized anxiety disorder. Other research has found that people with chemical intolerance have increased rates of a wide variety of other health problems, including heart problems, asthma, autoimmune diseases, sinusitis, migraine, fibromyalgia, ME/CFS, and food intolerances.

The higher rate of mood disorders would, of course, be taken by those who consider the condition to be psychogenic as evidence of its psychiatric etiology. But experts on chemical intolerance suggest the causal arrow goes the other way—and not only because it's common for people with any chronic illness to become depressed or anxious. They think that the chemical exposures are producing the psychiatric symptoms. Indeed, there's no evidence that treating psychiatric symptoms in chemically intolerant patients helps without addressing the chemical intolerance. In one 2003 study that asked patients to rate the effectiveness of various conventional and alternative treatments, avoiding chemicals was the single most helpful thing, while prescription drugs like antidepressants and antianxiety meds were the very least.

Miller suggests that TILT may represent a whole new theory of disease, comparable to germ theory. In other words, chemical intolerance may not in fact be properly understood as a disease itself. It could be the underlying cause behind a whole class of diseases, explaining at least some cases of a wide range of chronic conditions—from asthma to migraine to depression to ME/CFS. It may seem audacious to predict that one of the most marginalized medical conditions holds the key to a game-changing paradigm shift in our understanding of disease. But the history of medicine suggests that may actually be a wise bet.

New theories of disease, Miller points out, have always arisen when medicine "observed patterns of illness that did not fit accepted explanations for disease at that time"—and then discovered a new mechanism that did explain them. The fact that chemical intolerance "does not fit already accepted mechanisms for disease is often offered as evidence that the condition does not exist," she writes. "However, the same criticism would have applied to the germ and immune theories of disease when they first were proposed." In fact, the same criticism *was* applied to them; medicine has consistently greeted new theories of disease with great skepticism initially. If TILT does end up being the next disease theory, the controversy and resistance it has faced for decades is par for the course.

"A NIGHTMARE SCENARIO"

Six years later, Brea is improved but still disabled by her illness. "I can leave my house now, but I can't walk more than fifty feet at a time, so I need to use a wheelchair. And I basically don't go out that much, because I always feel worse. If I go out for more than two hours in a day, I'll pay for it." In 2015, she cofounded #MEAction, an online platform for ME/CFS advocacy efforts. For the last four years, she's been working on a documentary about living with ME/CFS, called *Unrest*, featuring her own story and those of other patients around the world, which she directed mostly from her bed via Skype. The Sundance award–winning film had its theatrical release in 2017.

The neglect of ME/CFS by the medical community for three decades feels personal to Brea. "I was two years old when the Incline Village outbreak happened," she says. "I feel like there was a gunshot that went off during that outbreak. This disease has been with us for a very long time, but [that epidemic] was the first one to really raise it to the level of national consciousness in the U.S., and it was a real opportunity to start the race. And that didn't happen. Imagine what twenty-six years of research could have done. I feel like the hell that I've been through the last six years was completely preventable."

We should all be afraid of what the story of contested illnesses like ME/CFS, chronic Lyme, and chemical intolerance says about the medical system's ability (or inability) to recognize and respond to emerging diseases. Indeed, Johnson says she never wrote *Osler's Web* just for ME/CFS patients, although that's largely who has read the seven-hundred-page tome. She wrote it for the general public. "What I wanted to get across was that doctors really need to start listening to patients instead of simply running their practices by lab tests." Because even though doctors are taught to look for horses, not zebras, "every once in a while, there is a zebra." And those zebras will be missed—systematically overlooked by the millions—if doctors don't trust their patients "when they come in and say, 'I'm sick, I can't walk, I can't think.'"

There is little doubt that the gender of the majority of the patients with these contested diseases has contributed to that lack of trust. Time and time again, the fact that they are more common in women has been used as a reason to dismiss them and to suggest that they are just fashionable new labels for women's age-old hysteria. As Johnson says, "When you've got a new disease with an 80 percent attack rate in women, plus this reluctance of doctors to keep their eyes open for zebras, it's just a nightmare scenario." When science finally does fully explain ME/CFS, POTS, chronic Lyme, chemical intolerance, and other "medically unexplained symptoms"— which it surely will eventually—we should remember how many millions of women were dismissed and disbelieved during this interim period. After all, those who forget their history are destined to keep repeating it. And in a constantly changing world, with rising temperatures and shifting habitats and ever more environmental toxins, there will always be new diseases waiting around the next corner.

CONCLUSION

OVARIAN CANCER IS A rare disease, ranking fifth after lung, breast, colorectal, and pancreatic cancers when it comes to cancer deaths among women. But it's one of the deadliest. Each year, more than 22,000 Americans are diagnosed with the disease, and about 14,000 die of it. Overall, only about one-third of those diagnosed will survive for ten years or more. The main reason for the low survival rate is that most cases are caught when the disease is already quite advanced. If found and treated before the cancer has spread outside the ovary, 92 percent of patients will survive five years. But only 15 percent of cases are detected at this stage, and once it has spread beyond the pelvis to a distant part of the body, that five-year survival figure drops below 30 percent.

One reason ovarian cancer is difficult to catch early is that there's no routine screening method, comparable to a mammogram to detect breast cancer or a pap smear for cervical cancer, to test for the disease. When it's suspected, doctors will do a manual pelvic exam to feel for a growth, an ultrasound to view it, and a blood test known as CA-125 that measures a cancer antigen that's often elevated when you have the disease, but surgery is required to confirm that a tumor is cancerous.

Furthermore, for most of the past century, medicine has believed that the disease doesn't cause any symptoms, at least not until its later stages, when it is too late to cure. Until recently, it was known as a "silent killer," an "insidious" disease that offered little hope of defeat through prompt detection. In 1942, gynecologist Harry Sturgeon Crossen described the disease, with its "symptomless onset and symptomless progress," as a "creeping death which defies early discovery."

This fatalistic attitude has shaped our approach to fighting the disease ever since the "war on cancer" took off during the postwar period. At that time, some doctors suggested just removing the healthy ovaries of all postmenopausal women as a preventive measure, while others recommended frequent pelvic exams of middle-aged patients in a desperate but largely unrealistic bid at early detection. But as historian Patricia Jasen has explained, the possibility that there might be early symptoms that the patient herself, not the doctor, could notice was rarely considered. "The 'silent killer' image was now firmly associated with the disease," she writes, "and some standard textbooks said nothing at all about its symptoms at any stage, thus leaving medical students and practitioners without a basis for recognizing possible signs of ovarian cancer experienced by their patients." The patients themselves were left in the dark too; ovarian cancer wasn't included in public awareness campaigns that, in pursuit of early detection, urged women to recognize the symptoms of and seek care for other cancers.

Despite the "silent killer" stereotype, as far back as the 1930s some doctors had been asking their ovarian cancer patients about their symptoms, and many said that they'd noticed abdominal discomfort and digestive problems, and sometimes even reported it to doctors, in the months, sometimes years, before the cancer was found. Sure, compared to the lump or unexplained bleeding of breast and uterine cancer respectively, these symptoms could be considered fairly vague and nonspecific, but the pattern was common enough that, British gynecologist Stanley Way argued in 1951, they should be considered to be "of diagnostic importance." He called for all women over forty who complained of such symptoms to be fully examined. Yet three decades later, the idea that ovarian cancer had no symptoms was still firmly entrenched. "All too often," gynecologist Hugh Barber lamented, an ovarian cancer patient complaining of early symptoms "is considered a middle-aged crock who goes to too many cocktail parties and eats too many hors d'oeuvres."

Even as concern about ovarian cancer grew along with rising rates of the disease between the 1960s and 1990s, medicine paid little attention to better understanding the symptoms. A prominent gynecology textbook in 1988 reminded students, "Ovarian cancer, is unfortunately, very insidious and 'silent' in terms of signs and symptoms." Instead, better epidemiological research in the eighties finally helped identify genetic and environmental risk factors for the disease. Meanwhile, considerable effort was put toward coming up with a mass screening method that could be used in all women. It wasn't until that goal began to look unlikely (while a combination of a pelvic exam, ultrasound imaging, and the CA-125 blood test are helpful in detecting the disease, they aren't accurate enough to be useful for routine screening) that some within the medical community finally accepted that there was one further option to explore: as one research team put it in 1996, "We have to rely on the woman and her initiative in order to achieve an early diagnosis."

The women had, in fact, been suggesting that for quite some time. Throughout the eighties and nineties ovarian cancer patients increasingly told their stories, first in the media and eventually on the Internet, and a common theme emerged that thoroughly challenged the notion that the disease was a "silent" menace. Many women had symptoms before being diagnosed that either they themselves or their doctors had dismissed, or else misdiagnosed as things like acid reflux, a bladder infection, gallstones, depression, menopause, or IBS. Advocacy groups began to insist that, contrary to its reputation, ovarian cancer was actually "the disease that whispers" with early symptoms that women could hear if only they—and, importantly, their doctors—would "listen." In fact, some argued, often the disease was actually shouting.

Beth, who was diagnosed with ovarian cancer in 1987, was active in one of the earliest online ovarian cancer support groups. "We talked about how so many of us had very similar experiences: we'd go to doctors with a list of worrisome symptoms, some even concerned about ovarian cancer because they had relatives who'd had it, but were told that it couldn't possibly be ovarian cancer because ovarian cancer has no symptoms; it was 'the silent killer,'" she says. "Eventually, diagnosis would occur, and then the patient would say to the doctor that 'see, they had symptoms!' And the doctor would reply that 'no, they had the silent killer, so what they were experiencing couldn't possibly have been symptoms.'" This kind of circular reasoning was maddening. "Women were shouting to be heard, but the louder we shouted, the more we were told we were silent or speaking nonsense."

A turning point finally came at a survivor conference in 1998. During the Q&A after a presentation on ovarian cancer, a member of the audience asked the speaker, a Harvard physician, to elaborate on the early symptoms of the disease. He replied with the standard line: well, there are none. By all accounts, he touched a nerve among the crowd of mostly ovarian cancer survivors. "They simultaneously decided they were mad as hell and weren't going to take it anymore," Beth says. They stood up and started shouting, approaching the stage in "an almost theatrical embodiment of an outraged mob."

Dr. Barbara Goff, a young gynecologic oncologist, happened to witness this eruption. "I sat in the back of the room, thinking, 'I'm glad I didn't give this talk, because I probably would have answered the question the same way,'" she says. "Throughout my fairly prestigious Ivy League education—an Ivy League college, an Ivy League medical school, an Ivy League residency—I had been taught that ovarian cancer is a silent killer." After the survivors-turned-outraged-mob settled down, Goff met some of them, and they asked her why the medical community wouldn't listen to them. "I said, well, there's this expert opinion and it's in every single textbook. The only way you're going to change that is by having some research that debunks this myth." The survivors asked if she could help make that happen, and she agreed.

Goff teamed with a prominent patient activist, Cindy Melancon, who ran a newsletter for ovarian cancer patients, to conduct a study of women's experiences getting diagnosed. They sent out 1,500 surveys, and they got a response rate of more than 100 percent, as patients forwarded it on to others, a testament, Goff says, to how much "pent-up demand to explain their stories" there was among the patient community. Published in the American Cancer Society's journal *Cancer* in 2000, the study concluded that "the majority of women with ovarian carcinoma are symptomatic and frequently have delays in diagnosis." And not just the patients with more advanced disease: nearly 90 percent of women with early-stage cancer (those patients who had between a 70 and 90 percent chance of survival) had symptoms prior to diagnosis.

The study also suggested that it was their doctors, more than the women themselves, who weren't hearing the "whispers" of the disease. While the patients did wait for an average of two to three months after their symptoms began to see a doctor, only about a fifth said the fact that they ignored their symptoms was the main barrier to getting a prompt diagnosis. Instead, about a third said the main problem was that they'd been misdiagnosed. Most had initially been given a wrong diagnosis or gotten some version of "it's all in your head": 15 percent were told they had IBS, 13 percent said that their doctors just told them "nothing was wrong," 12 percent got a label of "stress," and 6 percent were diagnosed with depression. Thirty percent had actually been given a prescription medication for another condition. Only 20 percent were told that they might have ovarian carcinoma.

There were limitations with that first study, including possible selection bias since the survey was sent out through a survivor newsletter, but it was a start. Goff and others went on to do more research on the topic and eventually developed a symptom index. In 2007, the American Cancer Society, the Gynecologic Cancer Foundation, and the Society of Gynecologic Oncologists officially retired the "silent killer" moniker. In a national consensus statement, they declared that four symptoms (bloating, pelvic or abdominal pain, difficulty eating or feeling full quickly, and urinary symptoms such as urgent or frequent feelings of needing to go) could indicate early ovarian cancer. The vast majority of the time, of course, they won't. But if the symptoms are new, occur nearly every day, and increase in severity for more than a few weeks, women should see a doctor for further evaluation.

"For years, women have known that ovarian cancer was not the silent killer it was said to be," the Ovarian Cancer Research Fund Alliance now declares on its website. "Over the past decade, science has confirmed what women have long known: ovarian cancer has symptoms."

The symbolism in this tale—the long struggle for women's voices to finally overturn an entrenched medical myth of a "silent" disease—is almost too pat.

Still, I was inclined to at least be optimistic about the happy ending. It may have taken a century, but the empowered patients had eventually found doctor-researchers who listened to them, and the result was a fruitful collaboration that pushed medical knowledge forward. Goff is more circumspect. "I'll tell you, there are still a lot of people who think that identifying ovarian cancer through symptoms is basically rubbish [and that] my research is a waste of time." While she and I may see it as a heartening example of partnership between the scientific and the patient communities, "because the advocates were involved, there are still scientists who think it's kind of 'soft' science."

According to Goff, there are also some "who say we shouldn't be teaching women about the symptoms of a potentially deadly disease, because all it does is cause them to worry." Since ovarian cancer is rare and its symptoms are common, critics argued that "women would be flooding their doctors' offices, that they'd be having anxiety, that they'd be having all sorts of unnecessary tests." The research suggests that the concern about over-testing is unfounded, but it's a revealing fear. Back in the sixties, during congressional hearings on the safety of the first birth control pill, doctors admitted that they didn't mention the side effects to their patients, because they didn't want to "plant seeds" in suggestible women: "If you tell them the symptoms they have them by the next day." More than half a century later, women are still thought to be such suggestible hypochondriacs that they'll work themselves into a tizzy over every minor, transient symptom.

This stereotype has no basis in reality. "Sure, we all have bloating from time to time," Goff says. "But women are smart; women know the difference between what they occasionally have, say, when they eat the wrong food or they're having their period, versus something that's not right for their body. They have busy lives, and they're not going to go running off to the doctor every two seconds when they have a little bit of abnormal bloating. Women don't do that; if anything, we tend to underestimate our problems."

Other researchers have suggested that improving the recognition of the symptoms won't necessarily lead to early enough diagnoses to significantly improve survival rates, and the best hope is still a screening method that can accurately detect the disease in symptomless women. At this point, the research to determine how better symptom recognition may affect survival rates just hasn't been done, but given how much better the odds are when ovarian cancer is caught early, it's worth a shot. And, as Goff says, "If you can diagnose a cancer earlier, why *wouldn't* you want to do that? Who would say, 'Oh no, let's diagnose her cancer later'?"

Besides, at this point, without a screening test, the symptoms are simply all we've got. "The best way to make a diagnosis is for physicians to have a high index of suspicion in symptomatic patients," Goff says. "So whether people like it or not, we make the diagnosis based on symptoms, so we need to be keyed into them." Which means we need to listen to women.

CHALLENGING THE POWER OF MEDICINE

The circular logic that ovarian cancer patients were up against is one so many women know all too well: The women with MS told that the pain they felt was simply impossible because MS doesn't cause pain. The teens whose endometriosis has gone undiagnosed because that's a "career women's disease." While science may, at its best, be self-correcting, medical facts can be stubbornly self-fulfilling—at least in a medical system that has an alternative explanation for any symptoms in women that it can't explain. Once accepted, medical myths tend to create their own reality. Were it not for patient advocacy, IC no doubt could have remained a rare psychosomatic condition of postmenopausal women, the millions of patients who didn't fit the profile dismissed to suffer their unexplained symptoms alone. For over a century, ovarian cancer *was* a silent killer. After all, do symptoms that medicine can't hear really make a sound?

It's not a surprise that the first step toward overturning the silent-killer myth came when ovarian cancer survivors began sharing their common experiences with each other online. It's hard to overstate how much the Internet has changed things for so many women patients, as the patient advocates I spoke to who first fell ill in the eighties and nineties attested to. Perhaps most obviously, thanks to the greater accessibility of medical information, it is far easier to diagnose yourself when the medical system fails to. "If we had the Internet back when I got sick," says Cynthia Toussaint, whose CRPS was undiagnosed for thirteen years, "I would have known what I had the day I got it." It's also easier for patients today to share practical advice with each other and organize for more research and greater awareness.

But the Internet has provided something even more basic for many women patients, particularly for those with diseases that medicine doesn't understand: the assurance that they are not alone and that they are not crazy. "I can't even tell you how isolating it was," Paula Kamen says of the years she spent searching for help for her chronic headache in the nineties. "You feel like you're the only one not being cured. When you go to a doctor, they make you feel like you're such an unusual case." It wasn't until she published her book in 2006 and started hearing from other headache patients that she truly realized she wasn't a "freak." "I was exactly the same as so many others."

This, in and of itself, can serve as an antidote to the delegitimization of women's experiences that is so pervasive within the medical system. Medicine has an enormous power: the authority, as Susan Wendell puts it, "to confirm or deny the reality of everyone's bodily experience"—to determine which symptoms are "explained" and which are "unexplained," to judge who is a sick person deserving of care and sympathy and who is a "heartsink patient" trying to get the "secondary gains" of the "sick role." But when women patients get together and see that their own experiences are also others' experiences, they can take some of that power back. As Amy Berkowitz, the writer with vulvodynia and fibromyalgia, says, "Whether or not fibromyalgia is a 'real' thing, we all have it."

I have to believe that most health care providers simply do not fully appreciate the harm they are capable of causing by doubting or belittling women's symptoms. When medicine denies the reality of your bodily experience, it is a deeply invalidating form of gaslighting: "What can I know if I can't know what I am feeling in my own body?" Wendell writes. "How can I remain connected to a world that denies I am in pain, or dizzy, or nauseated, when I myself cannot deny that I am?" For Berkowitz, finding other women online "who were feeling all the same experiences of shame and despair and literal pain" was, simply, lifesaving. "I honestly think that I would have killed myself if I'd been diagnosed with vulvodynia at age twenty-two after my first sexual experience and didn't have anyone to talk to about it."

I hope that this book has provided a basis for women to recognize that many of their experiences with the medical system are ones they share with other women across diseases. While the stories of a woman with ovarian cancer and a woman with an autoimmune disease may quickly diverge once they get diagnosed, until they are, they are often very similar. Though living with vulvodynia and living with ME/CFS are each difficult in their own unique ways, the reason that there is such a lack of awareness and so little research on these conditions is largely the same. While our diseases may be different, many of women's problems with the medical system are rooted in the same history and the same systemic problems.

Women's "doctor stories" are similar, even when they are quite different. A white Ivy league college student is more likely to be seen as anxiety-ridden, while a woman of color is more likely to be stereotyped as a drug seeker. "Educated white women" are seen as health-obsessed hypochondriacs who need to get off WebMD. But less-educated women may be seen as malingerers looking for a disability check. A thin woman is told she can't be seriously ill since she "looks so good!" while a fat woman is told all her symptoms are due to her weight. For most of our lives, we are "too young" to be sick anyway, and our symptoms can be blamed on menstrual cramps, pregnancy, motherhood, and menopause. By the time we're finally old enough to be seen as sick, we're so old that nobody cares if we are. Our intersecting identities may make the particular stereotypes that hurt us different—in some cases, even diametrically opposed—and yet somehow we so often end up in a similar place: fighting to have our reports of our symptoms trusted and taken seriously.

Of course, women have varying abilities to fight their way out of this place. Only some women have the enormous reserves of money and time required to see forty doctors over nine months to get properly diagnosed, as POTS sufferer Lauren Stiles did. Not all women of color are able to find doctors who will get on the phone for them in the middle of the night to ensure that the ER gatekeepers let them into the hospital, as Jackie eventually was. Only some women with Lyme disease have a retirement fund they can empty, as Sherrill did, in order to pay $12,000 out of pocket for treatment. Though it may be far easier for many women to diagnose themselves these days, as Ellen, Nicole, and Jen Brea did, not all women have the language skills and Internet savvy needed to do so. Too many trans women and overweight women find seeing a doctor so stressful and dehumanizing that they risk their health to avoid it altogether. And for many women, like Alexis, even when they finally find the quality medical care they need, it's out of their financial reach.

When I started researching this book, I expected that women's stories would be similar and rooted in the same systemic problems, but I didn't anticipate finding that our fates are so intimately intertwined. In a medical system with a tendency to assume that anything it can't explain is psychogenic, as long as women have more "medically unexplained symptoms" thanks to the knowledge gap, women will continue to find that they are stereotyped as stressed-out somaticizers and their symptoms are not taken as seriously as men's. All women, then, have a vested interest in seeing medicine finally explain the many "medically unexplained" syndromes that disproportionately affect women. As long as these syndromes remain functional diagnoses without biomarkers, doctors can continue to use them as diagnoses of exclusion, handed out prematurely when they haven't cracked the case. Women who have an autoimmune disease will continue to be told they have fibromyalgia. Women who are suffering from Lyme disease will continue to be labeled as having ME/CFS. Women with ovarian cancer will keep being misdiagnosed with IBS. And the women who actually have these poorly understood conditions will continue to suffer.

WOMEN ARE A SOURCE OF KNOWLEDGE

The story of ovarian cancer contains another lesson, though: while it may have been validating for the survivors to share their similar stories with each other online, overturning the entrenched expert opinion that the disease was a silent killer required a study by a physician. In an age of evidence-based medicine, the knowledge from a peer-reviewed study counts for far more than patient anecdotes—even thousands of them. This, too, is a common pattern. In 2006, a study demonstrated that roughly 10 percent of people who come down with a variety of acute infections develop ME/CFS, confirming the narrative that most ME/CFS patients had been telling for decades: they fell ill with a flu-like sickness and then never got better. Dr. Jose Montoya, an expert in ME/CFS at the Stanford University Medical Center, sums up: "Our patients were telling us that all along. And a study had to be done to prove that they were right."

This means that women need allies within medicine who have an alchemist's power to turn patient anecdotes into scientific research. We need more health care providers like Goff—as well as scientists at all levels of biomedical research—who see patients as partners in the quest for greater scientific knowledge and more effective medical care, not just as objects of study, let alone adversaries in a "contest" as the awful term *contested disease* implies. Like the ovarian cancer patients, women are eager to offer up their knowledge. And there is nothing "soft" about science that takes advantage of it.

Even as mere objects of study, women are a spring of untapped knowledge. Studying a disease in only half the population, or ignoring the possibility of differences between men and women, or neglecting some conditions altogether because they're assumed to be nothing more than the imaginary symptoms of neurotic women—these choices have created gaps in our medical knowledge that have impoverished us all. We know less about heart disease because we spent thirty-five years studying it almost exclusively in men. If curing the autoimmune epidemic were a bigger priority, we would know far more about the workings of the immune system, knowledge that could lead to breakthroughs in other realms—from cancer to infectious diseases. Our understanding of pain—the most common thing that brings people into the medical system—is in its infancy because for so long women's unexplained pain was assumed to be inexplicable. We would surely have a better understanding of how the toxic chemicals in our environment are affecting our health if medicine listened to the 11 million Americans who get sick from them every day.

Nowhere does medicine appear less like a science than in its approach to "medically unexplained symptoms." It's revealing that some of the most compelling journalistic investigations into medicine's treatment of "contested diseases" have come from longtime science writers who became patients. Used to seeing science as a force for truth, they frequently describe seeing medicine's approach to the "medically unexplained" as a shock and deep disappointment. Reading the PACE study claiming exercise and CBT helped ME/CFS patients—and the uncritical reporting of it in the media— Julie Rehmeyer "felt betrayed by the institutions of science and journalism." Encountering a medical establishment that, unable to explain her illness, had thrown up its hands and decided that it couldn't be explained, she "felt like a refugee, [her] citizenship in the land of science having been unceremoniously revoked."

WHAT CAN BE DONE?

I asked all the doctors and patient advocates I interviewed during my research for this book what message they'd want to get across to readers eager to do something to help effect change. All emphasized that women's advocacy can, as it did in the nineties, help quite a lot. "Don't think that there's nothing you can do. Because you can actually have more impact than you think," says Susan Wood, the former FDA official. Perhaps most concretely, you can tell your lawmakers to increase NIH funding for the neglected conditions discussed in this book that disproportionately affect women, that have been neglected largely *because* they disproportionately affect women, and that so desperately need more research.

Patient advocacy can only do so much to help bring about other necessary reforms, though. It is the funders, scientific journal editors, and researchers at all levels of biomedical research who need to help build a consensus within the research community that analyzing study results to detect potential sex/gender differences is just good science. And integrating the emerging knowledge of those differences into medical school curricula is a challenging task that requires the will of those within medicine. The same goes for reforms to give medical students more education about the implicit biases that can affect them and to ensure that doctors receive more sorely needed feedback on their diagnostic errors.

In short, those within the medical and research communities need to commit to fixing medicine's gender bias. And perhaps the best way that women, as patients, can help spur medicine to make that commitment is simply by telling their "doctor stories"—telling them in the media and on Facebook and to their friends, family, and colleagues working within medicine. The first step to fixing a problem, after all, is recognizing that it exists.

I also asked everyone I interviewed what advice they had for individual women navigating the medical system. I often heard *Listen to your body. Trust that you know when something is wrong. Don't second-guess yourself; get a second opinion instead.* This is good advice, but we should be very clear about why it is necessary advice: because all too often, when women enter the medical system, they encounter health care providers who do *not* listen to them, who do *not* trust that they know when something is wrong, who make them second-guess themselves and doubt the very reality of what they're feeling in their own bodies. As Brea says of pushing herself to walk home from her neurologist's office when her body was screaming out not to, "I let what the experts were telling me override my own instincts." Women should trust their instincts, yes, but medicine should not override them in the first place.

Many of the people I interviewed also encouraged women to become well-informed, educated health care consumers. They should do their own research on their conditions. They should seek out information about sex/gender differences—in everything from drug reactions to the symptoms of a heart attack. But, again, let's acknowledge that we are asking individual women to compensate for the medical system's failures. While some patients may *want* to be partners in their medical care, and the Internet has certainly made it easier for some patients to educate themselves, not all women have the vast resources required to become "empowered patients." And doing so should not be *mandatory*. As a society, we send doctors to school for many years, pay them good money, and confer on them the prestige and respect afforded to lauded experts; we should be able to be utterly uninformed, unempowered patients and still get quality medical care. "You can't just go to the doctor and rely on the fact that he or she is going to give you the correct diagnosis, assessment, and refer you to treatment. If you don't educate yourself and you don't empower yourself, you end up suffering," chronic pain advocate Chris Veasley says. "Is it the way it should be? No, that's not the way a medical system should work, but it is the way it is."

I also asked all the women I interviewed how their experiences of being misdiagnosed and dismissed and neglected by health care providers had changed their view of the medical system. And universally I heard the same refrain: *I have less trust in medicine now.* They said they saw now that health care providers were fallible and, worse, that they often failed to acknowledge that they were fallible. It is up to the medical community to earn back women's trust. And some of the changes needed are big systemic ones, ones that are difficult to implement and will no doubt take time, but there is one that is simple and can be accomplished tomorrow: Listen to women. Trust us when we say we're sick. Start there, and you'll find we have a lot of knowledge to share.

ACKNOWLEDGMENTS

THANK YOU, FIRST AND FOREMOST, to all the women who shared their "doctor stories" with me. Over a hundred women wrote to tell me about their experiences of gender bias in the medical system, and I interviewed dozens of them. Each and every story, whether or not it was mentioned in the book, shaped my thinking. One story is just an anecdote, but at a certain point, anecdotes become data.

Thanks to my editor, Julia Pastore, and the team at HarperOne. All credit for recognizing that people wanted and needed this book goes to her. On the basis of one article I wrote, she suspected that there was a whole book here—and, even more crazily, that perhaps I, a first-time author, should be the one to write it. I hope that ultimately, after many a missed deadline, I lived up to that confidence.

Thanks to the whole Feministing crew for holding down the fort while I took time off—especially to the brilliant and hardworking Lori Adelman. I owe you one. To Lori and Jos Truitt: working on this very solitary project has made me all the more grateful for our work together. Thanks, as always, to the extended Feministing family, whose example and mentorship is the foundation of my entire career.

Thanks to my fact-checkers, Erica Langston and Will Greenberg, for their thorough work.

Thanks to my dear friends, whose notes of encouragement I returned to frequently during this process. Thanks to Martha Polk for her thoughtful editorial feedback, which made this book so much better, and for her friendship, which makes everything so much better. I can't wait to edit your book. Thanks to my sister, Lisa Dusenbery, for being such a steady research assistant, sounding board, and hand-holder. You know better than anyone that this book wouldn't have gotten done without you. Thanks to my parents, Van Dusenbery and Liz Coville, for the home-cooked meals and patience these past months, as well as the high standards and financial subsidies these many years.

Finally, thanks to the experts—the doctors, researchers, and advocates—who shared their knowledge with me. They taught me so much and made me hopeful that medicine can become what it should be: a pursuit that is constantly self-critical and improving, that is always seeking to understand more and working to find better ways to ensure that knowledge helps us—all of us—be as healthy as we can be.

ABBREVIATIONS

AARDA	American Autoimmune Related Diseases Association
AHA	American Heart Association
AMA	American Medical Association
CAD	coronary artery disease
CDC	Centers for Disease Control and Prevention
CMD	coronary microvascular disease
COPD	chronic obstructive pulmonary disease
CPRA	Chronic Pain Research Alliance
CRPS	complex regional pain syndrome
DSM	*Diagnostic and Statistical Manual of Mental Disorders*
FDA	U.S. Food and Drug Administration
GAO	U.S. Government Accountability Office
HHS	U.S. Department of Health and Human Services
IBS	irritable bowel syndrome
IC	interstitial cystitis
ICA	Interstitial Cystitis Association
IOM	Institute of Medicine
MCS	multiple chemical sensitivity
ME/CFS	myalgic encephalomyelitis / chronic fatigue syndrome
MS	multiple sclerosis
NBME	National Board of Medical Examiners
NIH	National Institutes of Health
NVA	National Vulvodynia Association
OA	osteoarthritis

ORWH	Office of Research on Women's Health, National Institutes of Health
PBS	painful bladder syndrome
PID	pelvic inflammatory disease
POTS	postural orthostatic tachycardia syndrome
PTLDS	post-treatment Lyme disease syndrome
RA	rheumatoid arthritis
SGWHC	Sex and Gender Women's Health Collaborative
SSD	somatic symptom disorder
SWHR	Society for Women's Health Research
TILT	toxicant-induced loss of tolerance
TMD	temporomandibular disorder
TSH	thyroid-stimulating hormone
WISE	Women's Ischemia Syndrome Evaluation

NOTES

INTRODUCTION

1 *It's estimated that as many as 50 million* . . . American Autoimmune Related Diseases Association, "Autoimmune Disease Statistics," www.aarda.org/news -information/statistics/.

1 *and rates are on the rise* . . . Donna Jackson Nakazawa, *The Autoimmune Epidemic* (New York: Touchstone Books, 2008).

2 *According to a survey by the American Autoimmune Related Diseases Association* . . . American Autoimmune Related Diseases Association, "Do You Know Your Family AQ?," www.aarda.org/wp-content/uploads/2016/12/AARDA-Do_you _know_your_family_AQ-DoubleSided.pdf.

2 *women make up more than three-quarters* . . . American Autoimmune Related Diseases Association, "Autoimmune Disease in Women," www.aarda.org /autoimmune-information/autoimmune-disease-in-women/.

2 *while they constitute less than a third* . . . Aaron Young et al., "A Census of Actively Licensed Physicians in the United States, 2014," *Journal of Medical Regulation* 101, no. 2 (2015), www.fsmb.org/media/default/pdf/census/2014census.pdf.

3 *Women make up about two-thirds of people with Alzheimer's* . . . Karen Skelton and Angela Timashenka Geiger, "The Shriver Report Overview," *The Shriver Report*, 2010, www.alz.org/shriverreport/overview.html.

3 *which experts now consider the third* . . . Tara Bahrampour, "New Study Ranks Alzheimer's as Third Leading Cause of Death, after Heart Disease and Cancer," *The Washington Post*, March 5, 2014, www.washingtonpost.com/local/new-study -ranks-alzheimers-as-third-leading-cause-of-death-after-heart-disease-and -cancer/2014/03/05/8097a452-a48a-11e3-8466-d34c451760b9_story.html.

3 *They're at least twice as likely* . . . Mary Lou Ballweg et al., *Chronic Pain in Women: Neglect, Dismissal and Discrimination*, Campaign to End Chronic Pain in Women, May 2010, www.endwomenspain.org/Common/file?id=20.

3 *that affect 100 million* . . . Institute of Medicine, *Relieving Pain in America: A Blueprint for Transforming Prevention, Care, Education, and Research* (National Academy of Sciences, June 2011), www.nationalacademies.org/hmd/Reports/2011 /Relieving-Pain-in-America-A-Blueprint-for-Transforming-Prevention-Care -Education-Research.aspx.

3 *Then there are conditions like fibromyalgia* . . . Reva C. Lawrence et al., "Estimates of the Prevalence of Arthritis and Other Rheumatic Conditions in the United States, Part II," *Arthritis and Rheumatism* 58, no. 1 (January 2008), doi:10.1002 /art.23176.

3 *chronic fatigue syndrome* . . . Michele Reyes et al., "Prevalence and Incidence of Chronic Fatigue Syndrome in Wichita, Kansas," *Archive of Internal Medicine* 163, no. 13 (July 2003), doi:10.1001/archinte.163.13.1530.

3 *chronic Lyme disease* . . . Alison W. Rebman, Mark J. Soloski, and John N. Aucott, "Sex and Gender Impact Lyme Disease Immunopathology, Diagnosis and Treatment," in *Sex and Gender Differences in Infection and Treatments for Infectious Diseases*, eds. Sabra L. Klein and Craig W. Roberts (Cham, Switzerland: Springer International Publishing, 2015), doi:10.1007/978-3-319-16438-0_12.

3 *and multiple chemical sensitivities* . . . Stanley M. Caress and Anne C. Steinemann, "Prevalence of Multiple Chemical Sensitivities: A Population-Based Study in the Southeastern United States," *American Journal of Public Health* 94, no. 5 (May 2004), doi:10.2105/AJPH.94.5.746.

3 *While their numbers have increased since the early nineties* . . . National Institutes of Health: Office of Research on Women's Health, NIH Revitalization Act of 1993, S. Doc. No. 1, 103rd Congress (1993), https://orwh.od.nih.gov/resources/pdf /NIH-Revitalization-Act-1993.pdf.

4 *Women wait sixty-five minutes to men's forty-nine* . . . E. H. Chen et al., "Gender Disparity in Analgesic Treatment of Emergency Department Patients with Acute Abdominal Pain," *Academic Emergency Medicine* 15, no. 5 (May 2008), doi:10.1111/j.1553-2712.2008.00100.x.

4 *Young women are seven times more likely* . . . J. Hector Pope et al., "Missed Diagnoses of Acute Cardiac Ischemia in the Emergency Department," *The New England Journal of Medicine* 342, no. 16 (April 2000), doi:10.1056/NEJM200004203421603.

4 *Women face long delays* . . . Ruth Hadfield et al., "Delay in the Diagnosis of Endometriosis: A Survey of Women from the USA and the UK," *Human Reproduction* 11, no. 4 (April 1996), doi:10.1093/oxfordjournals.humrep.a019270.

4 *from brain tumors* . . . The Brain Tumour Charity, *Finding Myself in Your Hands: The Reality of Brain Tumor Treatment and Care* (Hampshire, UK: The Brain Tumour Charity, 2016), www.thebraintumourcharity.org/media/filer_public/b6 /db/b6dbb5d4-ce20-4169-a587-96f5195bd670/cfindingmyself_healthcarereport _rgb_finalc.pdf.

4 *to rare genetic disorders* . . . Anna Kole and François Faurisson, *The Voice of 12,000 Patients: Experiences and Expectations of Rare Disease Patients on Diagnosis and Care in Europe* (Paris: Eurordis, 2009), www.eurordis.org/IMG/pdf/voice_12000 _patients/EURORDISCARE_FULLBOOKr.pdf.

5 *"has often been told as an allegory of science* . . . Barbara Ehrenreich and Deirdre English, *For Her Own Good: Two Centuries of the Experts' Advice to Women* (1978; reprint, New York: Anchor Books, 2005), 37.

6 *One eighteenth-century commenter described* . . . William Cobbett, quoted in Ehrenreich and English, *For Her Own Good*, 52.

6 *By 1900, the number of female physicians had climbed* . . . *Women in Medicine: A Review of Changing Physician Demographics, Female Physicians by Specialty, State and Related Data* (Irving, TX: Staff Care, 2015), www.amnhealthcare .com/uploadedFiles/MainSite/Content/Staffing_Recruitment/Staffcare-WP -Women%20in%20Med.pdf.

6 *nineteen women's medical colleges and nine women's hospitals* . . . Eliza Lo Chin, "Looking Back Over the History of Women in Medicine," MOMMD, www .mommd.com/lookingback.shtml.

6 *"made their appearance, a general uprising of* . . . Dolores Burns, ed., *The Greatest Health Discovery: Natural Hygiene and Its Evolution, Past, Present, and Future* (Chicago: Natural Hygiene Press, 1972), 118.

7 *"They will raise the cry, 'She is out of her proper sphere'* . . . Gena Corea, *The Hidden Malpractice: How American Medicine Mistreats Women* (New York: HarperCollins, 1985), 27.

7 *In 1910, the resulting Flexner Report concluded* . . . Abraham Flexner, *Medical Education in the United States and Canada: A Report to the Carnegie Foundation for the Advancement of Teaching* (New York: The Carnegie Foundation for the Advancement of Teaching, 1910), http://archive.carnegiefoundation.org/pdfs /elibrary/Carnegie_Flexner_Report.pdf.

7 *"any strong demand for women physicians* . . . Flexner, *Medical Education.*

7 *By 1915, the portion of medical school graduates who* . . . Shari L. Barkin et al., "Unintended Consequences of the Flexner Report: Women in Pediatrics," *Pediatrics* 126, no. 6 (December 2010), doi:10.1542/peds.2010-2050.

8 *In 1970, when less than 10 percent* . . . Association of American Medical Colleges, "Medical Students, Selected Years, 1965–2013," table 1, www.aamc.org/download /411782/data/2014_table1.pdf.

8 *a survey of admissions officers found that nineteen of twenty-five American medical schools* . . . Leslie Laurence and Beth Weinhouse, *Outrageous Practices: How Gender Bias Threatens Women's Health* (1994; reprint, New Brunswick, NJ: Rutgers Univ. Press, 1997), 29.

8 *By the midseventies, the number of female medical* . . . Association of American Medical Colleges, "Medical Students," table 1.

8 *Since the mid-aughts, women have made up* . . . Association of American Medical Colleges, "Medical Students," table 1.

8 *For the last several years, about a third of practicing* . . . Aaron Young et al., "A Census of Actively Licensed Physicians in the United States, 2014," *Journal of Medical Regulation* 101, no. 2 (2015), www.fsmb.org/media/default/pdf/census/2014census.pdf.

8 *The proportion of practicing ob-gyns who are women* . . . Center for Workforce Studies, *2014 Physician Specialty Data Book* (Association of American Medical Colleges, November 2014), https://members.aamc.org/eweb/upload/Physician% 20Specialty%20Databook%202014.pdf.

8 *Currently, 60 percent of pediatricians are women* . . . Center for Workforce Studies, *2014 Physician Specialty Data Book.*

8 *In recent years, women have made up about* . . . Lyndra Vassar, "How Medical Specialties Vary by Gender," *AMA Wire*, February 18, 2015, https://wire.ama-assn .org/education/how-medical-specialties-vary-gender.

9 *There remain large segments of medicine where women are vastly outnumbered* . . . Center for Workforce Studies, *2014 Physician Specialty Data Book.*

9 *Women now make up 38 percent* . . . Diana M. Lautenberger et al., *The State of Women in Academic Medicine* (Association of American Medical Colleges, 2014), https://members.aamc.org/eweb/upload/The%20State%20of%20Women%20 in%20Academic%20Medicine%202013-2014%20FINAL.pdf, 2.

9 *In 2014, only 21 percent of full professors* . . . Lautenberger et al., *The State of Women,* 2.

9 *According to a 2015 analysis of data* . . . Anupam B. Jena et al., "Sex Differences in Academic Rank in US Medical Schools in 2014," *JAMA* 314, no. 11 (September 2015), doi:10.1001/jama.2015.10680.

9 *Only about 30 percent of researchers receiving NIH* . . . Sally Rockey, "Women in Biomedical Research," National Institutes of Health Office of Extramural Research, August 8, 2014, https://nexus.od.nih.gov/all/2014/08/08/women-in -biomedical-research/.

9 *A 2016 study published in* The BMJ *found that growth* . . . Giovanni Filardo et al., "Trends and Comparison of Female First Authorship in High Impact Medical Journals: Observational Study (1994–2014)," *The BMJ* 352, no. 847 (March 2016), doi:10.1136/bmj.i847.

9 *women make up just 17.5 percent* . . . K. Amrein et al., "Women Underrepresented on Editorial Boards of 60 Major Medical Journals," *Gender Medicine* 8, no. 6 (December 2011), doi:10.1016/j.genm.2011.10.007.

10 *According to a 2016 study published in* JAMA . . . Anupam B. Jena, Andrew R. Olenski, and Daniel M. Blumenthal, "Sex Differences in Physician Salary in US Public Medical Schools," *JAMA Internal Medicine* 176, no. 9 (September 2016), doi:10.1001/jamainternmed.2016.3284.

10 *In fact, some studies suggest that the gap has actually been increasing* . . . Anthony T. Lo Sasso et al., "The $16,819 Pay Gap for Newly Trained Physicians: The Unexplained Trend of Men Earning More Than Women," *Health Affairs* 30, no. 2 (February 2011), doi:10.1377/hlthaff.2010.0597.

10 *A 2000 study of over 3,000 full-time faculty* . . . P. L. Carr et al., "Faculty Perceptions of Gender Discrimination and Sexual Harassment in Academic Medicine," *Annals of Internal Medicine* 132, no. 11 (June 2000), www.ncbi.nlm.nih.gov /pubmed/10836916.

10 *In 2016, a* JAMA *study of over a thousand* . . . Jagsi Reshma et al., "Sexual Harassment and Discrimination Experiences of Academic Medical Faculty," *JAMA* 315, no. 19 (May 2016), doi:10.1001/jama.2016.2188.

10 *A 2013 Canadian study of 870 doctors* . . . Université de Montréal, "Female Doctors Better Than Male Doctors, but Males Are More Productive," *ScienceDaily*, October 17, 2013, www.sciencedaily.com/releases/2013/10/131017100601.htm.

10 *They tend to be more "patient-centered," expressing* . . . Debra L. Roter and Judith A. Hall, "Women Doctors Don't Get the Credit They Deserve," *Journal of General Internal Medicine* 30, no. 3 (March 2015), doi:10.1007/s11606-014-3081-9.

11 *As researchers, they are more likely than men* . . . Filardo et al., "Female First Authorship."

11 *investigators overwhelmingly use male cells* . . . Janine A. Clayton and Francis S. Collins, "Policy: NIH to Balance Sex in Cell and Animal Studies," *Nature* 509 (May 15, 2014), doi:10.1038/509282a.

11 *"We literally know less about every aspect of female* . . . Roni Caryn Rabin, "Health Researchers Will Get $10.1 Million to Counter Gender Bias in Studies," *The New York Times*, September 23, 2014, www.nytimes.com/2014/09/23/health/23gender .html?_r=1.

13 *Before it went into effect, approximately 20 percent* . . . Alina Salganicoff et al., *Women and Health Care in the Early Years of the ACA: Key Findings from the 2013 Kaiser Women's Heath Survey,* The Henry J. Kaiser Family Foundation, May 15, 2014, http://kff.org/womens-health-policy/report/women-and-health-care-in-the -early-years-of-the-aca-key-findings-from-the-2013-kaiser-womens-health-survey/.

13 *By 2015, that figure had dropped to about 11 percent . . .* The Henry J. Kaiser Family Foundation, *Women's Health Insurance Coverage,* The Henry J. Kaiser Family Foundation, October 21, 2016, http://kff.org/womens-health-policy/fact-sheet /womens-health-insurance-coverage-fact-sheet/.

13 *Health care reform also corrected . . .* Jessica Arons and Lucy Panza, "Top 10 Obamacare Benefits at Stake for Women," *ThinkProgress,* May 24, 2012, https:// thinkprogress.org/top-10-obamacare-benefits-at-stake-for-women-5ff541dfdf53 #.36n0gciws.

13 *Insurers are now required . . .* "Preventive Services Covered Under the Affordable Care Act," U.S. Department of Health and Human Services, September 23, 2010, www.hhs.gov/healthcare/facts-and-features/fact-sheets /preventive-services-covered-under-aca/.

14 *Still, 11.2 million women, many of them low-income women of color . . .* The Henry J. Kaiser Family Foundation, *Women's Health Insurance Coverage.*

14 *women have been especially impacted . . .* Rachel Garfield and Andy Damico, *The Coverage Gap: Uninsured Poor Adults in States That Do Not Expand Medicaid,* The Henry J. Kaiser Family Foundation, October 19, 2016, http://kff.org /uninsured/issue-brief/the-coverage-gap-uninsured-poor-adults-in-states-that -do-not-expand-medicaid/.

14 *According to a 2013 nationally representative survey . . .* Salganicoff, "Women and Health Care."

14 *For low-income women especially . . .* Salganicoff, "Women and Health Care."

15 *The result is that about a fifth of low-income women say . . .* Salganicoff, "Women and Health Care."

15 *even more report that they have a disability or chronic disease . . .* Salganicoff, "Women and Health Care."

16 *Most American women rely on contraception . . .* Guttmacher Institute, "Contraceptive Use in the United States," September 2016, www.guttmacher.org /fact-sheet/contraceptive-use-united-states.

16 *As many as one-quarter will at some point get an abortion . . .* Rachel K. Jones and Jenna Jerman, "Population Group Abortion Rates and Lifetime Incidence of Abortion: United States, 2008–2014," *American Journal of Public Health* 107, no. 12 (December 2, 2017), doi:10.2105/AJPH.2017.304042.

16 *80 percent will eventually have a child . . .* Gretchen Livingston and D'Vera Cohn, *Childlessness Up Among All Women; Down Among Women with Advanced Degrees,* Pew Research Center, June 25, 2010, www.pewsocialtrends.org/2010 /06/25/childlessness-up-among-all-women-down-among-women-with-advanced -degrees/2/.

16 *the provision of the procedure is often dictated by . . .* "Bad Medicine: How a Political Agenda Is Undermining Women's Health Care," National Partnership for Women & Families, 2016, www.nationalpartnership.org/research-library/repro /bad-medicine-download.pdf.

16 *In a country in which about a million abortions . . .* Guttmacher Institute, "Induced Abortion in the United States," September 2016, www.guttmacher.org /fact-sheet/induced-abortion-united-states.

16 *a 2005 survey of ob-gyn programs found that . . .* Mara Gordon, "The Scarcity of Abortion Training in America's Medical Schools," *The Atlantic,* June 9, 2015, www .theatlantic.com/health/archive/2015/06/learning-abortion-in-medical-school /395075/.

17 *While 97 percent of practicing ob-gyns have* . . . Gordon, "Scarcity of Abortion Training."

17 *which is used by 99 percent of sexually active women at some point* . . . Guttmacher Institute, "Contraceptive Use."

17 *Were we not stuck having such 1960s-era* . . . Ann Friedman, "Why Isn't Birth Control Getting Better?" *Good*, April 24, 2011, www.good.is/articles /why-isn-t-birth-control-getting-better.

17 *Many of the problems with reproductive health care* . . . Nina Martin and Renee Montagne, "Focus on Infants During Childbirth Leaves U.S. Moms in Danger," NPR.org and *ProPublica*, May 12, 2017, www.npr.org/2017/05/12/527806002 /focus-on-infants-during-childbirth-leaves-u-s-moms-in-danger.

17 *The United States is the only country in the developed world* . . . World Health Organization et al., *Trends in Maternal Mortality: 1990 to 2013* (Geneva: World Health Organization, 2014).

17 *At least half of maternal deaths* . . . Francine Coeytaux, Debra Bingham, and Nan Strauss, "Maternal Mortality in the United States: A Human Rights Failure," *Contraception Journal* 83, no. 3 (March 2011), doi:10.1016/j.contraception.2010 .11.013.

17 *black women are nearly four times as likely* . . . Centers for Disease Control and Prevention, "Pregnancy Mortality Surveillance System," last modified January 21, 2016, www.cdc.gov/reproductivehealth/maternalinfanthealth/pmss.html.

17 *In the last two decades, the C-section rate* . . . Coeytaux, Bingham, and Strauss, "Maternal Mortality."

17 *to more than three times the rate recommended* . . . World Health Organization and Human Reproduction Programme, "WHO Statement on Caesarean Section Rates: Executive Summary," 2015, www.who.int/reproductivehealth/publications /maternal_perinatal_health/cs-statement/en/.

17 *performed not out of medical need but for the* . . . Tina Rosenberg, "In Delivery Rooms, Reducing Births of Convenience," *The New York Times*, May 7, 2014, http://opinionator.blogs.nytimes.com/2014/05/07/in-delivery-rooms-reducing -births-of-convenience/.

18 *But with 4.5 million women lacking* . . . Jennifer J. Frost, Lori F. Frohwirth, and Mia R. Zolna, *Contraceptive Needs and Services, 2014 Update*, Guttmacher Institute, September 2016, www.guttmacher.org/report/contraceptive-needs-and -services-2014-update.

18 *nearly half of pregnancies in this country* . . . Guttmacher Institute, "Unintended Pregnancy in the United States," September 2016, www.guttmacher.org/fact-sheet /unintended-pregnancy-united-states.

18 *"Everyone had a 'doctor story'* . . . Kathy Davis, *The Making of Our Bodies, Ourselves: How Feminism Travels Across Borders* (Durham, NC: Duke Univ. Press, 2007), 21.

19 *But the gap has been narrowing since the eighties* . . . Patricia P. Rieker and Chloe E. Bird, "Rethinking Gender Differences in Health: Why We Need to Integrate Social and Biological Perspectives," *The Journals of Gerontology Series B: Psychological Sciences and Social Sciences* 60, no. 2 (October 2005), doi:10.1093/geronb/60 .Special_Issue_2.S40.

19 *And the additional 4.8 years of life expectancy* . . . Centers for Disease Control and Prevention, National Center for Health Statistics, *Health, United States, 2015: With Special Feature on Racial and Ethnic Health Disparities*, 2016, www.cdc .gov/nchs/data/hus/hus15.pdf#015.

19 *Women report poorer health* . . . "Percent of Adults Reporting Fair or Poor Health Status, by Gender," Kaiser Family Foundation Analysis of the Centers for Disease Control and Prevention (CDC)'s Behavioral Risk Factor Surveillance System (BRFSS) 2013–2015 Survey Results, http://kff.org/other/state-indicator/percent-of-adults-reporting-fair-or-poor-health-by-gender/.

20 *When it comes to "active" life expectancy* . . . Vicki A. Freedman, Douglas A. Wolf, and Brenda C. Spillman, "Disability-Free Life Expectancy over 30 Years: A Growing Female Disadvantage in the US Population," *American Journal of Public Health* 106, no. 6 (June 2016), doi:10.2105/AJPH.2016.303089.

20 *women have higher rates of debilitating but not life-threatening chronic diseases* . . . Anne Case and Christina H. Paxson, "Sex Differences in Morbidity and Mortality," *Demography* 42, no. 2 (May 2005), doi:10.1353/dem.2005.0011.

20 *More than half of all American women have at least one chronic* . . . Jessie Gerteis et al., *Multiple Chronic Conditions Chartbook* (Rockville, MD: Agency for Healthcare Research and Quality, 2014).

CHAPTER 1. THE KNOWLEDGE GAP

24 *"the historical lack of research focus on women's health concerns* . . . U.S. Public Health Service, "Report of the Public Health Service Task Force on Women's Health Issues," *Public Health Reports* 100, no. 1 (January–February 1985), www.ncbi.nlm.nih.gov/pmc/articles/PMC1424718/.

24 *In 1990, the GAO released its findings* . . . U.S. General Accounting Office, "National Institutes of Health: Problems in Implementing Policy on Women in Study Populations," (Testimony by Mark V. Vadel before Subcommittee on Health and the Environment, Committee on Energy and Commerce, House of Representatives), GAO/T-HRD-90-38, June 18, 1990, http://archive.gao.gov/d48t13/141601.pdf.

25 *the cochairs of the Congressional Caucus for Women's Issues lambasted NIH leaders* . . . Gina Kolata, "N.I.H. Neglects Women, Study Says," *The New York Times*, June 19, 1990, www.nytimes.com/1990/06/19/science/nih-neglects-women-study-says.html.

25 *by the midseventies, a third would be taking them* . . . E. Barrett-Connor et al., "Heart Disease Risk Factors and Hormone Use in Postmenopausal Women," *JAMA* 24, no. 20 (May 1979), doi:10.1001/jama.1979.03290460031015.

25 *"Somehow, I find it hard to believe* . . . Quoted in Laurence and Weinhouse, *Outrageous Practices*, 62.

26 *Since 1977, the agency had had in place a policy* . . . U.S. Food and Drug Administration, "Gender Studies in Product Development: Historical Overview," May 20, 2016, www.fda.gov/ScienceResearch/SpecialTopics/WomensHealthResearch/ucm134466.htm.

26 *the GAO report found that women were underrepresented* . . . U.S. General Accounting Office, "FDA Needs to Ensure More Study of Gender Differences in Prescription Drugs Testing," GAO/HRD-93-17, October 1992, www.gao.gov/products/GAO/HRD-93-17.

26 *In fact, there were only three gynecologists on staff* . . . Laurence and Weinhouse, *Outrageous Practices*, 62.

27 *"The medical community has viewed women's health* . . . Nanette K. Wenger, "You've Come a Long Way, Baby: Cardiovascular Health and Disease in Women: Problems and Prospects," *Circulation* 109, no. 5 (February 9, 2004), doi:10.1161/01.CIR.0000117292.19349.D0.

27 *only 13.5 percent of the NIH's most recent budget* . . . Ruth L. Kirschstein, "Research on Women's Health," *American Journal of Public Health* 81, no. 3 (March 1991), www.ncbi.nlm.nih.gov/pmc/articles/PMC1405014/pdf/amjph00203-0021.pdf.

27 *the new office summed up the state of affairs in its first research agenda* . . . U.S. Department of Health and Human Services, Office of Research on Women's Health, *Report of the National Institutes of Health: Opportunities for Research on Women's Health: September 4–6, 1991* (Hunt Valley, MD: NIH Publication no. 92–3457, 1992).

28 *And, in part, women had been excluded* . . . Katherine A. Liu and Natalie A. Dipietro Mager, "Women's Involvement in Clinical Trials: Historical Perspective and Future Implications," *Pharmacy Practice* 14, no. 1 (January–March 2016), doi:10.18549/PharmPract.2016.01.708.

28 *In the aftermath, in the late seventies, the United States finally* . . . The National Commission for the Protection of Human Subjects of Biomedical and Behavioral Research, *The Belmont Report: Ethical Principles and Guidelines for the Protection of Human Subjects of Research*, DHEW Publication No. (OS) 78–0013 and No. (OS) 78–0014, April 18, 1979, www.hhs.gov/ohrp/regulations-and-policy /belmont-report/.

29 *At a few respected American academic medical institutions, doctors* . . . Barbara Seaman and Susan F. Wood, "Role of Advocacy Groups in Research on Women's Health," *Women and Health* (December 2000), doi:10.1016/B978-012288145-9 /50005-X.

29 *Companies seeking FDA approval for their drugs* . . . Suzanne White Junod, "FDA and Clinical Drug Trials: A Short History," U.S. Food and Drug Administration, last modified April 11, 2016, www.fda.gov/AboutFDA/WhatWeDo/Hi

30 *"one wonders what aspect of pregnancy renders women particularly vulnerable* . . . Tracy Johnson and Elizabeth Fee, "Women's Participation in Clinical Research: From Protectionism to Access," in *Women and Health Research: Ethical and Legal Issues of Including Women in Clinical Studies*, vol. 2 (Washington, DC: The National Academies Press, 1999), www.ncbi.nlm.nih.gov/books /NBK236577/.

30 *Meanwhile, the 1977 FDA policy didn't stop at excluding patients* . . . U.S. Department of Health and Human Services, *General Considerations for the Clinical Evaluation of Drugs in Infants and Children*, HEW (FDA) 77–3041, September 1977, www.fda.gov/downloads/drugs/guidancecomplianceregulatoryinformation /guidances/ucm071687.pdf.

31 *The research community tended to offer* . . . Vanessa Merton, "The Exclusion of Pregnant, Pregnable, and Once-Pregnable People (a.k.a. Women) from Biomedical Research," *American Journal of Law & Medicine* 19, no. 4 (1993), https://ssrn.com /abstract=1292951.

31 *This excuse looked especially suspect since* . . . Joan W. Scott, "How Did the Male Become the Normative Standard for Clinical Drug Trials," *Food and Drug Law Journal* 48, no. 2 (1993), http://hdl.handle.net/10822/749306.

32 *With hormone levels that vary depending on where they are in their* . . . Anna C. Mastroianni, Ruth Faden, and Daniel Federman, eds., *Women and Health Research: Ethical and Legal Issues of Including Women in Clinical Studies*, vol. 1 (Washington, DC: National Academies Press, 1994).

32 *"It defies logic for researchers to acknowledge gender difference* . . . Laurence and Weinhouse, *Outrageous Practices*, 71.

32 *"You want doctors to study what they're interested in*... Laurence and Weinhouse, *Outrageous Practices*, 5.

32 *As Rep. Schroeder put it in 1990*... Ellen Goodman, "Science and Sex: All-Male Research Bitter Pill for Women to Swallow," *The Boston Globe*, June 24, 1990, http://articles.chicagotribune.com/1990-06-24/features/9002210663_1_bias -in-health-research-women-in-clinical-trials-ovarian-cancer-and-osteoporosis.

33 *"Basically, we're trying to get the type of data*... Laurence and Weinhouse, *Outrageous Practices*, 79.

33 *In 1993, President Bill Clinton signed the NIH Revitalization Act*... NIH: Office of Research on Women's Health, NIH Revitalization Act of 1993.

33 *The same year, in the wake of its own GAO report, the FDA dropped the 1977 policy*... U.S. Food and Drug Administration, "Guideline for the Study and Evaluation of Gender Differences in the Clinical Evaluation of Drugs," *Federal Register* 58, no. 139 (July 1993), www.fda.gov/downloads/RegulatoryInformation/Guidances /UCM126835.pdf.

33 *In 2015, Carolyn M. Mazure*... Carolyn M. Mazure and Daniel P. Jones, "Twenty Years and Still Counting: Including Women as Participants and Studying Sex and Gender in Biomedical Research," *BMC Women's Health* 15, no. 94 (October 2015), doi:10.1186/s12905-015-0251-9.

34 *It was only in 2014 that the NIH announced a policy*... Clayton and Collins, "Policy: NIH to Balance."

34 *In 1998, the rule was strengthened*... U.S. Food and Drug Administration, "Investigational New Drug Applications and New Drug Applications," *Federal Register* 63, no. 28 (February 1998), www.fda.gov/ScienceResearch/SpecialTopics /WomensHealthResearch/ucm133181.htm.

34 *In a 2000 review of how well the NIH*... U.S. General Accounting Office, "NIH Has Increased Its Efforts to Include Women in Research," GAO/HEHS-00-96, May 2000, www.gao.gov/archive/2000/he00096.pdf.

34 *The next year, the GAO gave a similar evaluation*... U.S. General Accounting Office, "Women Sufficiently Represented in New Drug Testing, but FDA Oversight Needs Improvement," GAO-01-754, July 2001, www.gao.gov/new.items/d01754.pdf.

35 *of the FDA-approved drugs that had been pulled from the market between*... Janet Heinrich, "Drug Safety: Most Drugs Withdrawn in Recent Years Had Greater Health Risks for Women," U.S. General Accounting Office, January 19, 2001, www .gao.gov/assets/100/90642.pdf.

35 *All told, women now make up a majority of patients*... U.S. General Accounting Office, "Better Oversight Needed to Help Ensure Continued Progress Including Women in Health Research," GAO-01-754, October 2015, www.gao.gov/assets /680/673276.pdf.

35 *"By not examining more detailed data on enrollment*... U.S. General Accounting Office, "Better Oversight."

35 *A review of federally funded randomized controlled trials*... Stacie E. Geller, Marci Goldstein Adams, and Molly Carnes, "Adherence to Federal Guidelines for Reporting of Sex and Race/Ethnicity in Clinical Trials," *Journal of Women's Health* 15, no. 10 (December 2006), doi:10.1089/jwh.2006.15.1123.

35 *When the researchers redid the analysis*... Stacie E. Geller et al., "Inclusion, Analysis, and Reporting of Sex and Race/Ethnicity in Clinical Trials: Have We Made Progress," *Journal of Women's Health* 20, no. 3 (March 2011), doi:10.1089 /jwh.2010.2469.

35 *"Women and racial/ethnic minorities," the authors concluded* ... Kat Kwiatkowski et al., "Inclusion of Minorities and Women in Cancer Clinical Trials, a Decade Later: Have We Improved?" *Cancer* 119, no. 16 (August 15, 2013), doi:10.1002/cncr.28168.

36 *"When an NIH staff member brought this up in a meeting* . . . Nancy Reame, quoted in Laurence and Weinhouse, *Outrageous Practices*, 79.

36 *In 2010, a review of 150 recent studies* . . . Andrea H. Weinberger, Sherry A. McKee, and Carolyn M. Mazure, "Inclusion of Women and Gender-Specific Analyses in Randomized Clinical Trials of Treatments for Depression," *Journal of Women's Health* 19, no. 9 (September 2010), doi:10.1002/cncr.28168.

36 *A 2011 review of 750 studies focused* . . . Basmah Safdar et al., "Inclusion of Gender in Emergency Medicine Research," *Academic Emergency Medicine* 18, no. 2 (February 2011), doi:10.1111/j.1553-2712.2010.00978.x.

36 *There was a sense in the nineties that just getting women* . . . All quotes from author's interview with Jan Werbinski (executive director of the Sex and Gender Women's Health Collaborative).

36 *"It's still a struggle to get the pharma companies to analyze* . . . All quotes from author's interview with Phyllis Greenberger (former president of the Society for Women's Health Research).

37 *While most of the seventy-two applications they reviewed* ... U.S. Food and Drug Administration, *Collection, Analysis, and Availability of Demographic Subgroup Data for FDA-Approved Medical Products*, August 2013, www.fda.gov/downloads /RegulatoryInformation/Legislation/SignificantAmendmentstotheFDCAct /FDASIA/UCM365544.pdf.

37 *"You just have to include what you have* . . . All quotes from author's interview with Susan Wood (former director of the FDA's Office of Women's Health).

37 *The FDA concluded that there was room for improvement* ... U.S. Food and Drug Administration, *FDA Action Plan to Enhance the Collection and Availability of Demographic Subgroup Data*, August 2014, www.fda.gov/downloads/Regulatory Information/Legislation/SignificantAmendmentstotheFDCAct/FDASIA /UCM410474.pdf.

37 *To that end, it launched the Drug Trials Snapshots initiative* . . . U.S. Food and Drug Administration, "Drug Trials Snapshots," last modified November 28, 2016, www.fda.gov/Drugs/InformationOnDrugs/ucm412998.htm.

37 *Though advocates applauded the move, they noted* ... Nancy A. Brown et al., "Re: [Docket No. FDA—2014-N-1818] Comments on FDA Drug Trials Snapshots" (letter to Margaret Hamburg, Commissioner of Food and Drugs, U.S. Food and Drug Administration), January 23, 2015, www.heart.org/idc/groups/ahaecc -public/@wcm/@adv/documents/downloadable/ucm_471897.pdf.

37 *"We found great resistance for many years for some reason* . . . All quotes from author's interview with Vivian Pinn (former director of the Office of Research on Women's Health).

37 *They offered various justifications: they didn't want to take* . . . Theresa M. Wizemann, *Sex-Specific Reporting of Scientific Research: A Workshop Summary* (Washington, DC: The National Academies Press, 2012).

38 *In 2010, the SWHR did an informal survey* . . . Society for Women's Health Research, "XX or XY: Medical Journals Must Report Sex Differences," *HuffPost*, February 9, 2015, www.huffingtonpost.com/society-for-womens-health-research /xx-or-xy-medical-journals_b_6288960.html.

38 *The same year, in a progress report on women's health research* . . . Institute of

Medicine, *Women's Health Research: Progress, Pitfalls, and Promise* (Washington, DC: The National Academies Press, 2010), doi:10.17226/12908.

38 *Today, according to Stanford University's Gendered Innovations project* . . . Gendered Innovations, "Sex and Gender Analysis Policies of Peer-Reviewed Journals," https://genderedinnovations.stanford.edu/sex-and-gender-analysis -policies-peer-reviewed-journals.html.

38 *There's one group of women that has been entirely left out* . . . Julia Belton, "The Desperate Need to Include Pregnant Women in Clinical Research: Proposed Recommendations to Increase Enrollment of Pregnant Women in Research," *Law School Student Scholarship* 660 (2015), http://scholarship.shu.edu/student _scholarship/660.

38 *In 1994, the IOM recommended that pregnant women* . . . Institute of Medicine (U.S.) Committee on Ethical and Legal Issues Relating to the Inclusion of Women in Clinical Studies, "Women's Participation in Clinical Studies" in *Women and Health Research: Ethical and Legal Issues of Including Women in Clinical Studies*, vol. 1 (Washington, DC: The National Academies Press, 1994), www.ncbi.nlm.nih .gov/books/NBK236540/.

38 *In a 2013 analysis, 95 percent of industry-sponsored* . . . K. E. Shields and A. D. Lyerly, "Exclusion of Pregnant Women from Industry-Sponsored Clinical Trials," *Obstetrics & Gynecology* 122, no. 5 (November 2013), doi:10.1097/AOG .0b013e3182a9ca67.

39 *Only eight medications are currently approved* . . . Nina Martin, "Most Drugs Aren't Tested on Pregnant Women. This Anti-Nausea Cure Shows Why That's a Problem," *ProPublica*, May 26, 2016, www.propublica.org/article/most-drugs -not-tested-pregnant-women-anti-nausea-cure-why-thats-a-problem.

39 *"Pregnant women," a 2011 report by the ORWH declared* . . . Mary A. Foulkes et al., "Clinical Research Enrolling Pregnant Women: A Workshop Summary," *Journal of Women's Health* 20, no. 10 (October 2011), doi:10.1089/jwh.2011.3118.

39 *Each year, over 400,000 women in the United States battle* . . . The Second Wave Initiative, "Case Statement: Ending the Knowledge Gap of Treating Illness in Pregnant Women," 2016, http://secondwaveinitiative.org/Case_Statement.html.

39 *As bioethicist Françoise Baylis wrote* . . . Françoise Baylis, "Pregnant Women Deserve Better," *Nature* 465 (June 10, 2010), doi:10.1038/465689a.

39 *Indeed, 90 percent of women take some medication* . . . U.S. Department of Health and Human Services, Centers for Disease Control and Prevention, "Treating for Two," January 16, 2015, www.cdc.gov/pregnancy/meds/treatingfortwo/facts.html.

39 *The average woman receives 1.3 prescriptions* . . . Euni Lee et al., "National Patterns of Medication Use During Pregnancy," *Pharmacoepidemiology and Drug Safety* 15, no. 8 (August 2006), doi:10.1002/pds.1241.

39 *nearly two-thirds of women use* . . . National Institute of Child Health and Human Development, Request for applications for obstetric-fetal pharmacology research units (HD-03-017), 2003, http://grants.nih.gov/grants/guide/rfa-files /RFA-HD-03-017.html.

39 *The profound changes it causes to just about every system of the body* . . . Anne Drapkin Lyerly, Margaret Olivia Little, and Ruth Faden, "The Second Wave: Toward Responsible Inclusion of Pregnant Women in Research," *International Journal of Feminist Approaches to Bioethics* 1, no. 2 (Fall 2008), doi:10.1353/ijf.0.0047.

39 *Just as the average woman can't be considered* . . . Lyerly, Little, and Faden, "The Second Wave."

40 *"In the absence of information about the safety and efficacy of medications* . . . Lyerly, Little, and Faden, "The Second Wave."

40 *A 2011 analysis found that less than 10 percent* . . . Margaret P. Adam, Janine E. Polifka, and J. M. Friedman, "Evolving Knowledge of the Teratogenicity of Medications in Human Pregnancy," *American Journal of Medical Genetics Part C: Seminars in Medical Genetics* 157, no. 3 (August 2011), doi:10.1002/ajmg.c.30313.

40 *In 2004, one of the largest studies of drug use during pregnancy* . . . Susan E. Andrade et al., "Prescription Drug Use in Pregnancy," *American Journal of Obstetrics & Gynecology* 191, no. 2 (August 2004), doi:10.1016/j.ajog.2004.04.025.

40 *"We learn on the backs of [pregnant] women while* . . . Martin, "Most Drugs Aren't Tested on Pregnant Women."

40 *For drugs approved between 1980 and 2000, it took an* . . . Adam, Polifka, and Friedman, "Evolving Knowledge."

40 *As the Second Wave Initiative explains* . . . Lyerly, Little, and Faden, "The Second Wave."

41 *But untreated depression during pregnancy* . . . Lyerly, Little, and Faden, "The Second Wave."

41 *pregnant women sometimes receive inadequate care* . . . Anne Drapkin Lyerly et al., "Risk and the Pregnant Body," *The Hastings Center Report* 39, no. 6 (November–December 2009), www.ncbi.nlm.nih.gov/pmc/articles/PMC3640505/.

41 *The FDA has drafted guidelines* . . . U.S. Department of Health and Human Services, Food and Drug Administration, Center for Drug Evaluation and Research, *2004 Guidance for Industry Pharmacokinetics in Pregnancy—Study Design, Data Analysis, and Impact on Dosing and Labeling,* www.fda.gov/ScienceResearch /SpecialTopics/WomensHealthResearch/ucm133348.htm.

41 *has urged companies to set up pregnancy registries* . . . U.S. Department of Health and Human Services, Food and Drug Administration, *List of Pregnancy Exposure Registries,* www.fda.gov/ScienceResearch/SpecialTopics /WomensHealthResearch/ucm134848.htm.

41 *"The alternative to responsible research in pregnancy* . . . Lyerly, Little, and Faden, "The Second Wave."

42 *A study of nearly 40,000 women concluded* . . . Paul M. Ridker et al., "A Randomized Trial of Low-Dose Aspirin in the Primary Prevention of Cardiovascular Disease in Women," *The New England Journal of Medicine* 352, no. 13 (March 2005), doi:10.1056/NEJMoa050613.

42 *"In my own area of cardiology, trying to convince them* . . . All quotes from author's interview with Marianne Legato (founder of the Partnership for Gender-Specific Medicine).

42 *Women are two to ten times more likely to develop autoimmune diseases* . . . AARDA, "Autoimmune Disease in Women."

42 *Women are more likely than men to recover* . . . Institute of Medicine, *Exploring the Biological Contributions to Human Health: Does Sex Matter?* (National Academy of Sciences, 2001), www.nationalacademies.org/hmd/Reports/2001/Exploring -the-Biological-Contributions-to-Human-Health-Does-Sex-Matter.aspx.

42 *Women who have lung cancer are more* . . . Tiziana Vavalà and Silvia Novello, "Women and Lung Cancer: Literature Assumptions and News from Recent Publications," *European Medical Journal Oncology* 2 (November 2014), https:// doaj.org/article/87ab6df376464c2ba8ed1bd4075ccee8.

42 *Women more commonly do not have any chest pain* . . . John G. Canto et al.,

"Association of Age and Sex with Myocardial Infarction Symptom Presentation and In-Hospital Mortality," *JAMA* 307, no. 8 (February 2012), doi:10.1001/jama.2012.199.

42 *Differences have been found in the responses to many drugs* . . . O. P. Sodin and D. R. Mattison, "Sex Differences in Pharmacokinetics and Pharmacodynamics," *Clinical Pharmacokinetics* 48, no. 3 (2009), doi:10.2165/00003088-200948030-00001.

43 *"Paradoxically however, most drugs are not administered* . . . Emmanuel O. Fadiran and Lei Zhang, "Effects of Sex Differences in the Pharmacokinetics of Drugs and Their Impact on the Safety of Medicines in Women," in *Medicine for Women*, ed. Mira Harrison-Woolrych (Switzerland: Springer International Publishing, 2015), 42–43.

43 *In 2013, the FDA announced that it was requiring the recommended* . . . Sabrina Tavernise, "Drug Agency Recommends Lower Doses of Sleep Aids for Women," *The New York Times*, January 10, 2013, http://www.nytimes.com/2013/01/11/health/fda-requires-cuts-to-dosages-of-ambien-and-other-sleep-drugs.html.

44 *Dr. Sandra Kweder, deputy director of the FDA's Office of New Drugs, acknowledged* . . . Lesley Stahl, "Sex Matters: Drugs Can Affect Sexes Differently," *CBS Interactive Inc.*, February 9, 2014, https://www.cbsnews.com/news/sex-matters-drugs-can-affect-sexes-differently/.

44 *As ORWH director Clayton* . . . Roni Caryn Rabin, "The Drug-Dose Gender Gap," *The New York Times*, January 28, 2013, https://well.blogs.nytimes.com/2013/01/28/the-drug-dose-gender-gap/.

44 *women are 50 to 75 percent more likely* . . . Heather P. Whitley and Wesley Lindsey, "Sex-Based Differences in Drug Activity," *American Family Physician* 80, no. 11 (December 2009), www.aafp.org/afp/2009/1201/p1254.html.

44 *In 2001, the IOM compiled the emerging knowledge* . . . Institute of Medicine, *Does Sex Matter?*

45 *In a classic article, the feminist biologist Anne Fausto-Sterling* . . . Anne Fausto-Sterling, "The Bare Bones of Sex: Part 1—Sex and Gender," *Signs* 30, no. 2 (Winter 2005), doi:10.1086/424932.

46 *"Wanting to learn more about women and* . . . Marianne J. Legato, *Eve's Rib: The Groundbreaking Guide to Women's Health* (New York: Three Rivers Press, 2003).

47 *In 2002 and 2004, the two studies* . . . Women's Health Initiative, *Findings from the WHI Postmenopausal Hormone Therapy Trials*, last modified September 21, 2010, www.nhlbi.nih.gov/whi/.

47 *In its resulting report*, Women's Health Research: Progress, Pitfalls, and Promise . . . Institute of Medicine, *Women's Health Research.*

48 *"If anyone thinks women are going to keep paying half the cost of health care* . . . Laurence and Weinhouse, *Outrageous Practices*, 65.

48 *In 2011, in a study published in* Neuroscience & Biobehavioral Reviews . . . Annaliese K. Beery and Irving Zucker, "Sex Bias in Neuroscience and Biomedical Research," *Neuroscience & Biobehavioral Reviews* 35, no. 3 (January 2011), doi:10.1016/j.neubiorev.2010.07.002.

48 *Annaliese Beery, lead author of the study, explained to* HuffPost . . . Erin Schumaker, "Sexism in the Doctor's Office Starts Here," *HuffPost*, November 10, 2015, www.huffingtonpost.com/entry/women-are-excluded-from-clinical-trials_us_5637ad65e4b0c66bae5d36ba.

48 *In 2014, a review of over six hundred studies* . . . Dustin Y. Yoon et al., "Sex Bias Exists in Basic Science and Translational Surgical Research," *Surgery* 156, no. 3 (September 2014), doi:10.1016/j.surg.2014.07.001.

48 *For example, studies have found that skeletal muscle stem cells . . .* Sabra L. Klein et al., "Sex Inclusion in Basic Research Drives Discovery," *PNAS* 112, no. 17 (April 28, 2015), doi:10.1073/pnas.1502843112.

49 *But the widespread reliance on male animals seems to stem . . .* Irving Zucker and Annaliese K. Beery, "Males Still Dominate Animal Studies: Many Researchers Avoid Using Female Animals," *Nature* 465 (June 10, 2010), doi:10.1038/465690a.

49 *A 2014 meta-analysis of nearly three hundred articles . . .* Brian J. Prendergast, Kenneth G. Onishi, and Irving Zucker, "Female Mice Liberated for Inclusion in Neuroscience and Biomedical Research," *Neuroscience & Biobehavioral Reviews* 40 (March 2014), doi:10.1016/j.neubiorev.2014.01.001.

49 *As the authors of a 2009 review of the male bias . . .* Roger B. Fillingim et al., "Sex, Gender, and Pain: A Review of Recent Clinical and Experimental Findings," *The Journal of Pain: Official Journal of the American Pain Society* 10, no. 5 (May 2009), doi:10.1016/j.jpain.2008.12.001.

49 *Nevertheless, a 2005 study found that nearly 80 percent . . .* Jeffrey S. Mogil and Mona Lisa Chanda, "The Case for the Inclusion of Female Subjects in Basic Science Studies of Pain," *Pain* 117, nos. 1–2 (September 2005), doi:10.1016/j.pain.2005.06.020.

49 *That's "ethically indefensible," Dr. Jeffrey Mogil . . .* Kelly Oakes, "This Scientist Says Pain Research Must Include More Female Mice," *BuzzFeed*, July 13, 2016, www.buzzfeed.com/kellyoakes/pain-research-must-include-more-female-mice?utm_term=.wu091qBEWm#.ctgAdXpx4j.

49 *He recently called on his colleagues . . .* Jeffrey S. Mogil, "Perspective: Equality Need Not Be Painful," *Nature* 535, no. 7 (July 14, 2016), doi:10.1038/535S7a.

50 *Meanwhile, a 2007 study found that roughly 80 percent . . .* R. N. Hughes, "Sex Does Matter: Comments on the Prevalence of Male-Only Investigations of Drug Effects on Rodent Behaviour," *Behavioural Pharmacology* 18, no. 7 (November 2007), doi:10.1097/FBP.0b013e3282eff0e8.

50 *In 2014, the NIH announced . . .* Clayton and Collins, "Policy: NIH to Balance."

50 *that, since there'd been no . . .* Erika Check Hayden, "Sex Bias Blights Drug Studies," *Nature* 464 (March 2010), doi:10.1038/464332b.

50 *progress in correcting the male bias . . .* Chelsea Wald and Corinna Wu, "On Mice and Women: The Bias in Animal Models," *Science* 327, no. 5973 (March 26, 2010), doi:10.1126/science.327.5973.1571.

50 *"The overreliance on male animals and cells in preclinical" . . .* Clayton and Collins, "Policy: NIH to Balance."

50 *In addition, some feminist scientists and scholars have argued . . .* Azeen Ghorayshi, "Here's Why Some Feminists Have a Problem with the Feds' New Animal Testing Rules," *BuzzFeed*, November 26, 2015, www.buzzfeed.com/azeenghorayshi/fight-over-female-mice?utm_term=.gaKMWyabrQ#.mwEOkYWM31; Sarah S. Richardson et al., "Opinion: Focus on Preclinical Sex Differences Will Not Address Women's and Men's Health Disparities," *PNAS* 112, no. 44 (November 2015), doi:10.1073/pnas.1516958112.

51 *While there are certainly limitations to what animal studies . . .* Carolyn M. Mazure, "Our Evolving Science: Studying the Influence of Sex in Preclinical Research," *Biology of Sex Differences* 7 (February 2016), doi:10.1186/s13293-016-0068-8.

51 *help us understand disease mechanisms and develop new treatments . . .* Klein et al., "Sex Inclusion in Basic Research."

51 *In a 1995 report, the Council on Graduate Medical Education* ... U.S. Department of Health and Human Services, Council on Graduate Medicinal Education, *Fifth Report: Women and Medicine*, HRSA-P-DM-95-1, July 1995, www.hrsa.gov /advisorycommittees/bhpradvisory/cogme/Reports/fifthreportfull.pdf.

51 *In the midnineties, the Association of American Medical Colleges* ... U.S. Department of Health and Human Services et al., *Women's Health in the Medical School Curriculum, Report of a Survey and Recommendations* (Washington, DC: U.S. Department of Health and Human Services, Health Resources and Services Administration, and the National Institutes of Health, 1996).

52 *Subsequent medical school surveys have revealed* ... Alyson J. McGregor et al., "Advancing Sex and Gender Competency in Medicine: Sex & Gender Women's Health Collaborative," *Biology of Sex Differences* 4 (2013), doi:10.1186 /2042-6410-4-11.

52 *The proportion of schools* ... Janet B. Henrich, Catherine M. Viscoli, and Gallane D. Abraham, "Medical Students' Assessment of Education and Training in Women's Health and in Sex and Gender Differences," *Journal of Women's Health* 17, no. 5 (June 2008), doi:10.1089/jwh.2007.0589.

52 *A 2001 survey by the SWHR suggested that the number of schools* ... Sarah Knab Keitt et al., "Positioning Women's Health Curricula in US Medical Schools," *MedScape*, May 28, 2003, www.medscape.com/viewarticle/455372.

52 *Between 1996 and 2007, federal funding flowed* ... Carol S. Weisman and Gayle L. Squires, "Women's Health Centers: Are the National Centers of Excellence in Women's Health a New Model?" *Women's Health Issues* 10, no. 5 (September– October 2000), doi:10.1016/S1049-3867(00)00055-4.

54 *According to a 2011 survey of forty-four medical schools* ... Virginia M. Miller et al., "Embedding Concepts of Sex and Gender Health Differences into Medical Curricula," *Journal of Women's Health* 22, no. 3 (March 2013), doi:10.1089 /jwh.2012.4193.

54 *A 2006 study took a different approach* ... Janet B. Henrich and Catherine M. Viscoli, "What Do Medical Schools Teach About Women's Health and Gender Differences?" *Academic Medicine* 81, no. 5 (May 2006), doi:10.1097/01.ACM .0000222268.60211.fc.

55 *A 2012 case study assessed how well sex/gender-specific knowledge* ... Virginia M. Miller, Pricilla M. Flynn, and Keith D. Lindor, "Evaluating Sex and Gender Competencies in the Medical Curriculum: A Case Study," *Gender Medicine* 9, no. 3 (June 2012), doi:10.1016/j.genm.2012.01.006.

56 *It convened a group of thirty experts to review* ... "Programs & Projects," Sex and Gender Women's Health Collaborative, 2015, http://sgwhc.org/about /programs-and-projects/#sthash.39yCKNxO.dpbs.

57 *"We're really talking about a very short period of time* ... Carissa R. Violante, "The Long Road: Where Women's Health Has Been and Where It's Going," Yale School of Medicine, December 20, 2016, https://medicine.yale.edu/news/article .aspx?id=14132.

57 *A 2012 IOM report concluded* ... Wizemann, *Sex-Specific Reporting*.

58 *"Until recently, medical emphases on differences* ... Steven Epstein, *Inclusion: The Politics of Difference in Medical Research* (Chicago: The Univ. of Chicago Press, 2007), 13.

59 *"The essence of sex is not confined* ... Pierre Roussel, *Système physique et moral de la femme ou Tableau philosophique de la constitution, de l'état organique, du*

tempérament, des mœurs et des fonctions propres au sexe (Paris, 1775), quoted in Epstein, *The Politics of Difference*, 35.

59 *"more often than not, the abstract patient was* . . . W. F. Bynum, *Science and the Practice of Medicine in the Nineteenth Century* (Cambridge: Cambridge Univ. Press, 1994), 211, quoted in Carol S. Weisman, *Women's Health Care: Activist Traditions and Institutional Change* (Baltimore: Johns Hopkins Univ. Press, 1998), 34.

59 *"In contrast to the current view that medicine* . . . Weisman, *Women's Health Care*, 33.

CHAPTER 2. THE TRUST GAP

61 *The pain started on a Friday morning* . . . All quotes from author's interview with Maggie.

62 *Women are still interrupted more in professional settings* . . . Adrienne B. Hancock and Benjamin A. Rubin, "Influence of Communication Partner's Gender on Language," *Journal of Language and Social Psychology* 34, no. 1 (2015), doi:10.1177/0261927X14533197.

62 *They're still quoted less as experts by the media* . . . Women's Media Center, *The Status of Women in the U.S. Media 2015* (Women's Media Center, 2015), https://wmc.3cdn.net/83bf6082a319460eb1_hsrm680x2.pdf.

63 *Since a womb that "remains barren* . . . Plato, Timaeus, quoted in Mark S. Micale, *Approaching Hysteria: Disease and Its Interpretations* (Princeton, NJ: Princeton Univ. Press, 1995), 19.

64 *"The womb is the origin of all diseases* . . . The Hippocratic *Places in Man* 47 (L 6.344), quoted in Helen King, "Once Upon a Text: Hysteria from Hippocrates," in *Hysteria Beyond Freud*, ed. Sander L. Gilman et al. (Berkeley: Univ. of California Press, 1993), 12–13.

64 *During the medieval period, the uterine theory of hysteria* . . . Cecilia Tasca, "Women and Hysteria in the History of Mental Health," *Clinical Practice and Epidemiology in Mental Health* 8 (2012), doi:10.2174/1745017901208010110.

64 *"The hysterical female was interpreted* . . . Micale, *Approaching Hysteria*, 20.

64 *"which in the common opinion* . . . Edward Jorden, *A Briefe Discourse of a Disease Called the Suffocation of the Mother* (London: John Windet, 1603), quoted in Micale, *Approaching Hysteria*, 48.

64 *"When at any time* . . . Thomas Willis, *An Essay on the Pathology of the Brain and Nervous Stock* (London: Dring, Harper and Leigh, 1681), 76–8, quoted in Andrew Scull, *Hysteria: The Disturbing History* (Oxford: Oxford Univ. Press, 2011), 30.

64 *"the chief disorder is in the nervous system* . . . Willis, *Pathology*, 76–8, quoted in Scull, *Hysteria*, 31.

64 *"a more volatile, dissipable* . . . Richard Blackmore, *A Treatise of the Spleen and Vapours: Or, Hypochondriacal and Hysterical Affections* (London: Pemberton, 1726), 96, quoted in Scull, *Hysteria*, 40.

65 *"as one egg is to another* . . . *The Entire Works of Dr. Thomas Sydenham, Newly Made English*, ed. John Swan (London: Cave, 1742), 367–71, quoted in Scull, *Hysteria*, 32.

65 *"The functions of the brain* . . . George Man Burrows, *Commentaries on Insanity* (London: Underwood, 1828), 146, quoted in Gilman et al., *Hysteria Beyond Freud*, 252.

65 *"the controlling organ in* . . . Frederick Hollick, *The Diseases of Woman, Their*

Causes and Cure Familiarly Explained (New York: Excelsior Publishing House, 1849), quoted in Ehrenreich and English, *For Her Own Good*, 132.

65 "give woman all her characteristics . . . G. L. Austin, *Perils of American Women or A Doctor's Talk with Maiden, Wife, and Mother* (Boston: Lee and Shepard, 1883), quoted in Rita Arditti, "Women as Objects: Science and Sexual Politics," *Science for the People*, September 1974, 9.

65 *For a good decade leading up to the twentieth century* . . . Ben Barker-Benfield, "The Spermatic Economy: A Nineteenth Century View of Sexuality," *Feminist Studies* 1, no. 1 (Summer 1972), 45–74, quoted in Ehrenreich and English, *For Her Own Good*, 136.

65 "the destroyer of everything . . . Howard A. Kelly, "Conservatism in Ovariotomy," *Journal of the American Medical Association* 26 (February 1896), 251, quoted in Scull, *Hysteria*, 92.

66 "something fundamental in their nature . . . Paul Chodoff, "Hysteria and Women," *American Journal of Psychiatry* 139, no. 5 (May 1982), 546, quoted in Elaine Showalter, "Hysteria, Feminism, and Gender," in *Hysteria Beyond Freud*, ed. Sander L. Gilman et al. (Berkeley: Univ. of California Press, 1993), 286–287.

67 "It were better not to educate girls . . . Silas Weir Mitchell, *Wear and Tear, or Hints for the Overworked*, 5th ed. (Philadelphia: Lippincott, 1891), 56, quoted in Scull, *Hysteria*, 99.

67 *In the midst of debate* . . . Edward H. Clarke, *Sex in Education; or, A Fair Chance for the Girls* (Boston: Houghton, Mifflin and Company, 1884), quoted in Ehrenreich and English, *For Her Own Good*, 140.

67 "One shudders to think of the conclusions . . . John S. Haller Jr. and Robin M. Haller, *The Physician and Sexuality in Victorian America* (Urbana: Univ. of Illinois Press, 1974), 143–44, quoted in Ehrenreich and English, *For Her Own Good*, 123–124.

67 "The theory of female frailty . . . Ehrenreich and English, *For Her Own Good*, 123–124.

67 "I think, finally, it is in the increased attention . . . Mary Putnam Jacobi, "On Female Invalidism," in *Root of Bitterness: Documents of the Social History of American Women*, ed. Nancy F. Cott (New York: E. P. Dutton, 1972), 207, quoted in Ehrenreich and English, *For Her Own Good*, 127.

67 "The African negress, who toils . . . Lucien C. Warner, *A Popular Treatise on the Functions and Diseases of Woman* (New York: Manhattan Publishing Company, 1874), 109, quoted in Ehrenreich and English, *For Her Own Good*, 125–126.

68 "One finds an underlying logic . . . Ann Douglas Wood, "'Fashionable Diseases': Women's Complaints and Their Treatment in Nineteenth-Century America," *The Journal of Interdisciplinary History* 4, no. 1 (Summer 1973), doi:10.2307/202356.

68 *admitted the hysterical woman was* . . . Mitchell, *Wear and Tear*, 32, quoted in Scull, *Hysteria*, 99.

68 *One British doctor described the typical hysterical woman* . . . Robert Brudenell Carter, *On the Pathology and Treatment of Hysteria* (London: Churchill, 1853), 111, quoted in Scull, *Hysteria*, 69–70.

69 "Recognizably modern notions of specific . . . Charles E. Rosenberg, *Our Present Complaint: American Medicine, Then and Now* (Baltimore: Johns Hopkins Univ. Press, 2007), 18.

69 *psychoanalysis is "the child of the hysterical woman* . . . Carroll Smith-Rosenberg, *Disorderly Conduct: Visions of Gender in Victorian America* (1985; reprint, Oxford: Oxford Univ. Press, 1986), 197.

70 *"Under Freud's influence, the scalpel* . . . Barbara Ehrenreich and Deirdre English, *Complaints and Disorders* (New York: Feminist Press, 2011), 91.

70 *"shifted from 'physically sick'* . . . Ehrenreich and English, *Complaints and Disorders*, 148.

70 *"Hysteria is dead, that it is certain* . . . Étienne Trillat, *Histoire de l'hystérie* (Paris: Seghers, 1986), 274, quoted in Micale, *Approaching Hysteria*, 169.

71 the term *"came to mean so many different things that* . . . Micale, *Approaching Hysteria*, 220.

71 *In a process that Micale called "diagnostic drift,"* . . . Micale, *Approaching Hysteria*, 174.

72 *Anna O. perhaps would today be diagnosed with* . . . Richard Webster, "Freud, Charcot and Hysteria: Lost in the Labyrinth," excerpted from Webster, *Freud* (London: Weidenfeld & Nicolson, 2003), www.richardwebster.net/freudandcharcot.html.

72 *"A generation ago* . . . James R. Morrison, "Management of Briquet Syndrome (Hysteria)," *The Western Journal of Medicine* 128, no. 6 (June 1978), www.ncbi .nlm.nih.gov/pmc/articles/PMC1238186/.

72 *in the 1960s, a group of American researchers* . . . Carol North, "The Classification of Hysteria and Related Disorders: Historical and Phenomenological Considerations," *Behavioral Sciences* 5, no. 4 (November 2015), doi:10.3390/bs5040496.

73 *First coined in the 1920s* . . . Wilhelm Stekel, quoted in Z. J. Lipowski, "Somatization: A Borderland Between Medicine and Psychiatry," *CMAJ* 135, no. 6 (September 1986), doi:10.1016/S0196-0644(87)80335-9.

73 *Acknowledging that the idea was* . . . Lipowski, "Somatization: A Borderland."

73 *"Patients with persistent somatization* . . . Lipowski, "Somatization: A Borderland."

73 *psychological theories of illness "are always* . . . Susan Sontag, *Illness as Metaphor* (1977; reprint, New York: Farrar, Straus and Giroux, 1978), 55–57.

74 *"Does the patient accept herself as a woman?"* J. P. Greenhill, *Office Gynecology* (Chicago: Year Book Medical Publishers, 1971), quoted in Gena Corea, *The Hidden Malpractice: How American Medicine Mistreats Women* (New York: Harper Colophon Books, 1985), 80.

74 *"there was remarkable agreement* . . . S. Munch, "Gender-Biased Diagnosing of Women's Medical Complaints: Contributions of Feminist Thought, 1970–1995," *Women & Health* 40, no. 1 (2004), doi:10.1300/J013v40n01_06.

74 *in the late seventies studies began to document* . . . Jacqueline Wallen, Howard Waitzkin, and John Stoeckle, "Physician Stereotypes About Female Health and Illness: A Study of Patient's Sex and the Informative Process During Medical Interviews," *Women & Health* 4, no. 2 (Summer 1979), doi:10.1300/J013v04n02_03; Karen J. Armitage, Lawrence J. Schneiderman, and Robert A. Bass, "Response of Physicians to Medical Complaints in Men and Women," *JAMA* 241, no. 20 (May 1979), doi:10.1001/jama.1979.03290460050020.

74 *"The open and emotional behavioral style* . . . Barbara Bernstein and Robert Kane, "Physicians' Attitudes Toward Female Patients," *Medical Care* 19, no. 6 (June 1981), www.jstor.org/stable/3763923.

74 *"might be responding to current stereotypes* . . . Armitage, Schneiderman, and Bass, "Response of Physicians to Medical Complaints."

75 *"Following traditional linguistic convention* . . . Mary C. Howell, "What Medical Schools Teach About Women," *The New England Journal of Medicine* 291 (August 8, 1974), doi:10.1056/NEJM197408082910612.

75 *According to a 1973 survey* . . . Margaret A. Campbell, *Why Would a Girl Go into*

Medicine? Medical Education in the United States: A Guide for Women (New York: Feminist Press, 1973).

75 *A 1971 gynecology text warned that* . . . Greenhill, *Office Gynecology*, quoted in Corea, *The Hidden Malpractice*, 80.

75 *According to the textbook, in cases of dysmenorrhea* . . . Greenhill, *Office Gynecology*, quoted in Corea, *The Hidden Malpractice*, 80.

76 *Nausea during early pregnancy* . . . Greenhill, *Office Gynecology*, quoted in Corea, *The Hidden Malpractice*, 81.

76 *"somatoform disorders* . . . North, "The Classification of Hysteria."

76 *"The somatoform disorders have* . . . Z. J. Lipowski, "Somatization: The Concept and Its Clinical Application," *American Journal of Psychiatry* 145, no. 11 (November 1988), doi: 10.1176/ajp.145.11.1358.

77 *With the exception of hypochondriasis* . . . Arthur J. Barsky, Heli M. Peekna, and Jonathan F. Borus, "Somatic Symptom Reporting in Women and Men," *Journal of General Internal Medicine* 16, no. 4 (2001), doi:10.1046/j.1525-1497.2001.00229.x.

77 *The mnemonic aid* . . . E. Othmer and C. DeSouza, "A Screening Test for Somatization Disorder (Hysteria)," *American Journal of Psychiatry* 142, no. 10 (1985), doi:10.1176/ajp.142.10.1146.

77 *"'Functional' [is] the contemporary term* . . . David Edelberg, "Fibromyalgia Confounds Allopathic Habits of Mind," *AMA Journal of Ethics* 14, no. 4 (April 2012), http://journalofethics.ama-assn.org/2012/04/ecas2-1204.html.

77 *"The symptoms of somatizing patients* . . . Lipowski, "Somatization: The Concept."

77 *often used to imply a psychogenic origin* . . . Elizabeth M. Marks and Myra S. Hunter, "Medically Unexplained Symptoms: An Acceptable Term?" *British Journal of Pain* 9, no. 2 (May 2015), doi:10.1177/2049463714535372.

77 *In an analysis of seventy-five articles* . . . Annemarie Jutel, "Medically Unexplained Symptoms and the Disease Label," *Social Theory & Health* 8, no. 3 (November 2010), doi:10.1057/sth.2009.21.

77 *"following a frequently challenged* . . . Michael Sharpe, "Somatic Symptoms: Beyond 'Medically Unexplained,'" *The British Journal of Psychiatry* 203, no. 5 (November 2013), doi:10.1192/bjp.bp.112.122523.

78 *that's exactly how medicine thinks of them* . . . Jon Stone et al., "What Should We Say to Patients with Symptoms Unexplained by Disease? The 'Number Needed to Offend,'" *BMJ* 325 (December 2002), doi:10.1136/bmj.325.7378.1449.

78 *In one 2009 study* . . . Tim C. Olde Hartman et al., "Explanation and Relations. How Do General Practitioners Deal with Patients with Persistent Medically Unexplained Symptoms: A Focus Group Study," *BMC Family Practice* 10 (2009), doi:10.1186/1471-2296-10-68.

78 *Almost invariably patients* . . . Peter Salmon, Sarah Peters, and Ian Stanley, "Patients' Perceptions of Medical Explanations for Somatisation Disorders: Qualitative Analysis," *BMJ* 318, no. 7180 (February 1999), www.ncbi.nlm.nih.gov/pmc/articles/PMC27727/.

78 *In an afterword to his influential 2007 book* . . . Jerome Groopman, *How Doctors Think* (New York: Houghton Mifflin Harcourt, 2007), 276.

79 *In a biting critique* . . . Allen Frances, "The New Somatic Symptom Disorder in DSM-5 Risks Mislabeling Many People as Mentally Ill," *BMJ* 346 (March 2013), doi:10.1136/bmj.f1580.

79 *Studies have estimated* . . . Heather Huang and Robert M. McCarron, "Medically Unexplained Physical Symptoms: Evidence-Based Interventions," *Current*

Psychiatry 10, no. 7 (July 2011), www.mdedge.com/currentpsychiatry/article /64365/depression/medically-unexplained-physical-symptoms-evidence-based.

80 *"It is not unusual for physical diseases* ... Annemarie Goldstein Jutel, *Putting a Name to It: Diagnosis in Contemporary Society* (Baltimore: Johns Hopkins Univ. Press, 2011), 30.

80 *In treating "medically unexplained symptoms" as if* ... Jutel, *Putting a Name to It*, 82.

80 *And in attributing a psychogenic cause* ... Jutel, *Putting a Name to It*, 86.

80 *"the wastepaper basket of medicine* ... Charles Lasègue, quoted in Angela Kennedy, *Authors of Our Own Misfortune? The Problems with Psychogenic Explanations for Physical Illnesses* (New York: Village Digital Press, 2012), 17.

81 *Eliot Slater warned in a 1965 editorial* ... Eliot Slater, "Diagnosis of 'Hysteria,'" *British Medical Journal* 1, no. 5447 (May 1965), doi:10.1136/bmj.1.5447.1395.

82 *"The lack of an objective test* ... Laurie Endicott Thomas, "Are Your Patient's Medically Unexplained Symptoms Really 'All in Her Head'?" *Medical Hypotheses* 78, no. 4 (April 2012), doi:10.1016/j.mehy.2012.01.031.

82 *"a patient with somatization will often deny* ... Lipowski, "Somatization: A Borderland."

82 *"It is a diagnosis made* ... Jutel, *Putting a Name to It*, 83.

83 *The American Academy of Family Physicians* ... Oliver Omaya, Catherine Paltoo, and Julian Greengold, "Somatoform Disorders," *American Family Physician* 76, no. 9 (November 2007), www.aafp.org/afp/2007/1101/p1333.html.

83 *"out of a fear of overlooking a serious disease* ... Teus Kappen and Sandra van Dulmen, "General Practitioners' Responses to the Initial Presentation of Medically Unexplained Symptoms: A Quantitative Analysis," *Biopsychosocial Medicine* 2 (November 2008), doi:10.1186/1751-0759-2-22.

83 *In a 2016 Dutch study* ... Madelon den Boeft, "Recognition of Patients with Medically Unexplained Physical Symptoms by Family Physicians: Results of a Focus Group Study," *BMC Family Practice* 17, no. 55 (May 2016), doi:10.1186 /s12875-016-0451-x.

83 *A 2000 British study* ... C. Nimnuan, M. Hotopf, and S. Wessely, "Medically Unexplained Symptoms: How Often and Why Are They Missed?" *QJM* 93, no. 1 (January 2000), doi:10.1093/qjmed/93.1.21.

84 *"The vehemence with which many patients* ... Michael Sharpe, "ME. What Do We Know—Real Physical Illness or All in the Mind?" (lecture, University of Strathclyde, Glasgow, October 1999), quoted in Kennedy, *Authors of Our Own Misfortune?*, 158.

85 *"The difference between* ... Antoinette J. Church, "Myalgic Encephalitis: An Obscene Cosmic Joke?" *Medical Journal of Australia* 1, no. 7 (April 1980): 307–9, quoted in Robert A. Aronowitz, *Making Sense of Illness: Science, Society, and Disease* (Cambridge: Cambridge Univ. Press, 1998), 33.

85 *"In medicine, resistance to the notion of error* ... Diane O'Leary, "Re: The New Somatic Symptom Disorder in DSM-5 Risks Mislabeling Many People as Mentally Ill," *BMJ* 346 (2013), www.bmj.com/content/346/bmj.f1580/rr/638352.

85 *diagnostic errors are a* ... Mark L. Graber, "The Incidence of Diagnostic Error in Medicine," *BMJ Quality Safety* (June 15, 2013), doi:10.1136/bmjqs-2012 -001615.

85 *In 2015, an IOM report concluded* ... National Academies of Sciences, Engineering, and Medicine; Institute of Medicine; Board on Health Care

Services; Committee on Diagnostic Error in Health Care, *Improving Diagnosis in Health Care*, eds. Erin P. Balogh, Bryan T. Miller, and John R. Ball (Washington, DC: The National Academies Press, 2015), doi:10.17226/21794.

85 *The Society to Improve Diagnosis in Medicine estimates* . . . "About Diagnostic Error," Society to Improve Diagnosis in Medicine, www.improvediagnosis.org /page/AboutDiagnosticErr.

85 *A 2014 study concluded* . . . Hardeep Singh, Ashley N. D. Meyer, and Eric J. Thomas, "The Frequency of Diagnostic Errors in Outpatient Care: Estimations from Three Large Observational Studies Involving US Adult Populations," *BMJ Quality Safety* (April 17, 2014), doi:10.1136/bmjqs-2013-002627.

85 *According to a conservative estimate* . . . Martin A. Makary and Daniel Michael, "Medical Error—The Third Leading Cause of Death in the US," *The BMJ* 353 (2016), doi:10.1136/bmj.i2139.

86 *"The concept that they* . . . Eta S. Berner and Mark L. Graber, "Overconfidence as a Cause of Diagnostic Error in Medicine," *The American Journal of Medicine* 121, no. 5 (May 2008), doi:10.1016/j.amjmed.2008.01.001.

86 *"It seems a remarkable coincidence* . . . Susan Wendell, "Old Women Out of Control: Some Thoughts on Aging, Ethics, and Psychosomatic Medicine" in *Mother Time: Women, Aging, and Ethics*, ed. Margaret U. Walker (Lanham, MD: Rowman and Littlefield; 1999), 140.

87 *As Angela Kennedy points out* . . . Kennedy, *Authors of Our Own Misfortune?*, 221.

88 *"borderland between psychiatry and medicine* . . . Lipowski, "Somatization: A Borderland."

88 *"old wine in new bottles"* . . . S. Wessely, "Old Wine in New Bottles: Neurasthenia and 'ME,'" *Psychological Medicine* 20, no. 1 (February 1990), www.ncbi.nlm.nih .gov/labs/articles/2181519/.

89 *"we are in a catch-22 situation* . . . Quoted in Martin Pall, *Explaining Unexplained Illnesses: Disease Paradigm for Chronic Fatigue Syndrome, Multiple Chemical Sensitivity, Fibromyalgia, Post-Traumatic Stress Disorder, Gulf War Syndrome and Others* (Boca Raton, FL: CRC Press, 2007), 113.

90 *In a 2016 article* . . . Carolyn E. Wilshire and Tony Ward, "Psychogenic Explanations of Physical Illness: Time to Examine the Evidence," *Perspectives on Psychological Science* 11, no. 5 (September 29, 2016), doi:10.1177/1745691616645540.

90 *"One of the great puzzles* . . . Pall, *Explaining Unexplained Illnesses*, 217.

90 *In a 1986 study* . . . B. L. Miller et al., "Misdiagnosis of Hysteria," *American Family Physician* 34, no. 4 (October 1986), http://europepmc.org/abstract/med/3766359.

91 *Women are about twice as likely to have a diagnosis of depression or anxiety disorder* . . . National Institute of Mental Health, "Major Depression Among Adults," 2015, www.nimh.nih.gov/health/statistics/prevalence/major-depression-among-adults .shtml; National Institute of Mental Health, "Any Anxiety Disorder Among Adults," www.nimh.nih.gov/health/statistics/prevalence/any-anxiety-disorder-among -adults.shtml.

91 *About one in five women in the United States* . . . Thomas J. Moore and Donald R. Mattison, "Adult Utilization of Psychiatric Drugs and Differences by Sex, Age, and Race," *JAMA Internal Medicine* 177, no. 2 (February 2017), doi:10.1001 /jamainternmed.2016.7507.

91 *And it's estimated that four out of five* . . . Ramin Mojtabai and Mark Olfson, "Proportion of Antidepressants Prescribed Without a Psychiatric Diagnosis Is Growing," *Health Affairs* 30, no. 8 (August 2011), doi:10.1377/hlthaff.2010.1024.

91 *Studies in the nineties suggested* . . . Bonnie J. Floyd, "Problems in Accurate Medical Diagnosis of Depression in Female Patients," *Social Science & Medicine* 44, no. 3 (February 1997), doi:10.1016/S0277-9536(96)00159-1.

92 *They warned their fellow mental health* . . . Elizabeth A. Klonoff and Hope Landrine, *Preventing Misdiagnosis of Women: A Guide to Physical Disorders That Have Psychiatric Symptoms* (Thousand Oaks, CA: SAGE Publications, 1997), xxii.

92 *"Ironically, medical misdiagnoses* . . . Floyd, "Problems in Accurate Medical Diagnosis."

92 *"psych-out error"* . . . Pat Croskerry, "The Importance of Cognitive Errors in Diagnosis and Strategies to Minimize Them," *Academic Medicine* 78, no. 8 (August 2003), http://journals.lww.com/academicmedicine/Fulltext/2003/08000 /The_Importance_of_Cognitive_Errors_in_Diagnosis.3.aspx.

94 *In an influential 2001 article entitled "The Girl Who Cried Pain* . . . Diane E. Hoffmann and Anita J. Tarzian, "The Girl Who Cried Pain: A Bias Against Women in the Treatment of Pain," *Journal of Law, Medicine & Ethics* 29 (2001), doi:10.1111/j.1748-720X.2001.tb00037.x.

94 *In the hospital setting, one study showed that women received* . . . B. S. Faherty and M. R. Grier, "Analgesic Medication for Elderly People Post-Surgery," *Nursing Research* 33, no. 6 (November–December 1984), www.ncbi.nlm.nih.gov/pubmed /6567868.

94 *Another found that after a coronary artery* . . . Karen L. Calderone, "The Influence of Gender on the Frequency of Pain and Sedative Medication Administered to Post-operative Patients," *Sex Roles* 23, no. 11 (December 1990), doi:10.1007/BF00289259.

94 *The difference started early* . . . Judith E. Beyer et al., "Patterns of Postoperative Analgesic Use with Adults and Children Following Cardiac Surgery," *Pain* 17, no. 1 (September 1983), doi:10.1016/0304-3959(83)90129-X.

94 *Studies of metastatic cancer* . . . Hoffmann and Tarzian, "The Girl Who Cried Pain."

94 *and AIDS patients found that women were overrepresented* . . . William Breitbart et al., "The Undertreatment of Pain in Ambulatory AIDS Patients," *Pain* 65, nos. 2–3 (May 1996), doi:10.1016/0304-3959(95)00217-0.

94 *In the late eighties and early nineties, pain researchers* . . . Roger B. Fillingim et al., "Sex, Gender, and Pain: A Review of Recent Clinical and Experimental Findings."

95 *A 2008 study of nearly a thousand people* . . . Ester H. Chen et al., "Gender Disparity in Analgesic Treatment of Emergency Department Patients with Acute Abdominal Pain," *Academic Emergency Medicine* 15, no. 5 (May 2008), doi:10.1111/j.1553-2712.2008.00100.x.

96 *Public health researcher Kate Hunt* . . . Kate Hunt et al., "Do Women Consult More Than Men? A Review of Gender and Consultation for Back Pain and Headache," *Journal of Health Services Research & Policy* 16, no. 2 (April 2011), doi:10.1258 /jhsrp.2010.009131.

98 *In a 2014 study that found female heart attack* . . . Roxanne Pelletier et al., "Sex-Related Differences in Access to Care Among Patients with Premature Acute Coronary Syndrome," *CMAJ: Canadian Medical Association Journal* 186, no. 7 (April 2014), doi:10.1503/cmaj.131450.

99 *Take Lauron's experience* . . . All quotes from author's interview with Lauron.

100 *"Patients with persistent somatization* . . . Lipowski, "Somatization: A Borderland."

100 *"These labels express the frustration* . . . Lipowski, "Somatization: The Concept."

100 *article from the late eighties that coined the term "heartsink patients"* . . . T. C. O'Dowd, "Five Years of Heartsink Patients in General Practice," *BMJ* 297, no. 6647

(August 1988), www.ncbi.nlm.nih.gov/pmc/articles/PMC1840368/pdf/bmj00300 -0038.pdf.

100 *As Dr. Lisa Sanders . . .* Lisa Sanders, *Every Patient Tells a Story: Medical Mysteries and the Art of Diagnosis* (New York: Broadway Books, 2009), 183.

100 *As one article on "medically unexplained symptoms" noted . . .* Laurence J. Kirmayer et al., "Explaining Medically Unexplained Symptoms," *Canadian Journal of Psychiatry* 49, no. 10 (October 2004), https://ww1.cpa-apc.org/Publications /Archives/CJP/2004/october/kirmayer.asp.

101 *"The communication of somatic complaints . . .* Lipowski, "Somatization: The Concept."

101 *In one 1978 article . . .* James R. Morrison, "Management of Briquet Syndrome (Hysteria)," *Western Journal of Medicine* 128, no. 6 (June 1978), www.ncbi.nlm.nih .gov/pmc/articles/PMC1238186/pdf/westjmed00262-0032.pdf.

102 *"Clinicians behaved as though . . .* Chloë Atkins, *My Imaginary Illness: A Journey into Uncertainty and Prejudice in Medical Diagnosis* (Ithaca, NY: Cornell Univ. Press, 2010), 149.

103 *"a cultural artifact masquerading as a medical truth . . .* Atkins, *My Imaginary Illness*, 126.

CHAPTER 3. HEART DISEASE AND OTHER LIFE-THREATENING EMERGENCIES

109 *On a spring morning in 2008, Carolyn Thomas . . .* All quotes from author's interview with Carolyn Thomas.

110 *Advertised "for women only," it was called . . .* Laurence and Weinhouse, *Outrageous Practices*, 85–86.

110 *In 2016, the association released its first official scientific . . .* Laxmi S. Mehta et al., "Acute Myocardial Infarction in Women: A Scientific Statement from the American Heart Association," Circulation 133, no. 9 (March 1, 2016), doi:10.1161 /CIR.0000000000000351.

111 *About one in three deaths among women each . . .* American Heart Association, "Women and Cardiovascular Diseases," last modified 2015, www.heart.org /idc/groups/heart-public/@wcm/@sop/@smd/documents/downloadable/ucm _472913.pdf.

111 *"diagnostic and therapeutic strategies . . .* C. Noel Bairey Merz, "The Single Biggest Health Threat Women Face," TEDxWomen, December 2011, www.ted.com/talks /noel_bairey_merz_the_single_biggest_health_threat_women_face?language =en#t-858816.

111 *The result was that since 1984, more women than men . . .* Lori Mosca, Elizabeth Barrett-Connor, and Nanette Wenger, "Sex/Gender Difference in Cardiovascular Disease Prevention," *Circulation* 124, no. 19 (November 2011), doi:10.1161 /CIRCULATIONAHA.110.968792.

111 *26 percent of women versus 19 percent of men . . .* Mehta et al., "Acute Myocardial Infarction."

111 *In 1991, Dr. Bernadine Healy . . .* Bernadine Healy, "The Yentl Syndrome," *The New England Journal of Medicine* 325 (July 1991), doi:10.1056/NEJM199107253250408.

112 *In 1997, only 30 percent of American . . .* Lori Mosca et al., "Twelve-Year Follow-Up of American Women's Awareness of Cardiovascular Disease Risk and Barriers to Heart Health," *Circulation: Cardiovascular Quality and Outcomes* 3, no. 2 (March 2010), doi:10.1161/CIRCOUTCOMES.109.915538.

112 *by 2009, that figure . . .* Mosca et al., "Twelve-Year Follow-Up."

112 *Still, as recently as 2005, only 8 percent* . . . Lori Mosca et al., "National Study of Physician Awareness and Adherence to Cardiovascular Disease Prevention Guidelines," *Circulation* 111 (February 2011), doi:10.1161/01.CIR .0000154568.43333.82.

112 *And according to a 2017 survey, only 22 percent* . . . C. Noel Bairey Merz et al., "Knowledge, Attitudes, and Beliefs Regarding Cardiovascular Disease in Women," *Journal of the American College of Cardiology* 70, no. 2 (July 2017), doi:10.1016/j .jacc.2017.05.024.

112 *Meanwhile, a 2015 meta-analysis* . . . Aimee Galick, Elizabeth D'Arrigo-Patrick, and Carmen Knudson-Martin, "Can Anyone Hear Me? Does Anyone See Me? A Qualitative Meta-Analysis of Women's Experiences of Heart Disease," *Qualitative Health Research* 25, no. 8 (August 2015), doi:10.1177/1049732315584743.

113 *In a 2008 experiment* . . . M. Bönte et al., "Women and Men with Coronary Heart Disease in Three Countries: Are They Treated Differently?" *Women's Health Issues* 18, no. 3 (May–June 2008), doi:10.1016/j.whi.2008.01.003.

113 *In 2005, the AHA tested* . . . Mosca et al., "National Study of Physician Awareness."

114 *But a young and healthy woman* . . . Jan C. Frich, Kristi Malterud, and Per Fugelli, "Women at Risk of Coronary Heart Disease Experience Barriers to Diagnosis and Treatment: A Qualitative Interview Study," *Scandinavian Journal of Primary Health Care* 24, no. 1 (2006), doi:10.1080/02813430500504305.

114 *"I talked to the nurse practitioner and told her* . . . Jean C. McSweeney, Leanne L. Lefler, and Beth F. Crowder, "What's Wrong with Me? Women's Coronary Heart Disease Diagnostic Experiences," *Progress in Cardiovascular Nursing* 20, no. 2 (Spring 2005), doi:10.1111/j.0889-7204.2005.04447.x.

114 *seventy-two years compared to sixty-five years for men* . . . Dariush Mozaffarian et al., "Heart Disease and Stroke Statistics—2015 Update: A Report from the American Heart Association," *Circulation* 131 (December 2015), doi:10.1161 /CIR.0000000000000152.

114 *and at every age up until seventy-five* . . . Mosca, Barrett-Connor, and Wenger, "Sex/Gender."

114 *Still, about 40,000 women under age fifty-five are hospitalized* . . . American Heart Association, "Most Young Women Don't Recognize Heart Attack Warning Signs," *ScienceDaily*, May 11, 2007, www.sciencedaily.com/releases /2007/05/070510160957.htm.

114 *Heart disease, in fact, kills more women at every age than* . . . Bairey Merz, "Biggest Health Threat."

114 *Studies in the nineties showed that younger female* . . . Viola Vaccarino et al., "Sex-Based Differences in Early Mortality After Myocardial Infarction," *The New England Journal of Medicine* 341, no. 4 (July 22, 1999), doi:10.1056 /NEJM199907223410401.

114 *a mortality gap that has just recently begun to narrow* . . . Viola Vaccarino et al., "Sex Differences in Mortality After Acute Myocardial Infarction: Changes from 1994 to 2006," *Archives of Internal Medicine* 169, no. 19 (October 2009), doi:10.1001 /archinternmed.2009.332.

114 *In fact, despite the overall downward* . . . Mehta et al., "Acute Myocardial Infarction."

114 *"I can clearly remember the distress I felt* . . . Frich, Malterud, and Fugelli, "Women at Risk."

115 *Indeed, in a study published in* The New England Journal of Medicine . . . J. Hector Pope et al., "Missed Diagnoses of Acute Cardiac Ischemia in the Emergency

Department," *The New England Journal of Medicine* 342, no. 16 (April 20, 2000), doi:10.1056/NEJM200004203421603.

115 *a "knowledge-mediated bias"* . . . K. Hamberg, "Gender Bias in Medicine," *Women's Health* 4, no. 3 (May 2008), doi:10.2217/17455057.4.3.237.

116 *Between 1980 and 2000, women's mortality rates* . . . MeiLan K. Han et al., "Gender and Chronic Obstructive Pulmonary Disease," *American Journal of Respiratory and Critical Care Medicine* 176, no. 12 (December 15, 2007), doi:10.1164/rccm .200704-553CC.

116 *In a 2001 study, researchers suggested that COPD* . . . Kenneth R. Chapman, Donald P. Tashkin, and David J. Pye, "Gender Bias in the Diagnosis of COPD," *Chest Journal* 119, no. 6 (June 2001), doi:10.1378/chest.119.6.1691.

116 *Today, despite now officially having* . . . American Lung Association, *Taking Her Breath Away: The Rise of COPD in Women*, June 2013, www.lung.org/assets /documents/research/rise-of-copd-in-women-summary.pdf.

117 *like autism and attention deficient disorder* . . . Maia Szalavitz, "New Research Suggests the Disorder Often Looks Different in Females, Many of Whom Are Being Misdiagnosed and Missing Out on the Support They Need," *Scientific American,* March 1, 2016, https://www.scientificamerican.com/article/autism -it-s-different-in-girls/; Jenny Anderson, "Decades of Failing to Recognize ADHD in Girls Has Created a 'Lost Generation' of Women," *Quartz,* January 19, 2016, https://qz.com/592364/decades-of-failing-to-recognize-adhd-in-girls-has-created -a-lost-generation-of-women/.

117 *It took Mae six doctor's visits* . . . All quotes from author's interview with Mae.

117 *in the sixties, it was estimated at 6:1* . . . G. C. Manzoni, "Gender Ratio of Cluster Headache over the Years: A Possible Role of Changes in Lifestyle," *Cephalalgia* 18, no. 3 (April 1998), doi:10.1046/j.1468-2982.1998.1803138.x.

119 *For example, while high total cholesterol is* . . . Mehta et al., "Acute Myocardial Infarction."

119 *Having type 2 diabetes increases* . . . Mehta et al., "Acute Myocardial Infarction."

119 *In 2011, the AHA declared for the first time that pregnancy complications* . . . Lori Mosca et al., "Effectiveness-Based Guidelines for the Prevention of Cardiovascular Disease in Women—2011 Update: A Guideline from the American Heart Association," *Circulation* 123, no. 11 (March 2011), doi:10.1161/CIR.0b013e31820faaf8.

119 *In the future, women's risk scores* . . . Pamela Ouyang et al., "Strategies and Methods to Study Female-Specific Cardiovascular Health and Disease: A Guide for Clinical Scientists," *Biology of Sex Differences* 7 (March 2016), doi:10.1186/s13293-016-0073-y.

120 *Yet in 1996, a national survey* . . . Martha Weinman Lear, "The Woman's Heart Attack," *The New York Times,* September 20, 2014, www.nytimes.com/2014/09/28 /opinion/sunday/womens-atypical-heart-attacks.html?_r=1.

120 *And a 2012 survey of American women found that less than* . . . Lori Mosca et al., "Fifteen-Year Trends in Awareness of Heart Disease in Women: Results of a 2012 American Heart Association National Survey," *Circulation* 127, no. 11 (March 19, 2013), doi: 10.1161/CIR.0b013e318287cf2f.

120 *A 2012 study that tracked more than 1.1 million* . . . John G. Canto, "Association of Age and Sex with Myocardial Infarction Symptom Presentation and In-Hospital Mortality," *JAMA* 307, no. 8 (February 2012), doi:10.1001/jama.2012.199.

120 *A study published in* The BMJ . . . Anoop S. V. Shah et al., "High Sensitivity Cardiac Troponin and the Under-Diagnosis of Myocardial Infarction in Women: Prospective Cohort Study," *The BMJ* 350 (February 2015), doi:10.1136/bmj.g7873.

121 *In a 2015 qualitative study* . . . Judith H. Lichtman et al., "Symptom Recognition and Healthcare Experiences of Young Women with Acute Myocardial Infarction," *Circulation: Cardiovascular Quality and Outcomes* 9, no. 6 (November 2016), doi:10.1161/CIRCOUTCOMES.114.001612.

122 *"Doctors think that men have heart attacks* . . . C. J. Lisk and L. Grau, "Perceptions of Women Living with Coronary Heart Disease: An Overview of Study Findings," *American Journal of Geriatric Cardiology* 8, no. 4 (July 1999), doi:10.1300 /J013v29n01_03.

122 *A series of studies* . . . Gabrielle Rosina Chiaramonte, "Physicians' Gender Bias in the Diagnosis, Treatment, and Interpretation of Coronary Heart Disease Symptoms," (Ph.D. diss., Stony Brook Univ., 2007), https://dspace.sunyconnect .suny.edu/bitstream/handle/1951/44285/000000052.sbu.pdf?sequence=2.

122 *The presence of stress, the researchers explained* . . . Cardiovascular Research Foundation, "Signs of Heart Disease Are Attributed to Stress More Frequently in Women Than Men," *ScienceDaily*, October 14, 2008, www.sciencedaily.com /releases/2008/10/081012121314.htm.

123 *A 2014 study that tracked* . . . Pelletier et al., "Sex-Related Differences in Access to Care Among Patients with Premature Acute Coronary Syndrome."

124 *That's what was suggested by a 2009 study* . . . Nancy N. Maserejian et al., "Disparities in Physicians' Interpretations of Heart Disease Symptoms by Patient Gender: Results of a Video Vignette Factorial Experiment," *Journal of Women's Health* 18, no. 10 (October 2009), doi:10.1089/jwh.2008.1007.

124 *Chest pain is the second most common* . . . Basmah Safdar and Gail D'Onofrio, "Women and Chest Pain: Recognizing the Different Faces of Angina in the Emergency Department," *The Yale Journal of Biology and Medicine* 89, no. 2 (June 2016), www.ncbi.nlm.nih.gov/pmc/articles/PMC4918863/.

124 *One cardiologist put it* . . . Denise Dador, "'Medical Sexism': Women's Heart Disease Symptoms Often Dismissed," *ABC Eyewitness News*, November 2, 2011, http://abc7.com/archive/8416664/.

125 *While survival rates increase by half* . . . Debra K. Mosner et al., "Reducing Delay in Seeking Treatment by Patients with Acute Coronary Syndrome and Stroke: A Scientific Statement from the American Heart Association Council on Cardiovascular Nursing and Stroke Council," *Circulation* 114, no. 2 (July 2006), doi:10.1161/CIRCULATIONAHA.106.176040.

125 *and multiple studies have shown that women* . . . Mehta et al., "Acute Myocardial Infarction."

125 *According to a 2014 study* . . . C. Kreatsoulas et al., "The Symptomatic Tipping Point: Factors That Prompt Men and Women to Seek Medical Care," *Canadian Journal of Cardiology* 30, no. 10 supp. (October 2014), www.onlinecjc.ca/article /S0828-282X(14)00661-8/pdf.

125 *That certainly seems to be part of the story, according to the 2015 study* . . . Judith H. Lichtman, "Symptom Recognition and Healthcare Experiences of Young Women with Acute Myocardial Infarction," *Circulation: Cardiovascular Quality and Outcomes* 9, no. 6 (February 2015), doi:10.1161/CIRCOUTCOMES.114.001612.

126 *Patti is one woman* . . . Unless otherwise noted, all Patti Digh quotes are from the author's interview with Digh.

128 *"The sad fact is that I waited* . . . Patti Digh, "No, You Are Not an Hysterical Female, and This Is Not Just Anxiety," *HuffPost*, January 29, 2017, www.huffingtonpost .com/patti-digh/no-you-are-not-an-hysteri_b_9110982.html.

128 *"It's amazing and really alarming to see that cardiac arrest . . .* All quotes from author's interview with Alyson McGregor (director of the Division of Sex and Gender in Emergency Medicine at the Warren Alpert Medical School of Brown University).

128 *Indeed, in 2014, the first large-scale study . . .* David E. Newman-Toker et al., "Missed Diagnosis of Stroke in the Emergency Department: A Cross-Sectional Analysis of a Large Population-Based Sample," *Diagnosis* 1, no. 2 (April 2014), doi:10.1515/dx-2013-0038.

128 *between 50,000 and 100,000 missed stroke diagnoses . . .* Johns Hopkins Medicine, "ER Doctors Commonly Miss More Strokes Among Women, Minorities and Younger Patients," April 3, 2014, http://www.hopkinsmedicine.org/news/media /releases/er_doctors_commonly_miss_more_strokes_among_women_minorities _and_younger_patients.

129 *A 2016 analysis . . .* Luke K. Kim et al., "Sex-Based Disparities in Incidence, Treatment, and Outcomes of Cardiac Arrest in the United States, 2003–2012," *Journal of the American Heart Association* 5, no. 6 (June 2016), doi:10.1161 /JAHA.116.003704.

129 *After adjusting for other factors . . .* "Gender Gap Found in Cardiac Arrest Care, Outcomes," American Heart Association, June 22, 2016, http://newsroom.heart .org/news/gender-gap-found-in-cardiac-arrest-care-outcomes.

130 *In a 2014 AHA scientific statement . . .* "Gender-Specific Research Improves Accuracy of Heart Disease Diagnosis in Women," American Heart Association, June 16, 2014, http://newsroom.heart.org/news/gender-specific-research-improves-accuracy -of-heart-disease-diagnosis-in-women.

131 *Studies suggest that 60 to 70 percent of women . . .* Carl J. Pepine et al., "Emergence of Nonobstructive Coronary Artery Disease: A Woman's Problem and Need for Change in Definition on Angiography," *Journal of the American College of Cardiology* 66, no. 17 (October 2015), doi:10.1016/j.jacc.2015.08.876.

131 *Small observational studies since the sixties . . .* Kamakki Banks et al., "Angina in Women Without Obstructive Coronary Artery Disease," *Current Cardiology Reviews* 6, no. 1 (February 2010), doi:10.2174/157340310790231608.

131 *In 1996, the National Heart, Lung, and Blood Institute . . .* Raffaele Bugiardini and C. Noel Bairey Merz, "Angina with 'Normal' Coronary Arteries," *JAMA* 293, no. 4 (January 2005), doi:10.1001/jama.293.4.477.

132 *Over the course of a lifetime, the researchers estimated, the health care costs . . .* Leslee J. Shaw et al., "The Economic Burden of Angina in Women with Suspected Ischemic Heart Disease: Results from the National Institutes of Health– National Heart, Lung, and Blood Institute–Sponsored Women's Ischemia Syndrome Evaluation," *Circulation* 114, no. 9 (August 2006), doi:10.1161 /CIRCULATIONAHA.105.609990.

132 *Furthermore, by the mid-aughts, results from the WISE project . . .* Martha Gulati et al., "Adverse Cardiovascular Outcomes in Women with Nonobstructive Coronary Artery Disease: A Report from the Women's Ischemia Syndrome Evaluation Study and the St James Women Take Heart Project," *Archives of Internal Medicine* 169, no. 9 (May 2009), doi:10.1001/archinternmed.2009.50.

132 *After ten years, 6.7 percent of the symptomatic patients with . . .* Barry Sharaf et al., "Adverse Outcomes Among Women Presenting with Signs and Symptoms of Ischemia and No Obstructive Coronary Artery Disease: Findings from the NHLBI- Sponsored Women's Ischemia Syndrome Evaluation (WISE) Angiographic

Core Laboratory," *American Heart Journal* 166, no. 1 (July 2013), doi:10.1016/j .ahj.2013.04.002.

132 *The WISE study found that 10 to 25 percent* . . . Bugiardini and Bairey Merz, "Angina."

132 *Autopsy studies also show that while about three-quarters* . . . Mehta et al., "Acute Myocardial Infarction."

132 *Among the WISE women, nearly half* . . . S. E. Reis et al., "Coronary Microvascular Dysfunction Is Highly Prevalent in Women with Chest Pain in the Absence of Coronary Artery Disease: Results from the NHLBI WISE Study," *American Heart Journal* 141, no. 5 (May 2001), www.ncbi.nlm.nih.gov/pubmed/11320360.

133 *A 2015 study of patients with chest pain* . . . Bong-Ki Lee et al., "Invasive Evaluation of Patients with Angina in the Absence of Obstructive Coronary Artery Disease," *Circulation* (February 20, 2015), doi:10.1161/CIRCULATIONAHA.114.012636.

133 *According to a 2016 article by emergency room physicians* . . . Safdar and D'Onofrio, "Women and Chest Pain."

134 *In fact, the growing appreciation that alternate mechanisms* . . . Filippo Crea, Paolo G. Camici, and Cathleen Noel Bairey Merz, "Coronary Microvascular Dysfunction: An Update," *European Heart Journal* 35, no. 17 (May 1, 2014), doi:10.1093/eurheartj/eht513.

134 *including the fact that nearly a third of patients* . . . Pepine et al., "Emergence of Nonobstructive Coronary Artery Disease."

134 *"We've been working on this for fifteen years"* . . . Bairey Merz, "Biggest Health Threat."

134 *"Is it widespread? I would say not quite yet* . . . All quotes from author's interview with Dr. C. Noel Bairey Merz.

134 *A review of the AHA's 2007 prevention guidelines for women* . . . Chiara Melloni et al., "Representation of Women in Randomized Clinical Trials of Cardiovascular Disease Prevention," *Circulation: Cardiovascular Quality and Outcomes* 3, no. 2 (March 2010), doi:10.1161/CIRCOUTCOMES.110.868307.

135 *Women made up about one-third of participants* . . . Sanket S. Dhruva, Lisa A. Bero, and Rita F. Redberg, "Gender Bias in Studies for Food and Drug Administration Premarket Approval of Cardiovascular Devices," *Circulation: Cardiovascular Quality and Outcomes* 4, no. 2 (March 2011), doi:10.1161 /CIRCOUTCOMES.110.958215.

CHAPTER 4. AUTOIMMUNE DISEASE AND THE LONG SEARCH FOR A DIAGNOSIS

137 *Jackie was sixteen the first time she fell ill* . . . All quotes from author's interview with Jackie.

138 *But experts and advocacy groups, like the AARDA* . . . American Autoimmune Related Diseases Association, "Autoimmune Disease Statistics."

138 *In the United States, autoimmune disease makes the top ten* . . . Stephen J. Walsh and Laurie M. Rau, "Autoimmune Diseases: A Leading Cause of Death Among Young and Middle-Aged Women in the United States," *American Journal of Public Health* 90, no. 9 (September 2000), doi:10.2105/AJPH.90.9.1463.

139 *tripling over the last few decades* . . . Nakazawa, *The Autoimmune Epidemic*, xv.

139 *Today, that's increased only slightly to 15 percent* . . . American Autoimmune Related Diseases Association, "AARDA Launches 'My Autoimmune Story' Video Series," www.aarda.org/video-series-autoimmune-story/.

139 *One of the key reasons for the lack of awareness* . . . Warwick Anderson and Ian R.

Mackay, *Intolerant Bodies: A Short History of Autoimmunity* (Baltimore: Johns Hopkins Univ. Press, 2014) and Nakazawa, *The Autoimmune Epidemic.*

140 *"Twenty-two million"*... Nakazawa, *The Autoimmune Epidemic*, 37.

140 *"mimic all the physical diseases*... Thomas Sydenham, quoted in Katherine A. Phillips, ed., *Somatoform and Factitious Disorders* (Washington, DC: American Psychiatric Publishing, 2001), 103.

140 *This shift, as researcher Colin L. Talley has shown*... C. L. Talley, "The Emergence of Multiple Sclerosis, 1870–1950: A Puzzle of Historical Epidemiology," *Perspectives in Biology and Medicine* 48, no. 3 (Summer 2005), doi:10.1353/pbm .2005.0079.

141 *"physicians interpreted increasing numbers*... Talley, "Multiple Sclerosis."

141 *"the frequent mistaking*... quoted in Talley, "Multiple Sclerosis."

141 *Larger epidemiological studies questioned that, until finally*... Talley, "Multiple Sclerosis."

141 *"considerable resentment on the part*... Marilyn R. Kassirer and Donald H. Osterberg, "Pain in Chronic Multiple Sclerosis," *Journal of Pain and Symptom Management* 2, no. 2 (Spring 1987), doi:10.1016/S0885-3924(87)80022-2.

141 *Finally, in the mideighties, various researchers decided to survey*... Kassirer and Osterberg, "Pain in Chronic Multiple Sclerosis."

142 *A 2003 Israeli study*... Netta Levin, Michal Mor, and Tamir Ben-Hur, "Patterns of Misdiagnosis of Multiple Sclerosis," *Israeli Medical Association Journal* 5, no. 7 (July 2003), www.ima.org.il/FilesUpload/IMAJ/0/54/27188.pdf.

143 *"you must have had something terrible happen in your life*... All quotes from author's interview with Virginia Ladd (executive director of the AARDA).

143 *"self-sacrificing, masochistic, conforming*... Rudolf H. Moos, "Personality Factors Associated with Rheumatoid Arthritis: A Review," *Journal of Chronic Diseases* 17, no. 1 (January 1964), doi:10.1016/0021-9681(64)90038-4.

144 *According to the most recent survey by the AARDA*... American Autoimmune Related Diseases Association, "News Briefing for Autoimmune Disease Awareness Month 2014," www.aarda.org/news-briefing-for-autoimmune-disease -awareness-month-2014/.

144 *Almost three-quarters said the education they'd received*... Alicia Ault, "Autoimmune Disease Coalition Seeks to Increase Physician Knowledge," *Clinical Endocrinology News*, March 18, 2014, www.mdedgecom/clinicalendocrinologynews /article/81050/multiple-sclerosis/autoimmune-disease-coalition-seeks.

146 *"As a patient, you have to meet their narrow*... Liz Welch, "Autoimmune Epidemic: The Medical Experts," *Self*, March 31, 2015, www.self.com/story /autoimmune-epidemic-doctors-working-toward-answers.

146 *"In my own practice, I started seeing a lot of patients*... Welch, "Autoimmune Epidemic."

147 *"Many were told that their symptoms were 'in their heads'*... American Autoimmune Related Diseases Association, "Do You Know Your Family AQ?"

147 *"they should not describe their fatigue as fatigue"*... American Autoimmune Related Diseases Association, *Highlights from "The State of Autoimmune Disease: A National Summit"* (Eastpointe, MI: American Autoimmune Related Diseases Association, 2015), www.aarda.org/wp-content/uploads/2017/04/HighlightsFrom SummitMarch20151-1.pdf.

147 *Katie was in college the first time*... All quotes from author's interview with Katie Ernst.

148 *"even as late as 2000, mental health professionals were often the first to make . . .*
     Charles W. Schmidt, "Questions Persist: Environmental Factors in Autoimmune
     Disease," *Environmental Health Perspectives* 119, no. 6 (June 2011), doi:10.1289
     /ehp.119-a248.

148 *A 2010 Chinese study . . .* Jin-Bao Feng et al., "Gender and Age Influence on Clinical
     and Laboratory Features in Chinese Patients with Systemic Lupus Erythematosus:
     1,790 Cases," *Rheumatology International* 30, no. 8 (June 2010), doi:10.1007
     /s00296-009-1087-0.

148 *A 2014 Finnish study . . .* V. Fuchs et al., "Factors Associated with Long Diagnostic
     Delay in Celiac Disease," *Scandinavian Journal of Gastroenterology* 49, no. 11
     (November 2014), doi:10.3109/00365521.2014.923502.

148 *A 2013 survey . . .* The Centre for International Economics, *The Cost to Patients
     and the Community of Myasthenia Gravis* (prepared for Myasthenia Gravis Asso-
     ciation of Queensland), November 2013, www.thecie.com.au/wp-content/uploads
     /2014/06/Final-report_Economic-Impact-of-Myasthenia-Gravis-08112013.pdf.

148 *According to a 2010 German study . . .* Benjamin Bleicken et al., "Delayed
     Diagnosis of Adrenal Insufficiency Is Common: A Cross-Sectional Study in 216
     Patients," The American Journal of the Medical Sciences 339, no. 6 (June 2010),
     doi:10.1097/MAJ.0b013e3181db6b7a.

149 *For example, a 2001 study . . .* L. R. Lard et al., "Delayed Referral of Female
     Patients with Rheumatoid Arthritis," *The Journal of Rheumatology* 28, no. 10
     (October 2001), www.ncbi.nlm.nih.gov/pubmed/11669154.

149 *A 2005 study of RA patients in Norway . . .* E. Purinszky and O. Palm, "Women
     with Early Rheumatoid Arthritis Are Referred Later Than Men," *Annals of the
     Rheumatic Diseases* 64, no. 8 (August 2005), doi:10.1136/ard.2004.031716.

149 *RA, for one, is . . .* K. Forslind, I. Hafström, and M. Ahlmén, "Sex: A Major Predictor
     of Remission in Early Rheumatoid Arthritis?" *Annals of the Rheumatic Diseases*
     66, no. 1 (January 2007), doi:10.1136/ard.2006.056937.

150 *In 2015, inspired by her struggle to get diagnosed . . .* Katie Ernst, *Miss•Treated*
     (blog), www.misstreated.org/.

151 *In 2016, the Brain Tumour Charity released a report . . .* The Brain Tumour
     Charity, *Finding Myself in Your Hands.*

152 *A 2015 study revealed . . .* Nafees U. Din, "Age and Gender Variations in Cancer
     Diagnostic Intervals in 15 Cancers: Analysis of Data from the UK Clinical Practice
     Research Datalink," *PLOS One* 10, no. 5 (May 15, 2015), doi:10.1371/journal
     .pone.0127717.

152 *A 2013 study, for example, concluded that more than twice . . .* Georgios
     Lyratzopoulos et al., "Gender Inequalities in the Promptness of Diagnosis of
     Bladder and Renal Cancer After Symptomatic Presentation: Evidence from
     Secondary Analysis of an English Primary Care Audit Survey," *BMJ Open* 3, no. 6
     (2013), doi:10.1136/bmjopen-2013-002861.

152 *Collectively, they affect one in ten . . .* National Organization for Rare Disorders,
     "News from NORD: An Update for Our Members and Friends," Fall 2010, http://
     rarediseases.org/wp-content/uploads/2014/12/NORD_Newsletter_Fall_2010
     .pdf.

152 *or 30 million people . . .* U.S. Department of Health and Human Services, National
     Institutes of Health, Genetic and Rare Diseases Information Center, "FAQs About
     Rare Diseases," August 11, 2016, https://rarediseases.info.nih.gov/about-ordr
     /pages/31/frequently-asked-questions.

152 *On average, it takes them over seven* . . . Shire, *Rare Disease Impact Report: Insights from Patients and the Medical Community*, April 2013, https://globalgenes.org /wp-content/uploads/2013/04/ShireReport-1.pdf.

153 *According to a survey of 12,000 patients with several rare* . . . Kole and Faurisson, *The Voice of 12,000 Patients.*

153 *Laurie Edwards, author of* . . . Laurie Edwards, "The Gender Gap in Pain," *The New York Times*, March 16, 2013, www.nytimes.com/2013/03/17/opinion/sunday /women-and-the-treatment-of-pain.html.

153 *"No matter how many times* . . . Laurie Edwards, *In the Kingdom of the Sick: A Social History of Chronic Illness in America* (New York: Bloomsbury USA, 2013), 72.

154 *One woman, diagnosed with anxiety* . . . Author unknown, "Story: Woman Committed Rather Than Treated," *Miss•Treated* (blog), December 17, 2015, www.misstreated.org/blog/2015/12/17/woman-is-committed-rather-than -getting-the-medical-care-she-needs.

156 *A growing body of research explores* . . . Elizabeth N. Chapman, Anna Kaatz, and Molly Carnes, "Physicians and Implicit Bias: How Doctors May Unwittingly Perpetuate Health Care Disparities," *Journal of General Internal Medicine* 28, no. 11 (November 2013), doi:10.1007/s11606-013-2441-1.

156 *A 2012 meta-analysis* . . . Salimah H. Meghani, Eeeseung Byun, and Rollin M. Gallagher, "Time to Take Stock: A Meta-Analysis and Systematic Review of Analgesic Treatment Disparities for Pain in the United States," *Pain Medicine* 13, no. 2 (February 2012), doi:10.1111/j.1526-4637.2011.01310.x.

156 *A 2015 study found that white children* . . . Monika K. Goyal et al., "Racial Disparities in Pain Management of Children with Appendicitis in Emergency Departments," *JAMA Pediatrics* 169, no. 11 (November 2015), doi:10.1001 /jamapediatrics.2015.1915.

157 *A 2016 study published in* Proceedings of the National Academy of Sciences . . . Kelly M. Hoffman et al., "Racial Bias in Pain Assessment and Treatment Recommendations, and False Beliefs About Biological Differences Between Blacks and Whites," *PNAS* 113, no. 16 (April 19, 2016), doi:10.1073/pnas.1516047113.

158 *They also tend to get it at younger ages and have more life-threatening* . . . Lupus Foundation, "Black Women Develop Lupus at Younger Age with More Life-Threatening Complications," October 24, 2013, www.lupus.org/general -news/entry/black-women-develop-lupus-younger-with-more-life-threatening -complications.

158 *As Meghan O'Rourke wrote in a 2013* New Yorker *article* . . . Meghan O'Rourke, "What's Wrong with Me?" *The New Yorker*, August 26, 2013, www.newyorker .com/magazine/2013/08/26/whats-wrong-with-me.

159 *The American Thyroid Association estimates that 20 million* . . . American Thyroid Association, "General Information/Press Room," www.thyroid.org/media-main /about-hypothyroidism/.

159 *Women have a one in eight* . . . American Thyroid Association, "General Information."

160 *"consider treatment for patients who test outside* . . . Mary Shomon, *Living Well with Hypothyroidism: What Your Doctor Doesn't Tell You* . . . *That You Need to Know*, rev. ed. (New York: William Morrow Paperbacks, 2005).

160 *But the new recommended range sparked great controversy* . . . Mary Shomon, "TSH (Thyroid Stimulating Hormone) Reference Range Wars," *Very Well*, November 04, 2016, www.verywell.com/tsh-thyroid-stimulating -hormone-reference-range-wars-3232912.

160   *"The implicit message is this . . .* Sara Gottfried, "Good Housekeeping's Thyroid Storm: A Case of Misogyny?" *Dear Thyroid,* August 2, 2011, http://dearthyroid.org/2011/08/02/good-housekeeping%E2%80%99s-thyroid-storm-a-case-of-misogyny/.

161   *In 2006, Dr. Anthony Weetman, a British endocrinologist, angered . . .* A. P. Weetman, "Whose Thyroid Hormone Replacement Is It Anyway?" *Clinical Endocrinology* 64, no. 3 (March 2006), doi:10.1111/j.1365-2265.2006.02478.x.

161   *"If we have obvious thyroid symptoms, and yet fall into one of these mathematical . . .* Mary Shomon, "Dear Endocrinologists: Time to Hear What Thyroid Patients Have to Say," *Very Well,* September 15, 2016, www.verywell.com/thyroid-care-feedback-from-patients-to-endocrinologists-3233126.

162   *"If fatigue were a sound made manifest by . . .* Nakazawa, *The Autoimmune Epidemic,* 24.

162   *In a recent survey the AARDA conducted of more than 7,800 . . .* American Autoimmune Related Diseases Association, *Highlights from "The State of Autoimmune Disease."*

163   *"utterly failed" to help . . .* Atul Gawande, "Letting Go," *The New Yorker,* August 2, 2010, www.newyorker.com/magazine/2010/08/02/letting-go-2.

163   *"Chronic illness has become . . .* Atul Gawande, "The Heroism of Incremental Care," *The New Yorker,* January 23, 2017, www.newyorker.com/magazine/2017/01/23/the-heroism-of-incremental-care.

167   *Despite doing "a million dollars' worth of tests . . .* Daniela J. Lamas, "When the Brain Is Under Attack," *The Boston Globe,* May 27, 2013, www.bostonglobe.com/lifestyle/health-wellness/2013/05/26/when-brain-attacks-newly-discovered-disease-can-mimic-psychosis/dyixxnwdHJJIUITsNYJC3O/story.html.

167   *Their symptoms, the researchers later wrote . . .* Roberta Vitaliani et al., "Paraneoplastic Encephalitis, Psychiatric Symptoms, and Hypoventilation in Ovarian Teratoma," *Annals of Neurology* 58, no. 4 (October 2005), doi:10.1002/ana.20614.

167   *In a 2007 article, he described . . .* Josep Dalmau et al., "Paraneoplastic Anti-*N*-Methyl-D-Aspartate Receptor Encephalitis Associated with Ovarian Teratoma," *Annals of Neurology* 61, no. 1 (January 2007), www.ncbi.nlm.nih.gov/pmc/articles/PMC2430743/.

168   *"My arms suddenly whipped . . .* Susannah Cahalan, *Brain on Fire: My Month of Madness* (New York: Free Press, 2012), 40.

169   *Even with proper treatment . . .* Maarten J. Titulaer et al., "Treatment and Prognostic Factors for Long-Term Outcome in Patients with Anti-*N*-Methyl-D-Aspartate (NMDA) Receptor Encephalitis: A Cohort Study," *Lancet Neurology* 12, no. 2 (February 2013), www.ncbi.nlm.nih.gov/pmc/articles/PMC3563251/.

169   *Three months after her symptoms began . . .* Josep Dalmau et al., "Clinical Experience and Laboratory Investigations in Patients with Anti-NMDAR Encephalitis," *Lancet Neurology* 10, no. 1 (January 2011), doi:10.1016/S1474-4422(10)70253-2.

170   *Her personal Dr. House estimated that . . .* Susannah Cahalan, "My Mysterious Lost Month of Madness," *New York Post,* October 4, 2009, https://nypost.com/2009/10/04/my-mysterious-lost-month-of-madness/.

170   *The fact that the number of cases . . .* Gregory S. Day and Harry E. Peery, "Autoimmune Synaptic Protein Encephalopathy Syndromes and the Interplay Between Mental Health, Neurology and Immunology," *Health Science Inquiry* 4, no. 1 (2013), www.researchgate.net/profile/Gregory_Day/publication/252323135_Autoimmune_synaptic_protein_encephalopathy_syndromes_and_the_interplay_between

_mental_health_neurology_and_immunology/links/0deec51f345d51dd84000000
.pdf?disableCoverPage=true.

170   *as Dalmau and a colleague write* . . . Matthew S. Kayser and Josep Dalmau, "The
      Emerging Link Between Autoimmune Disorders and Neuropsychiatric Disease,"
      The Journal of Neuropsychiatry and Clinical Neurosciences 23, no. 1 (Winter
      2011), doi:10.1176/appi.neuropsych.23.1.90.

170   *"A Case of Hysteria" reads the title of one article* . . . Heather R. Williams, Colette
      M. Gnade, and Colleen K. Stockdale, "A Case of Hysteria: Anti-*N*-Methyl-D-
      Aspartate Receptor Encephalitis Resulting from a Mature Ovarian Teratoma,"
      Proceedings in Obstetrics and Gynecology 6, no. 1 (March 2016), http://ir.uiowa
      .edu/pog/vol6/iss1/5/.

170   *"Not Hysteria" reads another* . . . Rachel Roberts et al., "Not Hysteria: Ovarian
      Teratoma-Associated Anti-*N*-Methyl-D-Aspartate Receptor Encephalitis," *Scot-
      tish Medical Journal* 57, no. 3 (August 2012), doi: 10.1258/smj.2012.012026.

170   *In fact, British psychiatrist Thomas A. Pollak suggested* . . . Thomas A. Pollak,
      "Hysteria, Hysterectomy, and Anti-NMDA Receptor Encephalitis: A Modern
      Perspective on an Infamous Chapter in Medicine," *BMJ* 346, no. f3756 (2013),
      doi:10.1136/bmj.f3756.

CHAPTER 5. CHRONIC PAIN: "PAIN IS REAL WHEN YOU GET OTHER PEOPLE TO BELIEVE IN IT"

176   *"I just felt like no one ever believed me* . . . All quotes from author's interview with
      Alexis.

176   *In 2011, the IOM released an influential report* . . . Institute of Medicine, *Relieving
      Pain.*

176   *That's a mere 5 percent of what goes to* . . . Chronic Pain Research Alliance, *Impact
      of Chronic Overlapping Pain Conditions on Public Health and the Urgent Need
      for Safe and Effective Treatment: 2015 Analysis and Policy Recommendations,*
      May 2015, www.chronicpainresearch.org/public/CPRA_WhitePaper_2015-FINAL
      -Digital.pdf.

176   *Students received, on average, eleven hours of instruction* . . . Department of
      Neurology, Johns Hopkins School of Medicine, "Pain Education in North American
      Medical Schools," *The Journal of Pain* 12, no. 12 (December 2011), doi:10.1016/j
      .jpain.2011.06.006.

176   *a national survey found that almost 30 percent* . . . D. Blumenthal et al.,
      "Preparedness for Clinical Practice: Reports of Graduating Residents at Academic
      Health Centers," *JAMA* 286, no. 9 (September 2001), doi:10.1001/jama.286.9.1027.

177   *And the 3,000 to 4,000 pain specialists nationwide* . . . Institute of Medicine,
      Relieving Pain.

177   *In surveys that ask respondents whether they've had pain in different parts* . . .
      Institute of Medicine, *Relieving Pain.*

177   *a 2008 study of tens of thousands of patients in over a dozen countries found* . . .
      Adley Tsang et al., "Common Chronic Pain Conditions in Developed and
      Developing Countries: Gender and Age Differences and Comorbidity with
      Depression-Anxiety Disorders," *Journal of Pain: Official Journal of the American
      Pain Society* 9, no. 10 (October 2008), doi:10.1016/j.jpain.2008.05.005.

177   *Many of the most prevalent chronic pain conditions* . . . Jeffrey S. Mogil, "Sex
      Differences in Pain and Pain Inhibition: Multiple Explanations of a Controversial
      Phenomenon," *Nature Reviews Neuroscience* 13, no. 12 (December 2012), doi:
      10.1038/nrn3360.

177 *Women are up to four times more likely* . . . Overlapping Conditions Alliance and Campaign to End Chronic Pain in Women, *Chronic Pain in Women: Neglect, Dismissal and Discrimination*, May 2010, www.endwomenspain.org/Common /file?id=20.

177 *"chronic pain is a disease in its own right* . . . David Niv, *EFIC's Declaration on Chronic Pain as a Major Healthcare Problem, a Disease in Its Own Right*, October 2001, www.iasp-pain.org/files/Content/ContentFolders/GlobalYearAgainstPain2 /20042005RighttoPainRelief/painasadisease.pdf.

179 *"If pain were a fire alarm, the nociceptive type would be activated* . . . Clifford J. Woolf, "What Is This Thing Called Pain?" *Journal of Clinical Investigation* 120, no. 11 (November 2010), doi:10.1172/JCI45178.

179 *"pain without lesion"* . . . Daniel Goldberg, "Pain Without Lesion: Debate Among American Neurologists, 1850–1900," *19: Interdisciplinary Studies in the Long Nineteenth Century* 15 (December 2012), doi:10.16995/ntn.629.

180 *"Those who suffered from unexplained chronic pain syndromes* . . . Marcia L. Meldrum, "A Capsule History of Pain Management," *JAMA* 290, no. 18 (November 2003), doi:10.1001/jama.290.18.2470.

181 *"very frustrating for the patients because they knew in their heart* . . . All quotes from author's interview with Daniel Clauw (director of the Chronic Pain and Fatigue Research Center).

182 *"I was dismissed to live* . . . Vicki Ratner, "The Interstitial Cystitis Association of America: Lessons Learned over the Past 30 Years," *Translational Andrology and Urology* 4, no. 5 (October 2015), doi:10.3978/j.issn.2223-4683.2015.09.02.

182 *"Ultimately, I had to make the diagnosis myself* . . . Unless otherwise noted, all quotes from author's interview with Vicki Ratner.

183 *an irritable bladder in an irritable patient* . . . Anthony Walsh, quoted in Jane M. Meijlink, "Interstitial Cystitis/Bladder Pain Syndrome: An Overview of Diagnosis & Treatment," International Painful Bladder Foundation, May 2016, www.painful -bladder.org/pdf/Diagnosis&Treatment_IPBF.pdf.

183 *"I spent the last two years of medical school in intense, unremitting pain* . . . Ratner, "Lessons Learned."

183 *"Patients had often seen five to ten physicians* . . . Ratner, "Lessons Learned."

184 *"The extreme pain and despair over chances for a cure* . . . Ratner, "Lessons Learned."

184 *According to a 1993 study* . . . D. C. Webster, "Interstitial Cystitis: Women at Risk for Psychiatric Misdiagnosis," *AWHONN's Clinical Issues in Perinatal and Women's Health Nursing* 4, no. 2 (1993), http://europepmc.org/abstract/med/8242045.

184 *in 2015, according to a WebMD poll* . . . Poncie Rutsch, "Why the Urologist Is Usually a Man, but Maybe Not for Long," NPR.org, April 29, 2015, www .npr.org/sections/health-shots/2015/04/29/402850925/why-the-urologist-is -usually-a-man-but-maybe-not-for-long.

185 *In 1987, the ICA teamed up with a urologist on the first epidemiological study* . . . Jane E. Brody, "Personal Health; Interstitial Cystitis: Help for a Puzzling Illness," *The New York Times*, January 25, 1995, www.nytimes.com/1995/01/25/us/personal -health-interstitial-cystitis-help-for-a-puzzling-illness.html.

185 *In 1987, encouraged by the ICA, the National Institute drew up a first consensus* . . . Meijlink, "Interstitial Cystitis."

186 *In 2011, researchers from the RAND Corporation came* . . . Sandra H. Berry et al., "Prevalence of Symptoms of Bladder Pain Syndrome/Interstitial Cystitis Among

Adult Females in the United States," *The Journal of Urology* 186, no. 2 (August 2011), doi:10.1016/j.jur0.2011.03.132.

186 *Strikingly, a follow-up study* . . . Katy S. Konkle et al., "Comparison of an Interstitial Cystitis/Bladder Pain Syndrome Clinical Cohort with Symptomatic Community Women from the RAND Interstitial Cystitis Epidemiology Study," *The Journal of Urology* 187, no. 2 (February 2012), doi:10.1016/j.jur0.2011.10.040.

186 *And while it was originally thought that IC affected nine times more women* . . . Konkle et al., "Interstitial Cystitis."

186 *Studies demonstrated an intriguing* . . . Clifford J. Woolf, "Central Sensitization: Implications for the Diagnosis and Treatment of Pain," *Pain* 152, no. 3 (March 2011), doi:10.1016/j.pain.2010.09.030

187 *"These notions were generally not very well received initially* . . . Woolf, "Central Sensitization."

188 *Cynthia Toussaint, founder of the organization For Grace,* . . . All quotes from author's interview with Cynthia Toussaint (founder of For Grace).

189 *In a 2002* New York Times *article* . . . Nancy Wartik, "In Search of Relief; Hurting More, Helping Less?" *The New York Times*, June 23, 2002, www.nytimes .com/2002/06/23/health/in-search-of-relief-hurting-more-helping-less.html.

190 *As the authors of a 2007 study of doctor-patient interactions* . . . Lisa Maria E. Frantsve and Robert D. Kerns, "Patient–Provider Interactions in the Management of Chronic Pain: Current Findings Within the Context of Shared Medical Decision Making," *Pain Medicine* 8, no. 1 (January–February 2007), doi:10.1111/j.1526-4637.2007.00250.x.

190 *As the title of a 2003 qualitative study* . . . Anne Werner and Kirsti Malterud, "It Is Hard Work Behaving as a Credible Patient: Encounters Between Women with Chronic Pain and Their Doctors," *Social Science and Medicine* 57, no. 8 (October 2003).

190 *A 1996 study found that patients judged "attractive" were perceived* . . . Thomas Hadjistarvropoulos, Bruce McMurty, and Kenneth D. Craig, "Beautiful Faces in Pain: Biases and Accuracy in the Perception of Pain," *Psychology and Health* 11, no. 3 (March 1996).

190 *In 2014, For Grace teamed up with the online news site* National Pain Report . . . Pat Anson, "Women in Pain Report Significant Gender Bias," *National Pain Report*, September 12, 2014, http://nationalpainreport.com/women-in-pain -report-significant-gender-bias-8824696.html.

191 *In journalist Judy Foreman's book* . . . Judy Foreman, *A Nation in Pain: Healing Our Biggest Health Problem* (New York: Oxford Univ. Press, 2014).

192 *As Dr. Sean Mackey, chief of the Stanford Division of Pain Medicine, recently* . . . German Lopez, "A Pain Doctor Explains How He Balances His Patients' Needs with the Opioid Epidemic's Lessons," *Vox*, May 2, 2017, https://www.vox.com /policy-and-politics/2017/5/2/15440000/sean-mackey-opioids-chronic-pain.

194 *According to an estimate by the Chronic Pain Research Alliance (CPRA), vulvody-nia* . . . Chronic Pain Research Alliance, *Impact.*

194 *One of their concerns was that patients* . . . Harold Merskey, "Pain Disorder, Hysteria or Somatization?" *Pain Research and Management* 9, no. 2 (Summer 2004), doi:10.1155/2004/605328.

195 *"Doctors in each era, including our own* . . . Paula Kamen, *All in My Head: An Epic Quest to Cure an Unrelenting, Totally Unreasonable, and Only Slightly Enlightening Headache* (Boston: De Capo Press, 2006), 109.

195 *"be attributed to experiences of unsatisfactory treatment* . . . Harold Merskey, "History of Psychoanalytic Ideas Concerning Pain," in *Personality Characteristics of Patients with Pain*, eds. Robert J. Gatchel and James N. Weisberg (Washington, DC: American Psychological Association, 2000), 25–35.

196 *According to this neuromatrix theory, though pain is often triggered by tissue injury* . . . Ronald Melzack, "Pain and the Neuromatrix in the Brain," *Journal of Dental Education* 65, no. 12 (December 2001), www.ncbi.nlm.nih.gov/pubmed /11780656.

197 *They also seem to share other abnormalities in common: dysregulation* . . . Chronic Pain Research Alliance, *Impact*.

197 *Approximately 20 to 30 percent of people with autoimmune diseases* . . . Daniel J. Clauw, "Round 35: Neurobiology of Chronic Pain: Lessons Learned from Fibromyalgia and Related Conditions," Johns Hopkins Arthritis Center, July 9, 2010, www.hopkinsarthritis.org/physician-corner/rheumatology-rounds/round -35-neurobiology-of-chronic-pain-lessons-learned-from-fibromyalgia-and -related-conditions/.

197 *In the last decade, larger studies* . . . Hong Chen et al., "Relationship Between Temporomandibular Disorders, Widespread Palpation Tenderness and Multiple Pain Conditions: A Case-Control Study," *The Journal of Pain: Official Journal of the American Pain Society* 13, no. 10 (October 2012), doi:10.1016/j.jpain.2012 .07.011.

197 *"there actually are more people* . . . All quotes from author's interview with Chris Veasley (director of the Chronic Pain Research Alliance).

199 *Fibromyalgia's history follows a familiar trajectory* . . . Fatma Inanici and Muhammad B. Yunus, "History of Fibromyalgia: Past to Present," *Current Pain and Headache Reports* 8, no. 5 (October 2004), doi:10.1007/s11916-996-0010-6; Howard B. Pikoff, "A Study in Psychological Mislabelling: The Rise and (Protracted) Fall of Psychogenic Fibromyalgia," *International Musculoskeletal Medicine* 32, no. 3 (2010), doi:10.1179/175361410X12798116924336.

199 *"pain in the muscles is so common that there is not* . . . Pierre Briquet, *Clinical and Therapeutic Treatise on Hysteria* (1859), quoted in David B. Morris, *The Culture of Pain* (Berkeley: Univ. of California Press, 1993), 110.

200 *In the 1930s, a Scottish doctor argued that chronic rheumatism* . . . James L. Halliday, "Psychological Factors in Rheumatism, Part I," *British Medical Journal* 1, no. 3969 (January 1937), www.ncbi.nlm.nih.gov/pmc/articles/PMC2092737/.

200 *In 1943, two US military physicians suggested* . . . Edward W. Boland and William P. Corr, "Psychogenic Rheumatism," *JAMA* 123, no. 13 (November 1943), doi: 10.1001/jama.1943.02840480005002.

200 *In 1968, one American physician described most of the features of fibromyalgia as* . . . Bret Stetka, "Fibromyalgia: Maligned, Misunderstood and (Finally) Treatable," *Scientific American*, May 27, 2014, www.scientificamerican.com /article/fibromyalgia-maligned-misunderstood-and-finally-treatable/.

200 *In 1990, the American College of Rheumatology released* . . . Frederick Wolfe et al., "Criteria for the Classification of Fibromyalgia," *Arthritis and Rheumatism* 33, no. 2 (February 1990), doi:10.1007/978-3-642-86812-2_2.

200 *When these criteria were revised in 2010* . . . Frederick Wolfe et al., "The American College of Rheumatology Preliminary Diagnostic Criteria for Fibromyalgia and Measurement of Symptom Severity," *Arthritis Care and Research* 62, no. 5 (May 2010), doi:10.1002/acr.20140.

201 *"The complexity of the pain transmission circuitry* . . . Joel Katz, Brittany N. Rosenbloom, and Samantha Fashler, "Chronic Pain, Psychopathology, and DSM-5 Somatic Symptom Disorder," *Canadian Journal of Psychiatry* 60, no. 4 (April 2015), doi:10.1177/070674371506000402.

201 *Yet as recently as 2008, skeptics questioned whether fibromyalgia exists* . . . Alex Berenson, "Drug Approved. Is Disease Real?" *The New York Times*, January 14, 2008, www.nytimes.com/2008/01/14/health/14pain.html.

201 *In a 2000 article in* The New Yorker . . . Jerome Groopman, "Hurting All Over: With So Many People in So Much Pain, How Could Fibromyalgia Not Be a Disease?" *The New Yorker*, November 13, 2000.

201 *And a significant subset of people with other "explained" pain conditions* . . . Daniel J. Clauw, "Chronic Pain: Is It All in Their Head?," presentation at the University of Michigan on December 5, 2013, www.youtube.com/watch?v=pgCfkA9RLrM.

202 *Three-quarters of doctors say* . . . David Edelberg, "Medical Sexism and Fibromyalgia," WholeHealth Chicago, December 5, 2011, http://wholehealthchicago .com/2011/12/05/medical-sexism-and-fibromyalgia/.

202 *Unsurprisingly, then, a 2012 population-based study that estimated* . . . Brian Walitt et al., "The Prevalence and Characteristics of Fibromyalgia in the 2012 National Health Interview Survey," ed. Mario D. Cordero, *PLOS One* 10, no. 9 (September 2015), doi:10.1371/journal.pone.0138024.

203 *a 2013 study based on a survey of 670 fibromyalgia patients* . . . Carroline P. Lobo et al., "Impact of Invalidation and Trust in Physicians on Health Outcomes in Fibromyalgia Patients," *The Primary Care Companion for CNS Disorders* 16, no. 5 (October 2014), doi:10.4088/PCC.14m01664.

203 *"a medical sexism that's hard to miss even if you're not looking closely* . . . Edelberg, "Medical Sexism."

203 *In her book* Tender Points, *writer Amy Berkowitz* . . . Amy Berkowitz, *Tender Points* (Oakland: Timeless, Infinite Light, 2015).

203 *"Fibromyalgia patients are those* . . . Frederick Wolfe and Brian Walitt, "Culture, Science and the Changing Nature of Fibromyalgia," *Nature Reviews Rheumatology* 9, no. 12 (December 2013), doi:10.1038/nrrheum.2013.96.

205 *"must rely on a person's ability to express* . . . Institute of Medicine, *Relieving Pain.*

205 *That means a whopping 18 percent of adult American* . . . Migraine Research Foundation, "Migraine Facts," https://migraineresearchfoundation.org/about -migraine/migraine-facts/.

205 *And it's estimated that 2.4 to 7.1 million Americans have chronic migraine* . . . Joanna Kempner, *Not Tonight: Migraine and the Politics of Gender and Health* (Chicago: The Univ. of Chicago Press, 2014).

205 *"That no one dies of migraine seems, to someone deep into an attack* . . . Joan Didion, *The White Album: Essays* (New York: Farrar, Straus and Giroux, 2009), 171.

205 *Cindy McCain famously said she could imagine her husband Senator* . . . Liz McNeil, "Cindy McCain's Secret Struggle with Migraines," *People*, September 2, 2006, http://people.com/celebrity/cindy-mccains-secret-struggle-with-migraines/.

206 *"For the past 100 years, migraine has been thought of as an imagined* . . . P. Phillips, "Migraine as a Woman's Issue—Will Research and New Treatments Help?" *JAMA* 280, no. 23 (December 1998), doi:10.1001/jama.280.23.1975-JMN1216-2-1.

206 *"We used to believe that migraine was a disorder of neurotic women* . . . Stephen Silberstein, quoted in Kempner, *Not Tonight*, 66.

206 *In both cases, those with a "nervous temperament* . . . Peter Wallwork Latham, *On Nervous or Sick-Headache: Its Varieties and Treatment* (Cambridge: Deighton, Bell and Co., 1873), 15.

207 *Though their perfectionist tendencies* . . . Helen Goodell, "Thirty Years of Headache Research in the Laboratory of the Late Dr. Harold G. Wolff," *Headache* 6 (1967), 162, quoted in Kempner, *Not Tonight*, 40.

207 *He claimed 80 percent of his female patients* . . . Harold Wolff, *Headache and Other Head Pain*, quoted in Kempner, *Not Tonight*, 40.

207 *"Whenever a woman is having three attacks of migraine* . . . Walter C. Alvarez, "The Migrainous Woman and All Her Troubles," *Alexander Blain Hospital Bulletin* 4 (1945): 3–8.

208 *"The discovery of sumatriptan confirmed* . . . Patrick P. A. Humphrey, "The Discovery and Development of the Triptans, a Major Therapeutic Breakthrough," *Headache* 48, no. 5 (May 2008), doi:10.1111/j.1526-4610.2008.01097.x.

208 *get an average of two to four hours of education* . . . Kempner, *Not Tonight*, 56.

208 *"Headache is the commonest symptom found in neurologic* . . . Madeline Drexler, *New Approaches to Neurological Pain: Planning for the Future* (Boston: The Dana Foundation, 2008), 3.

209 *According to a recent survey by the American Academy of Neurology* . . . Richard B. Lipton et al., "Migraine Practice Patterns Among Neurologists," *Neurology* 62, no. 11 (June 2004): 1926–31, cited in Kempner, *Not Tonight*, 8.

209 *That's shockingly little considering* . . . Todd J. Schwedt and Robert E. Shapiro, "Funding of Research on Headache Disorders by the National Institutes of Health," *Headache* 49, no. 2 (February 2009), doi:10.1111/j.1526-4610.2008.01323.x.

209 *Preventive treatments* . . . Domenico D'Amico and Stewart J. Tepper, "Prophylaxis of Migraine: General Principles and Patient Acceptance," *Neuropsychiatric Disease and Treatment* 4, no. 6 (December 2008), doi:10.2147/NDT.S3497.

210 *Maureen learned that a few years ago, when she had a migraine* . . . All quotes from author's interview with Maureen.

211 *"for a disease to be fully legitimated* . . . Kempner, *Not Tonight*, 12.

CHAPTER 6. THE CURSE OF EVE: WHEN BEING SICK IS "NORMAL"

213 *Ellen got her period at age eleven, and, after a few years* . . . All quotes from author's interview with Ellen.

214 *"As a general rule, all women* . . . Auguste Fabre, *L'hystérie viscérale—nouveaux fragments de clinique médicale* (Paris: A. Delahaye & E. Lecrosnier, 1883), 3, quoted in Elaine Showalter, "Hysteria, Feminism, and Gender," in *Hysteria Beyond Freud*, ed. Sander L. Gilman et al. (Berkeley: Univ. of California Press, 1993), 287.

214 *"Many a young life* . . . George Engelmann, quoted in Ehrenreich and English, *For Her Own Good*, 121.

214 *"The theories which guided* . . . Ehrenreich and English, *For Her Own Good*, 121.

215 *"Long walks, dancing, shopping* . . . W. C. Taylor, *A Physician's Counsels to Woman in Health and Disease* (Springfield: W. J. Holland and Co., 1871), 284–85, quoted in Ehrenreich and English, *For Her Own Good*, 122.

215 *One textbook in the 1970s declared that dysmenorrhea* . . . J. P. Greenhill, *Office Gynecology*, quoted in Corea, *The Hidden Malpractice*, 80.

215 *In 1966, Robert A. Wilson argued* . . . Robert A. Wilson, *Feminine Forever* (New York: Pocket Books, 1966), 17 and 20, quoted in Joan C. Callahan, "Menopause: Taking the Cures or Curing the Takes?" in *Mother Time: Women, Aging and Ethics*,

ed. Margaret Urban Walker (Lanham, MD: Rowman & Littlefield Publishers, 1999), 151.

215 *"Until menopause became big business* . . . Susan M. Love with Karen Lindsey, *Dr. Susan Love's Hormone Book* (New York: Random House, 1997), 20, quoted in Joan C. Callahan, "Menopause: Taking the Cures or Curing the Takes?" in *Mother Time: Women, Aging and Ethics*, ed. Margaret Urban Walker (Lanham, MD: Rowman & Littlefield Publishers, 1999), 161–62.

215 *"The movement is a breathtaking one* . . . Joan C. Callahan, "Menopause: Taking the Cures or Curing the Takes?" in *Mother Time: Women, Aging and Ethics*, ed. Margaret Urban Walker (Lanham, MD: Rowman & Littlefield Publishers, 1999), 161–62.

216 *A common, poorly understood disease that affects at least 6.3 million* . . . Endometriosis Association, "What Is Endometriosis?" www.endometriosisassn.org /endo.html.

216 *About a third of women with endometriosis are infertile* . . . Robert N. Taylor et al., "Pain and Endometriosis: Etiology, Impact, and Therapeutics," *Middle East Fertility Society Journal* 17, no. 4 (December 2012), doi:10.1016/j.mefs.2012.09.002.

217 *Some women with endometriosis have pain all the time* . . . Y. Ozawa et al., "Management of the Pain Associated with Endometriosis: An Update of the Painful Problems," *Tohoku Journal of Experimental Medicine* 210, no. 3 (November 2006), www.ncbi.nlm.nih.gov/pubmed/17077594.

217 *In the United States, on average, it takes ten* . . . N. Sinaii et al., "High Rates of Autoimmune and Endocrine Disorders, Fibromyalgia, Chronic Fatigue Syndrome and Atopic Diseases Among Women with Endometriosis: A Survey Analysis," *Human Reproduction* 17, no. 10 (October 2002), doi:10.1093/humrep/17.10.2715.

217 *to twelve years* . . . R. Hadfield et al., "Delay in the Diagnosis of Endometriosis: A Survey of Women from the USA and the UK," *Human Reproduction* 11, no. 4 (April 1996), doi:10.1093/oxfordjournals.humrep.a019270.

217 *which, for 60 percent of patients, is before age twenty* . . . I. Brosens, S. Gordts, and G. Benagiano, "Endometriosis in Adolescents Is a Hidden, Progressive and Severe Disease That Deserves Attention, Not Just Compassion," *Human Reproduction* 28, no. 8 (August 2013), doi: 10.1093/humrep/det243.

217 *"substantial, if not irrefutable, evidence that hysteria* . . . Camran Nezhat et al., "Endometriosis: Ancient Disease, Ancient Treatments," *Fertility and Sterility* 98, no. 6 (December 2012), doi:10.1016/j.fertnstert.2012.08.001.

218 *"explained that the 'violent' hysterical* . . . Nezhat et al., "Endometriosis."

218 *Touted as a remedy for "Nervous Breakdown,"* . . . Ella Shohat, "Lasers for Ladies: Endo Discourse and the Inscriptions of Science," *Camera Obscura* 10, no. 2 29 (May 1992), doi:10.1215/02705346-10-2_29-57.

218 *Mary Lou Ballweg, founder of the Endometriosis Association, pointed out* . . . Mary Lou Ballweg, "Blaming the Victim: The Psychologizing of Endometriosis," *Obstetrics and Gynecology Clinics of North America* 24, no. 2 (June 1997), doi: 10.1016/S0889-8545(05)70312-0.

219 *"It's bigger than just the physicians* . . . All quotes from author's interview with Mary Lou Ballweg (founder of the Endometriosis Association).

219 *A 2006 study of women who were eventually diagnosed* . . . Karen Ballard, Karen Lowton, and Jeremy Wright, "What's the Delay? A Qualitative Study of Women's Experiences of Reaching a Diagnosis of Endometriosis," *Fertility and Sterility* 86, no. 5 (November 2006), doi:10.1016/j.fertnstert.2006.04.054.

220 *Kate Seear, author of* The Makings of a Modern Epidemic: Endometriosis, Gender
     and Politics . . . Kate Seear, "The Etiquette of Endometriosis: Stigmatisation,
     Menstrual Concealment and the Diagnostic Delay," *Social Science and Medicine*
     69, no. 8 (October 2009), doi:10.1016/j.socscimed.2009.07.023.

221 *Advocates like Ballweg suggest we should question the entire notion* . . . Mary Lou
     Ballweg, "Primary Dysmenorrhea—Menstrual 'Cramps'—Matters!" National
     Women's Health Network, May 9, 2017, www.nwhn.org/primary-dysmenorrhea
     -menstrual-cramps-matters/.

221 *According to a 2006 estimate by the World Health Organization* . . . Pallavi Latthe
     et al., "WHO Systematic Review of Prevalence of Chronic Pelvic Pain: A Neglected
     Reproductive Health Morbidity," *BMC Public Health* 6, no. 177 (July 2006),
     doi:10.1186/1471-2458-6-177.

221 *According to a 2016 survey of over 59,000 American women* . . . M. J. Fuldeore
     and A. M. Soliman, "Prevalence and Symptomatic Burden of Diagnosed Endo-
     metriosis in the United States: National Estimates from a Cross-Sectional Survey
     of 59,411 Women," *Gynecologic and Obstetric Investigation* 82, no. 5 (2017),
     doi:10.1159/000452660.

222 *In the 1940s, Dr. Joe Vincent Meigs* . . . Joe Vincent Meigs, "Endometriosis—Its
     Significance," *Annals of Surgery* 114, no. 5 (November 1941), https://www.ncbi
     .nlm.nih.gov/pmc/articles/PMC1385984/pdf/annsurg00379-0069.pdf.

222 *"The patient is said to be mesomorphic but underweight, overanxious, intelligent* . . .
     Robert William Kistner, *Gynecology: Principals and Practice* (Chicago: Year Book
     Medical Publishers, 1971).

223 *"It's that type of individual who simply has to* . . . R. W. Kistner, quoted in Kate
     Seear, *The Makings of a Modern Epidemic: Endometriosis, Gender and Politics*
     (New York: Routledge, 2014), 114.

223 *"Over the last twenty years* . . . Niels H. Lauersen and Constance deSwann, *The
     Endometriosis Answer Book: New Hope, New Help* (New York: Rawson Associates/
     MacMillan, 1988), 20.

223 *the disease came to be imagined as a "product of women's inappropriate* . . . Kate
     Seear, *The Makings of a Modern Epidemic: Endometriosis, Gender and Politics*
     (New York: Routledge, 2014), 43.

223 *It likely won't surprise you* . . . Stephen Kennedy, "Who Gets Endometriosis?"
     Women's Health Medicine 2, no. 1 (January 2005), doi:10.1383/wohm.2.1.18.58876.

223 *Endometriosis expert Dr. Marc Laufer put it simply* . . . Shannon Cohn, *Endo
     What?*, www.endowhat.com/.

223 *One 1993 study suggested that up to 40 percent* . . . Carolyn Carpan, "Representation
     of Endometriosis in the Popular Press: 'The Career Woman's Disease,'" *Atlantis* 27,
     no. 2 (Spring/Summer 2003), http://journals.msvu.ca/index.php/atlantis/article
     /view/1317.

224 *Yet studies suggest that about 70 percent* . . . Taylor et al., "Pain and Endometriosis."

224 *On average, women see seven health care professionals* . . . Taylor et al., "Pain and
     Endometriosis."

224 *"I write this article as a plea to our profession* . . . Robert Albee Jr., "Is Endometriosis
     All in Your Head?" Endometriosis.org, http://endometriosis.org/news/opinion
     /albee-is-endometriosis-all-in-your-head/.

224 *About half of women with unexplained infertility have endometriosis* . . . Cohn,
     Endo What?

224 *A 2003 study confirmed that women who complained to doctors of infertility* . . .

M. S. Arid et al., "Time Elapsed from Onset of Symptoms to Diagnosis of Endometriosis in a Cohort Study of Brazilian Women," *Human Reproduction* 18, no. 4 (April 2003), doi:10.1093/humrep/deg136.

224 *"The greatest loss associated with endometriosis is the loss of children* . . . Lisa M. Sammiguel, "What's Wrong with This Picture? Comparing Lived Experience and Textual Representations of Endometriosis," in Norman K. Denzin, ed., *Cultural Studies*, vol. 1 (Bingley, UK: Emerald Publishing Group, 1996).

225 *even postdiagnosis, women often continue to find their reports* . . . Emma Whelan, "Staging and Profiling: The Constitution of the Endometriotic Subject in Gynecological Discourse," *Alternate Routes* 14 (1997), www.alternateroutes.ca /index.php/ar/article/view/20326.

225 *Some experts now think that it's how chemically active the tissue is* . . . Emma Whelan, "Negotiating Science and Experience in Medical Knowledge: Gynecologists on Endometriosis," *Social Science and Medicine* 68, no. 8 (April 2009), doi:10.1016/j.socscimed.2009.01.032.

225 *Some have even listed somatization* . . . Cara E. Jones, "Wandering Wombs and 'Female Troubles': The Hysterical Origins, Symptoms, and Treatments of Endometriosis," *Women's Studies: An Interdisciplinary Journal* 44, no. 8 (November 2015), doi:10.1080/00497878.2015.1078212.

225 *for decades, there was an assumption that "gynecology should focus* . . . Whelan, "Staging and Profiling."

226 *Back in the early eighties, when the NIH set aside a small chunk of funding* . . . Laurence and Weinhouse, *Outrageous Practices*, 3.

226 *"Endo is sorely underfunded* . . . All quotes from author's interview with Heather Guidone (surgical program director for the Center for Endometriosis Care).

226 *The lack of attention to endometriosis in the research community* . . . Ray Garry, "The Endometriosis Syndromes: A Clinical Classification in the Presence of Aetiological Confusion and Therapeutic Anarchy," *Human Reproduction* 19, no. 4 (April 2004), doi:10.1093/humrep/deh147.

227 *"My doctor told me having a baby would help my pain* . . . Sylvia Freedman, "With Endometriosis Shouldn't 'Let's Get You Well' Come Before 'Let's Get You Pregnant'?" *The Guardian*, February 18, 2016, www.theguardian.com/commentisfree /2016/feb/19/with-endometriosis-shouldnt-lets-get-you-well-come-before-lets -get-you-pregnant.

228 *"Endometriosis may be described as enigmas wrapped* . . . R. Jaffe, foreword to *Endometriosis: The Complete Reference for Taking Charge of Your Health*, eds. M. L. Ballweg and the Endometriosis Association (New York: McGraw-Hill Education, 2003), xv–xvii.

228 *Others question whether Sampson's theory is salvageable* . . . David B. Redwine and Endometriosis Institute of Oregon, *100 Questions & Answers About Endometriosis* (Sudbury, MA: Jones and Bartlett Publishers, 2009).

229 *"The conclusion that endometriosis is* . . . Shohat, "Lasers."

229 *"beyond the powers of mere mortals to solve* . . . Jones, "Wandering."

229 *At age eighteen, she was getting her first checkup with a gynecologist* . . . All quotes from author's interview with Nicole.

230 *"if a man had a disease that causes him to be unable to father a child, to have unbearable* . . . "Endo Under-Diagnosed and Difficult to Treat," DrDeMarco.com, www.drdemarco.com/charge/rq039.htm.

230 *The Endometriosis Association created a series of cartoons entitled* Joe with

Endo... Mary Lou Ballweg and the Endometriosis Association, *The Endometriosis Sourcebook* (Chicago: Contemporary Books, 1995).

231 *More than half of patients with endometriosis experience painful penetrative sex*... Alison Prior et al., "Irritable Bowel Syndrome in the Gynecological Clinic: Survey of 798 Referrals," *Digestive Diseases and Sciences* 34, no. 13 (December 1989), doi:10.1007/BF01536698.

231 *Up to 90 percent of IC patients*... Interstitial Cystitis Association, *Because You Care: Exploring the Unique Intimacy Issues of People with Interstitial Cystitis* (Rockville, MD: Interstitial Cystitis Association, 2006).

231 *In 2003, the first population-based prevalence estimate*... B. L. Harlow and E. G. Stewart, "Population-Based Assessment of Chronic Unexplained Vulvar Pain: Have We Underestimated the Prevalence of Vulvodynia?" *Journal of the American Medical Women's Association* 58, no. 2 (Spring 2003), www.ncbi.nlm.nih.gov /pubmed/12744420.

232 *Subsequent studies have yielded similar estimates*... Barbara D. Reed et al., "Prevalence and Demographic Characteristics of Vulvodynia in a Population-Based Sample," *American Journal of Obstetrics and Gynecology* 206, no. 2 (February 2012), doi:10.1016/j.ajog.2011.08.012.

232 *laid to rest the misperception that vulvodynia*... B. D. Reed et al., "Pain at the Vulvar Vestibule: A Web-Based Survey," *Journal of Lower Genital Tract Disease* 8, no. 1 (January 2004), www.ncbi.nlm.nih.gov/pubmed/15874837; R. J. Lavy, L. S. Hynan, and R. W. Haley, "Prevalence of Vulvar Pain in an Urban, Minority Population," *Journal of Reproductive Medicine* 52, no. 1 (January 2007), www.ncbi .nlm.nih.gov/pubmed/17286071.

232 *According to a 2012 study*... Reed et al., "Prevalence and Demographic Characteristics."

232 *"although fortunately not very frequent, is by*... T. G. Thomas, *Practical Treatise on the Diseases of Women* (Philadelphia: Henry C. Lea's Son, 1874), 115.

232 *After that, with the exception of one mention in the 1920s*... Marek Jantos, *A Psychophysiological Perspective on Vulvodynia* (thesis, Univ. of Adelaide, 2009), https://digital.library.adelaide.edu.au/dspace/bitstream/2440/61980/8/02whole .pdf.

232 *Thus, as sociologist Amy Kaler has shown in her analysis*... Amy Kaler, "Gendered Normativities and Shifting Metaphors of Vulvar Pain," paper presented at the annual meeting of the American Sociological Association, Montreal Convention Center, Montreal, Quebec, Canada, August 10, 2006, http://citation.allacademic .com/meta/p_mla_apa_research_citation/0/9/6/9/2/pages96925/p96925-1.php.

233 *"The dyspareunic patient must be helped to see for herself that the hyperesthesia*... J. Malleson, "Sex Problems in Marriage with Particular Reference to Coital Discomfort and the Unconsummated Marriage," *Practitioner* 172, no. 1030 (April 1954), www.ncbi.nlm.nih.gov/pubmed/13155342.

233 *"Sexual intercourse is a wonderful act that results*... Kaler, "Gendered Normativities."

233 *medical articles with titles like "Wives Who Refuse Their Husbands*... M. F. Weiner, "Wives Who Refuse Their Husbands," *Psychosomatics* 14, no. 5 (September– October 1973), doi:10.1016/S0033-3182(73)71320-7.

233 *On the other hand, while the condition had previously been seen as "a two party problem*... Weiner, "Wives Who Refuse."

233 *According to one influential 1978 article*... M. G. Dodson and E. G. Friedrich

Jr., "Psychosomatic Vulvovaginitis," *Obstetrics and Gynecology* 51, no. 1 supp. (January 1978), www.ncbi.nlm.nih.gov/pubmed/618469.

234 *"vaginismus is a conversion disorder which is a neurotic* . . . C. M. Duddle, "Etiological Factors in the Unconsummated Marriage," *Journal of Psychosomatic Research* 21, no. 2 (1977), doi:10.1016/0022-3999(77)90083-6.

234 *In interviews Kaler conducted in the mid-aughts with over a hundred women* . . . Amy Kaler, "Classifying Pain: What's at Stake for Women with Dyspareunia," *Archives of Sexual Behavior* 34, no. 1 (February 2005), doi:10.1007/s10508-005-7467-x.

235 *"in this imperfect world it is never possible to be* . . . P. Lynch, "Vulvodynia: A Syndrome of Unexplained Vulvar Pain, Psychological Disability and Sexual Dysfunction," *Journal of Reproductive Medicine* 31, no. 9 (September 1986), doi:10.1080/713846809.

235 *"was long thought to be an unusual* . . . Marilynne McKay, "Vulvodynia: A Multifactorial Clinical Problem," *Archives of Dermatology* 125, no. 2 (February 1989), doi:10.1001/archderm.1989.01670140108021.

236 *"The only reason NIH started looking at vulvodynia* . . . All quotes from author's interview with Phyllis Mate (former executive director of the National Vulvodynia Association).

236 *Many vulvodynia experts argued that it didn't make sense to list dyspareunia* . . . Caroline F. Pukall, "Pain Measurement in Vulvodynia," *Journal of Sex and Marital Therapy* 29, no. 1 (February 2003), doi:10.1080/713847136.

236 *One 1992 study gave patients a series of quantitative tests of psychological distress* . . . L. R. Schover, David D. Youngs, and Ruth Cantata, "Psychosexual Aspects of the Evaluation and Management of Vulvar Vestibulitis," *American Journal of Obstetrics and Gynecology* 167, no. 3 (September 1992), doi:10.1016/S0002-9378(11)91562-2.

237 *The stereotypes were so prevalent that in a 1994 article* . . . R. Basson, "Vulvar Vestibulitis Syndrome: A Common Condition Which May Present as Vaginismus," *Journal of Sexual and Marital Therapy* 9, no. 3 (1994), doi:10.1080/02674659408409587.

237 *Indeed, as late as 2007 dissenters tried to resurrect old-school* . . . Franco Mascherpa, "Vulvodynia as a Possible Somotoform Disorder: More Than Just an Opinion," *The Journal of Reproductive Medicine* 52, no. 2 (February 2007), www.ncbi.nlm.nih.gov/pubmed/17393771.

239 *A 2013 survey of eighty-five patients eventually diagnosed with* . . . Jennifer J. Connor, Cassandra M. Brix, and Stephanie Trudeau-Hern, "The Diagnosis of Provoked Vestibulodynia: Steps and Roadblocks in a Long Journey," *Sexual and Relationship Therapy* 28, no. 4 (2013), doi:10.1080/14681994.2013.842969.

240 *One of the only ones that has been done, funded* . . . U.S. Department of Health and Human Services, National Institutes of Health, Eunice Kennedy Shriver National Institute of Child Health and Human Development, *What Are the Treatments for Vulvodynia?*, www.nichd.nih.gov/health/topics/vulvodynia/conditioninfo/Pages/treatment.aspx.

240 *According to the NIH Research Plan on Vulvodynia, published* . . . U.S. Department of Health and Human Services, National Institutes of Health, Eunice Kennedy Shriver National Institute of Child Health and Human Development, *NIH Research Plan on Vulvodynia*, www.nichd.nih.gov/publications/pubs/documents/NIH_Vulvodynia_Plan_April2012.pdf.

241 *When she was seventeen, Rebecca came down* . . . All quotes from author's interview with Rebecca.

243 *But experts warn that treatable conditions* . . . Karin M. Ouchida and Mark S. Lachs, "Not for Doctors Only: Ageism in Healthcare," *Generations* (Fall 2015), www.asaging.org/blog/not-doctors-only-ageism-healthcare.

243 *As one older patient with severe OA* . . . Stephen Thielke, Joanna Sale, and M. Carrington Reid, "Aging: Are These 4 Pain Myths Complicating Care?" *The Journal of Family Practice* 61, no. 11 (November 2012), www.ncbi.nlm.nih.gov /pmc/articles/PMC4356472/.

243 *A 2011 study found that, on average, American medical students* . . . Juno Obedin-Maliver et al., "Lesbian, Gay, Bisexual, and Transgender-Related Content in Undergraduate Medical Education," *JAMA* 306, no. 9 (September 2011), doi:10.1001/jama.2011.1255.

243 *In a 2011 survey, a quarter of trans people in the United States* . . . Jaime M. Grant, Lisa A. Mottet, and Justin Tanis, *Injustice at Every Turn: A Report of the National Transgender Discrimination Survey* (Washington, DC: National Center for Transgender Equality and National Gay and Lesbian Task Force, 2011).

243 *coined the term "trans broken arm syndrome" to describe it* . . . Naith Payton, "Feature: The Dangers of Trans Broken Arm Syndrome," *PinkNews*, July 9, 2015, www.pinknews.co.uk/2015/07/09/feature-the-dangers-of-trans-broken-arm -syndrome/.

244 *Rebecca Puhl, an expert in weight stigma* . . . Harriet Brown, "For Obese People, Prejudice in Plain Sight," *The New York Times*, March 15, 2010, www.nytimes .com/2010/03/16/health/16essa.html.

244 *According to patient surveys* . . . Christopher N. Sciamanna et al., "Who Reports Receiving Advice to Lose Weight? Results from a Multistate Survey," *Archives of Internal Medicine* 160, no. 15 (August 2000), doi:10.1001/archinte.160.15.2334.

244 *A 2001 study found that doctors were more likely* . . . Caitlin Anderson et al., "Weight Loss and Gender: An Examination of Physician Attitudes," *Obesity* 9, no. 4 (April 2001), doi:10.1038/oby.2001.30.

244 *In one 2014 study, 53 percent of women reported* . . . Ryan Sean Darby, Nicole Henniger, Christine R. Harris, "Reactions to Physician-Inspired Shame and Guilt," *Basic and Applied Social Psychology* 36, no. 1 (February 2014), doi:10.1080 /01973533.2013.856782.

244 *"Smaller amounts of 'overweight' are taken much more seriously in women* . . . All quotations from the author's interview with Harriet Brown.

244 *According to a 2008 study from the Rudd Center* . . . R. M. Puhl, T. Andreyeva, and K. D. Brownell, "Perceptions of Weight Discrimination: Prevalence and Comparison to Race and Gender Discrimination in America," *International Journal of Obesity* 32, no. 6 (June 2008), doi:10.1038/ijo.2008.22.

244 *or sixty-eight pounds "overweight"* . . . Tara Parker-Pope, "Fat Bias Worse for Women," *The New York Times*, March 31, 2008, https://well.blogs.nytimes.com /2008/03/31/fat-bias-worse-for-women/.

245 *Studies consistently confirm that women* . . . Catherine M. Phillips et al., "Defining Metabolically Healthy Obesity: Role of Dietary and Lifestyle Factors," ed. Stephen L. Atkin, *PLOS One* 8, no. 10 (October 2013), doi:10.1371/journal .pone.0076188.

245 *According to a 2016 analysis, relying on BMI as a crude measure* . . . A. J. Tomiyama et al., "Misclassification of Cardiometabolic Health When Using

Body Mass Index Categories in NHANES 2005–2012," *International Journal of Obesity* 40, no. 5 (May 2016), doi:10.1038/ijo.2016.17.

245 *A 2008 study found that 57 percent of overweight women* . . . Rachel P. Wildman et al., "The Obese Without Cardiometabolic Risk Factor Clustering and the Normal Weight with Cardiometabolic Risk Factor Clustering: Prevalence and Correlates of 2 Phenotypes Among the US Population (NHANES 1999–2004)," *Archives of Internal Medicine* 168, no. 15 (August 2008), doi:10.1001/archinte.168.15.1617.

245 *According to a 2016 nationally representative survey* . . . American College of Cardiology, "Many Women Not Properly Informed of Heart Risk by Their Doctors: Survey Shows Women Are Less Likely to Get Recommended Monitoring, Often Told to Lose Weight," *ScienceDaily*, March 23, 2016, www.sciencedaily.com /releases/2016/03/160323185532.htm.

245 *In a 2002 study* . . . Christine Aramburu Alegría and Margaret Louis, "Exploring the Association Between Body Weight, Stigma of Obesity, and Health Care Avoidance," *Journal of the American Academy of Nurse Practitioners* 14, no. 12 (December 2002), doi:10.1111/j.1745-7599.2002.tb00089.x.

245 *A recent* New York Times *article highlighted the stories* . . . Gina Kolata, "Why Do Obese Patients Get Worse Care? Many Doctors Don't See Past the Fat," *The New York Times*, September 25, 2016, www.nytimes.com/2016/09/26/health/obese -patients-health-care.html.

246 *When Natalie was eleven years old* . . . All quotes from author's interview with Natalie.

248 *In a recent* BuzzFeed *article, women readers shared* . . . Lara Parker, "Here Are 29 Stories from Women Whose Doctors Did Not Take Their Pain Seriously," *BuzzFeed*, March 20, 2017, www.buzzfeed.com/laraparker/women-pain?utm _term=.voNVkreQA#.wgRD3wNov.

248 *like non-Hodgkin lymphoma* . . . Angela Epstein, "Do You Suffer from Night Sweats? Don't Blame the Menopause Just Yet: After Being Misdiagnosed by Doctors for Two Years, Wendy Discovered She Had Cancer," *Daily Mail*, December 5, 2016, www.dailymail.co.uk/health/article-4002952/Do-suffer-night-sweats-Don-t -blame-menopause-just-misdiagnosed-doctors-two-years-Wendy-discovered -cancer.html.

248 *like uterine* . . . Julissa Catalan (as told to), "Doctors Told Me My Uterine Cancer Was Menopause," *Prevention*, June 7, 2016, www.prevention.com/health/doctors -told-me-my-uterine-cancer-was-menopause.

248 *everything from brain tumors* . . . Spotted Quoll, comment on Soraya Chemaly, "How Sexism Affects Women's Health Every Day," *Role Reboot*, June 23, 2015, www.rolereboot.org/culture-and-politics/details/2015-06-how-sexism-affects -womens-health-every-day/#comment-2096176555.

248 *to hepatitis C* . . . notmymonkees, comment on the thread "How Doctors Take Women's Pain Less Seriously (theatlantic.com)," in the subreddit "TwoXChromosomes," Reddit, October 15, 2015, www.reddit.com/r /TwoXChromosomes/comments/3ouv3t/how_doctors_take_womens_pain_less _seriously/cw0u5vw/.

249 *in a 2015 article in* The Telegraph, *a twenty-four-year-old British woman* . . . Radhika Sanghani, "'It's Just Lady Pains': Are Doctors Not Taking Women's Agony Seriously Enough?" *The Telegraph*, October 22, 2015, www.telegraph.co.uk /women/womens-life/11948057/Lady-pains-Are-doctors-not-taking-womens -pain-seriously-enough.html.

CHAPTER 7. CONTESTED ILLNESSES: WHEN DISEASES ARE "FASHIONABLE"

251 *In 2011, Jen Brea was traveling with her then boyfriend* . . . All quotes from author's interview with Jen Brea.

252 *"In our culture, a disease does not exist as* . . . Charles E. Rosenberg and Janet Golden, eds., *Framing Disease: Studies in Cultural History* (New Brunswick, NJ: Rutgers Univ. Press, 1992), xiii.

253 *According to a 1997 article by one physician, somatizing patients* . . . Charles V. Ford, "Somatization and Fashionable Diagnoses: Illness as a Way of Life," *Scandinavian Journal of Work, Environment and Health* 23, no. 3 (1997), www .jstor.org/stable/40966698.

254 *By 1988, studies concluding that ME/CFS patients were actually suffering* . . . Hillary Johnson, *Osler's Web: Inside the Labyrinth of the Chronic Fatigue Syndrome Epidemic* (Lincoln, NE: Backinprint.com, 2006), 269.

254 *"Chronic Fatigue Is Often Mental Illness"* . . . Larry Thompson, "Chronic Fatigue Is Often Mental Illness," *The Washington Post*, May 10, 1988, www.highbeam.com /doc/1P2-1256027.html.

254 *"Fatigue: Fact or Figment?"* . . . Loraine O'Connell, "Fatigue: Fact or Figment?" *Orlando Sentinel*, June 14, 1988, http://articles.orlandosentinel.com/1988-06-14 /lifestyle/0040450292_1_fatigue-researchers-chronic.

254 *The next year, the same conclusion was reached by an NIH study* . . . M. J. Kruesi, J. Dale, and S. E. Straus, "Psychiatric Diagnoses in Patients Who Have Chronic Fatigue Syndrome," *Journal of Clinical Psychiatry* 50, no. 2 (February 1989), www.ncbi.nlm.nih.gov/pubmed/2536690.

254 *Patients have compared it to "permanently having the flu* . . . Center for Drug Evaluation and Research and U.S. Food and Drug Administration, *Chronic Fatigue Syndrome and Myalgic Encephalomyelitis*, September 2013, www.fda .gov/downloads/ForIndustry/UserFees/PrescriptionDrugUserFee/UCM368806 .pdf.

255 *In 2015, the IOM issued a three-hundred-page report* . . . Committee on the Diagnostic Criteria for Myalgic Encephalomyelitis/Chronic Fatigue Syndrome, *Beyond Myalgic Encephalomyelitis/Chronic Fatigue Syndrome: Redefining an Illness* (Washington, DC: The National Academies Press, 2015).

255 *The economic burden of ME/CFS in lost productivity and medical costs* . . . Jin-Mann S. Lin et al., "The Economic Impact of Chronic Fatigue Syndrome in Georgia: Direct and Indirect Costs," *Cost Effectiveness and Resource Allocation* 9, no. 1 (January 2011), doi:10.1186/1478-7547-9-1.

255 *Less than one-third of medical schools include ME/CFS* . . . Committee on the Diagnostic Criteria, *Beyond Myalgic Encephalomyelitis*.

255 *only 40 percent of medical textbooks* . . . Leonard A. Jason et al., "Frequency and Content Analysis of CFS in Medical Text Books," *Australian Journal of Primary Health* 16, no. 2 (2010), www.ncbi.nlm.nih.gov/pmc/articles/PMC3691015/.

255 *According to a 2011 study by researchers from the CDC, 85 percent* . . . E. Unger et al., "CFS Knowledge and Illness Management Behavior Among U.S. Healthcare Providers and the Public" (paper, IACFS/ME conference, Ottawa, CA, 2011).

256 *Patient surveys have found that* . . . The CFIDS Association of America, *ME/ CFS Road to Diagnosis Survey*, conducted January 2014, http://solvecfs.org/wp -content/uploads/2014/01/IOM_RoadtoDiagnosisSurveyReport.pdf; "A Profile of ME/CFS Patients: How Many Years and How Many Doctors?" *ProHealth*, May 16, 2008, www.prohealth.com/library/showarticle.cfm?libid=13672.

256 *The vast majority* . . . Committee on the Diagnostic Criteria, *Beyond Myalgic Encephalomyelitis.*

256 *"million-dollar workups on neurotic women* . . . Carol Jessop, quoted in Johnson, *Osler's Web,* 3.

257 *"[He] saw ten women* . . . Jessop, in Johnson, *Osler's Web,* 69.

257 *A 1996 Australian study of fifty patients eventually diagnosed* . . . Dorothy H. Broom and Roslyn V. Woodward, "Medicalisation Reconsidered: Toward a Collaborative Approach to Care," *Sociology of Health and Illness* 18, no. 3 (June 1996), doi:10.1111/1467-9566.ep10934730.

257 *"There was such clear evidence of extraordinary bias* . . . All quotes from author's interview with Hillary Johnson.

258 *In 1970, however, a couple psychiatrists* . . . Colin P. McEvedy and A. W. Beard, "Royal Free Epidemic of 1955: A Reconsideration," *British Medical Journal* 1, no. 5687 (February 1970), doi:10.1136/bmj.1.5687.7.

258 *They suggested that many of the other fifteen epidemics of ME* . . . Colin P. McEvedy and A. W. Beard, "Concept of Benign Myalgic Encephalomyelitis," *British Medical Journal* 1, no. 5687 (January 1970), www.ncbi.nlm.nih.gov/pmc /articles/PMC1700895/pdf/brmedj02268-0023.pdf.

259 *The subtitle of a 1987* Time *piece* . . . Dick Thompson, "Medicine: Stealthy Epidemic of Exhaustion," *Time,* June 29, 1987, http://content.time.com/time /magazine/article/0,9171,964813,00.html.

259 *A CBS segment that same year described* . . . *West 57th,* CBS, December 10, 1987, quoted in Johnson, *Osler's Web,* 232–233.

260 *"The one absolutely clear-cut clinical feature* . . . "Transcript of *Frontline* Documentary on ME from 1993," *Indigo Jo Blogs,* www.blogistan.co.uk/blog /articles/transcript_of_frontline_documentary_on_me_from_1993.

260 *According to two cardiologists featured in a 1988 article* . . . Patricia de Wolfe, "ME: The Rise and Fall of a Media Sensation," *Medical Sociology Online* 4, no. 1 (June 2009), www.medicalsociologyonline.org/oldsite/archives/issue41/pdwolfe.html.

260 *ME/CFS represented a "culturally sanctioned" flight* . . . S. E. Abbey and P. E. Garfinkel, "Neurasthenia and Chronic Fatigue Syndrome: The Role of Culture in the Making of a Diagnosis," *American Journal of Psychiatry* 148, no. 12 (December 1991), doi:10.1176/ajp.148.12.1638.

260 *"'Liberated' by feminism to enter previously all-male occupations* . . . N. C. Ware and A. Kleinman, "Culture and Somatic Experience: The Social Course of Illness in Neurasthenia and Chronic Fatigue Syndrome," *Psychosomatic Medicine* 54, no. 5 (September–October 1992), doi:10.1097/00006842-199209000-00003.

261 *The influence of the antifeminist backlash occurring at the time* . . . Judith A. Richman et al., "Feminist Perspectives on the Social Construction of Chronic Fatigue Syndrome," *Health Care for Women International* 14, no. 4 (2000), doi:10.1080/073993300245249.

261 *In a 1988 article, the NIH's resident* . . . S. E. Strauss et al., "Allergy and the Chronic Fatigue Syndrome," *Journal of Allergy and Clinical Immunology* 81, no. 5 (May 1988), www.ncbi.nlm.nih.gov/pubmed/2836490.

261 *an upper-middle-class housewife who'd been bedridden for ten years before finding her way to them, she'd spent* . . . Johnson, *Osler's Web,* 253.

262 *In 1991, researchers knocked on doors* . . . S. A. Daugherty et al., "Chronic Fatigue Syndrome in Northern Nevada," *Reviews of Infectious Diseases* 13, no. 1 (January–February 1991), www.ncbi.nlm.nih.gov/pubmed/1850542.

262 *In 1999, researchers surveyed nearly 30,000 people* . . . Leonard A. Jason, "A Community-Based Study of Chronic Fatigue Syndrome," *Archives of Internal Medicine* 159, no. 18 (October 1999), doi:10.1001/archinte.159.18.2129.

262 *In 1987, the media even reported* . . . Philip M. Boffey, "Fatigue 'Virus' Has Experts More Baffled and Skeptical Than Ever," *The New York Times*, July 28, 1987, www .nytimes.com/1987/07/28/science/fatigue-virus-has-experts-more-baffled-and -skeptical-than-ever.html?pagewanted=all.

262 *Her sister, who'd been a healthy young woman when* . . . All quotes from author's interview with Lucinda Bateman.

263 *"Are we to believe that just because symptoms are strange* . . . Thomas L. English, "Skeptical of Skeptics," *JAMA* 265, no. 8 (February 1991), doi:10.1001/jama.1991 .03460080032011.

266 *"I get constant jokes about this* . . . Johnson, *Osler's Web*, 264.

266 *"I am SICK . . . I am so tired it took me 6 days to dictate* . . . Johnson, *Osler's Web*, 154.

266 *One of the revelations Johnson reported in* Osler's Web . . . David Tuller, "Chronic Fatigue Syndrome and the CDC: A Long, Tangled Tale," *Virology Blog*, November 23, 2011, www.virology.ws/2011/11/23/chronic-fatigue-syndrome -and-the-cdc-a-long-tangled-tale/.

266 *In 1999, an audit by the U.S. Department of Health* . . . June Gibbs Brown, "Audit of Costs Charged to the Chronic Fatigue Syndrome Program at the Centers for Disease Control and Prevention," Department of Health and Human Services, May 10, 1999, https://oig.hhs.gov/oas/reports/region4/49804226.pdf.

266 *In 2000, the GAO reported* . . . U.S. General Accounting Office, "Chronic Fatigue Syndrome: CDC and NIH Research Activities Are Diverse, but Agency Coordination Is Limited," GAO/HEHS-00-98, June 2000, www.gao.gov/new .items/he00098.pdf.

267 *By 2000, in fact, the NIH* . . . Cort Johnson, "Former NIH Official Says Chronic Fatigue Syndrome Program Must Move in Order to Succeed," Health Rising, March 11, 2015, www.healthrising.org/blog/2015/03/11/former-nih-official-says -chronic-fatigue-program-must-move/.

267 *"[He] couldn't find out what was causing this illness* . . . Johnson, *Osler's Web*, 260.

267 *He began opening his lectures at medical schools* . . . Johnson, *Osler's Web*, 287.

268 *One article in the early nineties, noting the "striking resemblance"* . . . Susan E. Abbey and Paul E. Garfinkel, "Neurasthenia and Chronic Fatigue Syndrome: The Role of Culture in the Making of a Diagnosis," *American Journal of Psychiatry* 148, no. 12 (December 1991), doi:10.1176/ajp.148.12.1638.

268 *Another influential article that compared the two* . . . Wessely, "Old Wine in New Bottles."

268 *A 2013 article arguing that fibromyalgia* . . . Wolfe and Walitt, "Culture, Science and the Changing Nature of Fibromyalgia."

269 *"To claim [ME/CFS] as an incarnation of neurasthenia* . . . Dorothy Wall, *Encounters with the Invisible: Unseen Illness, Controversy, and Chronic Fatigue Syndrome* (Dallas: Southern Methodist Univ. Press, 2005), 95.

270 *In 2015, the NIH announced that it would "ramp up"* . . . Jennie Spotila, "2015 NIH Spending on ME/CFS Studies," *Occupy M.E.*, February 17, 2016, www .occupycfs.com/2016/02/17/2015-nih-spending-on-mecfs-studies/.

270 *"given the seriousness of the condition, I don't think we have* . . . Olga Khazan, "A Boost for Chronic Fatigue Syndrome Research," *The Atlantic*, October 29,

2015, www.theatlantic.com/health/archive/2015/10/a-boost-for-chronic-fatigue
-syndrome-research/413008/.

270 *For years, prominent British mental health professionals* . . . Mary Burgess and
Trudie Chalder, *PACE Manual for Therapists: Cognitive Behaviour Therapy for
CFS/ME* (PACE Trial Management Group, MREC version 2.1, December 8,
2004), www.wolfson.qmul.ac.uk/images/pdfs/3.cbt-therapist-manual.pdf.

271 *Its conclusions, first published in* The Lancet *in 2011* . . . P. D. White et al.,
"Comparison of Adaptive Pacing Therapy, Cognitive Behaviour Therapy, Graded
Exercise Therapy, and Specialist Medical Care for Chronic Fatigue Syndrome
(PACE): A Randomised Trial," *The Lancet* 377, no. 9768 (March 2011), doi:10.1016
/S0140-6736(11)60096-2.

271 *"Got ME? Just Get Out* . . . Jeremy Laurance, "Got ME? Just Get Out and Exercise,
Say Scientists," *The Independent*, February 18, 2011, www.independent.co.uk
/life-style/health-and-families/health-news/got-me-just-get-out-and-exercise-say
-scientists-2218377.html.

271 *a detailed exposé was published on the science site* Virology Blog . . . David Tuller,
"Trial by Error: The Troubling Case of the PACE Chronic Fatigue Syndrome Study,"
Virology Blog, October 21, 2015, www.virology.ws/2015/10/21/trial-by-error-i/.

271 *an open letter declared that "such flaws* . . . Ronald W. Davis et al., "An Open Letter
to Dr. Richard Horton and *The Lancet*," *Virology Blog*, November 13, 2015, www
.virology.ws/2015/11/13/an-open-letter-to-dr-richard-horton-and-the-lancet/.

272 *only 20 percent of patients* . . . Julie Rehmeyer and David Tuller, "Getting It Wrong
on Chronic Fatigue Syndrome," *The New York Times*, March 18, 2017, www
.nytimes.com/2017/03/18/opinion/sunday/getting-it-wrong-on-chronic-fatigue-
syndrome.html.

272 *"The researchers' modest results in fact offered compelling evidence* . . . Julie
Rehmeyer, *Through the Shadowlands: A Science Writer's Odyssey into an Illness
Science Doesn't Understand* (New York: Rodale Books, 2017), 95.

272 *"protect patients from ineffective and possibly* . . . Dharam V. Ablashi et al.,
"An Open Letter to Psychological Medicine About 'Recovery' and the PACE
Trial," *Virology Blog*, March 13, 2007, www.virology.ws/2017/03/13/an-open
-letter-to-psychological-medicine-about-recovery-and-the-pace-trial/.

273 *Normally, when we stand up, the autonomic nervous system* . . . Satish R. Raj,
"The Postural Tachycardia Syndrome (POTS): Pathophysiology, Diagnosis &
Management," *Indian Pacing and Electrophysiology Journal* 6, no. 2 (April–June
2006), www.ncbi.nlm.nih.gov/pmc/articles/PMC1501099/.

273 *Orthostatic intolerance is the umbrella term for conditions* . . . Peter C. Rowe,
"General Information Brochure on Orthostatic Intolerance and Its Treatment,"
Dysautonomia International, March 2014, www.dysautonomiainternational.org
/pdf/RoweOIsummary.pdf.

273 *Researchers have found POTS patients to be as impaired* . . . Lisa M. Benrud-
Larson et al., "Quality of Life in Patients with Postural Tachycardia Syndrome,"
Mayo Clinic Proceedings 77, no. 6 (June 2002), doi:10.4065/77.6.531.

273 *Approximately 25 percent of them are unable* . . . D. S. Goldstein et al., "Dys-
autonomias: Clinical Disorders of the Autonomic Nervous System," *Annals of
Internal Medicine* 137, no. 9 (November 2002), doi:10.7326/0003-4819-137-9
-200211050-00011.

274 *"We think part of the reason it's neglected is* . . . All quotes from author's interview with Lauren Stiles (cofounder of Dysautonomia International).

275 *In a 2016 study from the Mayo Clinic* . . . R. Bhatia et al., "Outcomes of Adolescent-Onset Postural Orthostatic Tachycardia Syndrome," *The Journal of Pediatrics* 173 (June 2016), doi:10.1016/j.jpeds.2016.02.035.

275 *can much more convincingly be traced back* . . . Oglesby Paul, "Da Costa's Syndrome or Neurocirculatory Asthenia," *British Heart Journal* 58, no. 4 (October 1987), www.ncbi.nlm.nih.gov/pmc/articles/PMC1277260/pdf/brheartj00094-0008.pdf.

276 *In 1941, American physician Dr. Paul Wood argued* . . . Paul Wood, "Da Costa's Syndrome: Aetiology. Lecture III," *British Medical Journal* 1, no. 4196 (June 1941), www.ncbi.nlm.nih.gov/pmc/articles/PMC2162062/.

276 *They estimated that it affected 2 to 5 percent of the population* . . . Mandel E. Cohen and Paul D. White, "Life Situations, Emotions, and Neurocirculatory Asthenia (Anxiety Neurosis, Neuroasthenia, Effort Syndrome)," *Psychosomatic Medicine* 13, no. 6 (November–December 1951), doi:10.1097/00006842 -195111000-00001.

276 *"It is possible that the curious lack of recognition of Da Costa's syndrome* . . . Paul Wood, "Da Costa's Syndrome (or Effort Syndrome)," *British Medical Journal* #1, no. 4194 (May 1941), www.ncbi.nlm.nih.gov/pmc/articles/PMC2161922/pdf /brmedj04094-0003.pdf.

276 *"diminished interest in Da Costa's* . . . Paul, "Da Costa's Syndrome."

277 *A 2008 study found that a group of POTS* . . . Vidya Raj et al., "Psychiatric Profile and Attention Deficits in Postural Tachycardia Syndrome," *Journal of Neurology, Neurosurgery, and Psychiatry* 80, no. 3 (March 2009), doi:10.1136 /jnnp.2008.144360.

278 *In the early nineties, researchers from Mayo Clinic coined* . . . R. Schondorg and P. A. Low, "Idiopathic Postural Orthostatic Tachycardia Syndrome: An Attenuated Form of Acute Pandysautonomia?" *Neurology* 43, no. 1 (January 1993), doi:10.1212 /WNL.43.1_Part_1.132.

278 *"a 20-year-old woman who appears* . . . David Robertson, "The Epidemic of Orthostatic Tachycardia and Orthostatic Intolerance," *The American Journal of the Medical Sciences* 317, no. 2 (February 1999), doi:10.1016/S0002-9629 (15)40480-X.

278 *Dysautonomia International recently teamed up with* . . . Lauren Stiles, "Quantifying the POTS Patient Experience," presentation, Beth Israel Deaconess Medical Center, 2016, www.dysautonomiainternational.org/pdf/Quantifying _POTS.pdf.

278 *One study explained the challenge of diagnosing POTS* . . . Lesley Kavi et al., "Postural Tachycardia Syndrome: Multiple Symptoms, but Easily Missed," *The British Journal of General Practice* 62, no. 599 (June 2012), doi:10.3399 /bjgp12X648963.

279 *The newest estimate is 1 to 3 million* . . . Dysautonomia International, "Postural Orthostatic Tachycardia Syndrome," www.dysautonomiainternational.org/page .php?ID=30.

280 *In the last few years, though, multiple research teams* . . . Hongliang Li et al., "Autoimmune Basis for Postural Tachycardia Syndrome," *Journal of the American Heart Association* 3, no. 1 (January 2014), doi:10.1161/JAHA.113.000755; Divyanshu Dubey, Steve Hopkins, and Steven Vernino, "M1 and M2 Muscarinic Receptor Antibodies Among Patients with Postural Orthostatic Tachycardia Syndrome," Dysautonomia International, www.dysautonomiainternational.org /pdf/Vernino_Muscarinic_Abstract.pdf.

281 *In the late eighties, Sherrill went to see . . .* All quotes are from author's interview with Sherrill.

282 *The CDC now estimates . . .* Centers for Disease Control and Prevention, "CDC Provides Estimate of Americans Diagnosed with Lyme Disease Each Year," 2013, www.cdc.gov/media/releases/2013/p0819-lyme-disease.html.

282 *"You, know, Mrs. Murray, some people subconsciously . . .* Pamela Weintraub, *Cure Unknown: Inside the Lyme Epidemic* (New York: St. Martin's Griffin, 2009), 44.

283 *Here's what everyone basically agrees . . .* Centers for Disease Control and Prevention, "CDC Provides Estimate."

284 *According to one study, over half of patients eventually diagnosed with Lyme . . .* John Aucott et al., "Diagnostic Challenges of Early Lyme Disease: Lessons from a Community Case Series," *BMC Infectious Diseases* 9 (June 2009), doi:10.1186/1471-2334-9-79.

284 *In a 2015 study, researchers tested over a hundred . . .* Allison Rebman et al., "Characteristics of Seroconversion and Implications for Diagnosis of Post-Treatment Lyme Disease Syndrome: Acute and Convalescent Serology Among a Prospective Cohort of Early Lyme Disease Patients," *Clinical Rheumatology* 34, no. 3 (March 2015), doi:10.1007/s10067-014-2706-z.

286 *According to one 1993 article in* Science *. . .* Alan G. Barbour and Durland Fish, "The Biological and Social Phenomenon of Lyme Disease," *Science* 260, no. 5114 (June 1993), www.wc4eb.org/wp-content/documents/BarbourFish.pdf

286 *Another study claimed to find a link between "severe psychological trauma . . .* Sanford P. Solomon et al., "Psychological Factors in the Prediction of Lyme Disease Course," *Arthritis and Rheumatism* 11, no. 5 (October 1998), doi:10.1002/art.1790110514.

286 *By the early nineties, skeptics of chronic Lyme . . .* Leonard H. Sigal, "Summary of the First 100 Patients Seen at a Lyme Disease Referral Center," *American Journal of Medicine* 88, no. 6 (June 1990), doi:10.1016/0002-9343(90)90520-N.

287 *As science journalist Pamela Weintraub writes in her 2009 book . . .* Weintraub, *Cure Unknown*, 131.

287 *"We would all be better off without . . .* George E. Ehrlich, quoted in Weintraub, *Cure Unknown*, 12.

287 *In a 2002 article, one prominent proponent of the mainstream view of Lyme . . .* Leonard H. Sigal and Afton L. Hassett, "Contributions of Societal and Geographical Environments to 'Chronic Lyme Disease': The Psychopathogenesis and Aporology of a New 'Medically Unexplained Symptoms' Syndrome," *Environmental Health Perspectives* 110, no. 4 (August 2002), www.ncbi.nlm.nih.gov/pmc/articles/PMC1241213/pdf/ehp110s-000607.pdf.

288 *In its 2006 guidelines, the Infectious Diseases Society of America . . .* Gary P. Wormser et al., "The Clinical Assessment, Treatment, and Prevention of Lyme Disease, Human Granulocytic Anaplasmosis, and Babesiosis: Clinical Practice Guidelines by the Infectious Diseases Society of America," *Clinical Infectious Diseases* 43, no. 9 (November 2006), doi:10.1086/508667.

288 *"a market for somatic labels exists in the large pool . . .* Robert A. Aronowitz, *Making Sense of Illness: Science, Society, and Disease* (Cambridge: Cambridge Univ. Press, 1998), 73.

289 *As researchers from the Johns Hopkins Lyme Disease Research Center explain . . .* John N. Aucott, Ari Seifter, and Alison W. Rebman, "Probable Late Lyme Disease: A Variant Manifestation of Untreated Borrelia Burgdorferi Infection," *BMC Infectious Diseases* 12 (August 2012), doi:10.1186/1471-2334-12-173.

289 *Mainstream experts blamed "sensationalist"* . . . Sigal and Hassett, "Contributions of Societal and Geographical Environments to 'Chronic Lyme Disease.'"

289 *in a 2005 article, two experts worried* . . . Leonard H. Sigal and Afton L. Hassett, "Commentary: 'What's in a Name? That Which We Call a Rose by Any Other Name Would Smell as Sweet.' Shakespeare W. Romeo and Juliet, II, ii(47–48)," *International Journal of Epidemiology* 34, no. 6 (December 2005), doi:10.1093/ije /dyi180.

289 *hypochondriacal, affluent women obsessed* . . . Sigal and Hasset, "Contributions of Societal and Geographical Environments to 'Chronic Lyme Disease.'"

289 *In 1991, a satirical column in* Annals of Internal Medicine . . . Ludwig A. Lettau, quoted in Weintraub, *Cure Unknown*, 132.

290 *In a 2009 article entitled "Implications of Gender* . . . Gary P. Wormser and Eugene D. Shapiro, "Implications of Gender in Chronic Lyme Disease," *Journal of Women's Health* 18, no. 6 (June 2009), doi:10.1089/jwh.2008.1193.

291 *"What happened to all the women?* . . . Maryalice Yakutchik, "Science of the Sexes," Johns Hopkins Bloomberg School of Public Health (Spring 2011), http:// magazine.jhsph.edu/2011/spring/features/science_of_the_sexes/.

291 *But it could also be that the women with late Lyme are more likely* . . . Alison W. Rebman, Mark J. Soloski, John N. Aucott, "Sex and Gender Impact Lyme Disease Immunopathology, Diagnosis, and Treatment," in *Sex and Gender Difference in Infection and Treatments for Infectious Diseases*, eds. Sabra L. Klein and Craig W. Roberts (New York: Springer International Publishing, 2015), 337–60.

292 *Several years ago, research program coordinator Alison Rebman* . . . All quotes from author's interview with Alison Rebman (research program coordinator for the Johns Hopkins Lyme Disease Research Center).

292 *in 2012, they conducted the first prospective study* . . . John N. Aucott et al., "Post-Treatment Lyme Disease Syndrome Symptomatology and the Impact on Life Functioning: Is There Something Here?" *Quality of Life Research* 22, no. 1 (February 2013), www.hopkinsrheumatology.org/wp-content/uploads/2015/06 /aucott_et_al_qol_research.pdf.

293 *In 2010, the center's first study directly looking at sex/gender differences* . . . Alison Schwarzwalder et al., "Sex Differences in the Clinical and Serologic Presentation of Early Lyme Disease: Results from a Retrospective Review," *Gender Medicine* 7, no. 4 (August 2010), www.lymemd.org/pdf/Sex_differences.pdf.

293 *And a study they did in 2015 suggests that women may be especially* . . . Alison W. Rebman, "Characteristics of Seroconversion and Implications for Diagnosis of Post-Treatment Lyme Disease Syndrome: Acute and Convalescent Serology Among a Prospective Cohort of Early Lyme Disease Patients," *Clinical Rheumatology* 34, no. 3 (March 2015), doi:10.1007/s10067-014-2706-z.

293 *Weintraub points out that mainstream Lyme experts* . . . Weintraub, *Cure Unknown*, 372.

293 *"if we are rejecting patient anecdote* . . . Weintraub, *Cure Unknown*, 20.

293 *"The truth is that the mainstream experts* . . . Weintraub, *Cure Unknown*, 345.

296 *According to surveys, 13 percent of Americans report* . . . S. M. Caress and A. C. Steinemann, "Prevalence of Multiple Chemical Sensitivities: A Population-Based Study in the Southeastern United States," *American Journal of Public Health* 94, no. 5 (May 2004), www.ncbi.nlm.nih.gov/pubmed/15117694?dopt=Abstract.

296 *Four percent say they become ill from them every day* . . . Pamela Reed Gibson, "An Introduction to Multiple Chemical Sensitivity and Electrical Sensitivity,"

The Environmental Illness Resource, November 9, 2015, www.ei-resource.org/articles/multiple-chemical-sensitivity-articles/an-introduction-to-multiple-chemical-sensitivity-and-electrical-sensitivity/.

296 *At least 13.5 percent of people with chemical intolerance* . . . Stanley M. Caress and Anne C. Steinemann, "A Review of a Two-Phase Population Study of Multiple Chemical Sensitivities," *Environmental Health Perspectives* 111, no. 12 (September 2003), www.ncbi.nlm.nih.gov/pmc/articles/PMC1241652/.

297 *A 2007 survey of physicians found that a little over half of respondents* . . . Pamela Reed Gibson and Amanda Lindberg, "Physicians' Perceptions and Practices Regarding Patient Reports of Multiple Chemical Sensitivity," portions of paper presented at the International Association for Chronic Fatigue Syndrome (IACFS) 8th International Conference on Chronic Fatigue Syndrome, Fibromyalgia and Other Related Illnesses, Fort Lauderdale, Florida, January 12–14, 2007, www.mcsresearch.net/journalpapers/Physiciansperceptions.pdf.

297 *Chemical intolerance expert Dr. Claudia Miller, who* . . . Jill Neimark, "Is the World Making You Sick?" *Nautilus*, July 24, 2014, http://nautil.us/issue/15/turbulence/is-the-world-making-you-sick.

297 *"Allergists had been accused by their colleagues of practicing witchcraft and 'voodoo'* . . . Claudia S. Miller, "White Paper: Chemical Sensitivity: History and Phenomenology," *Toxicology and Industrial Health* 10, nos. 4–5 (July–October 1994), www.ncbi.nlm.nih.gov/pubmed/7778099.

298 *Then there was the fact that most of the patients were women* . . . Pamela Reed Gibson, "Multiple Chemical Sensitivity, Culture and Delegitimization: A Feminist Analysis," *Feminism and Psychology* 7, no. 4 (November 1997), doi: 10.1177/0959353597074003.

298 *Many of the early outbreaks of "sick building syndrome"* . . . L. Soine, "Sick Building Syndrome and Gender Bias: Imperiling Women's Health," *Social Work in Health Care* 20, no. 3 (1995), doi:10.1300/J010v20n03_04.

298 *"In debates between experts over the reality* . . . Michelle Murphy, *Sick Building Syndrome and the Problem of Uncertainty* (Durham, NC: Duke Univ. Press, 2006), 5–6.

298 *In 1999, the first population-based survey* . . . Richard Kreutzer, Raymond R. Neutra, and Nan Lashuay, "Prevalence of People Reporting Sensitivities to Chemicals in a Population Based Survey," *American Journal of Epidemiology* 150, no. 1 (July 1999), doi:10.1093/oxfordjournals.aje.a009308.

299 *"It's a belief, not a disease* . . . Duff Wilson, "Crippling Illness or Just 'Hysteria'?—It 'Ruined My Life,' Says One Sufferer, a Doctor," *The Seattle Times*, January 5, 1994, http://community.seattletimes.nwsource.com/archive/?date=19940105&slug=1888139.

299 *As Murphy writes, MCS was seen as a "version of women's age-old ability to* . . . Michelle Murphy, "The 'Elsewhere Within Here' and Environmental Illness; or, How to Build Yourself a Body in a Safe Space," *Configurations* 8, no. 1 (Winter 2000), doi:10.1353/con.2000.0006.

299 *In the early nineties, the National Research Council* . . . National Research Council Steering Committee on Identification of Toxic and Potentially Toxic Chemicals for Consideration by the National Toxicology Program, *Toxicity Testing: Strategies to Determine Needs and Priorities* (Washington, DC: The National Academies Press, 1984).

299 *Meanwhile, the average American now spends 90 percent* . . . U.S. Environmental

Protection Agency, "The Inside Story: A Guide to Indoor Air Quality," last modified May 31, 2016, www.epa.gov/indoor-air-quality-iaq/inside-story -guide-indoor-air-quality.

300 *In 1997, Miller proposed the theory of toxicant-induced loss of tolerance* . . . Claudia S. Miller, "Toxicant-Induced Loss of Tolerance—An Emerging Theory of Disease?" *Environmental Health Perspectives* 105, no. 2 (March 1997), www .ncbi.nlm.nih.gov/pmc/articles/PMC1469811/pdf/envhper00327-0048.pdf.

300 *An Australian study that looked at the differences between physicians* . . . Tarryn Philips, "Debating the Legitimacy of a Contested Environmental Illness: A Case Study of Multiple Chemical Sensitivities," *Sociology of Heath and Illness* 32, no. 7 (November 2010), doi:10.1111/j.1467-9566.2010.01255.x.

301 *Perhaps the most popular is one that borrows* . . . Jill Neimark, "Extreme Chemical Sensitivity Makes Sufferers Allergic to Life," *Discover*, December 11, 2013, http:// discovermagazine.com/2013/nov/13-allergic-life.

301 *Laboratory studies have implicated both central nervous system* . . . Dominique Bel-pomme, Christine Campagnac, and Philippe Irigaray, "Reliable Disease Biomarkers Characterizing and Identifying Electrohypersensitivity and Multiple Chemical Sensitivity as Two Etiopathogenic Aspects of a Unique Pathological Disorder," *Reviews on Environmental Health* 30, no. 4 (2015), doi:10.1515/reveh-2015-0027.

301 *In a 2012 study published in* Annals of Family Medicine . . . David A. Katerndahl et al., "Chemical Intolerance in Primary Care Settings: Prevalence, Comorbidity, and Outcomes," *Annals of Family Medicine* 10, no. 4 (July–August 2012), doi:10 .1370/afm.1346.

302 *In one 2003 study that asked patients to rate the effectiveness* . . . Pamela Reed Gibson, Amy Nicole-Marie Elms, and Lisa Ann Ruding, "Perceived Treatment Efficacy for Conventional and Alternative Therapies Reported by Persons with Multiple Chemical Sensitivity," *Environmental Health Perspectives* 111, no. 12 (September 2003), www.ncbi.nlm.nih.gov/pmc/articles/PMC1241653/.

302 *New theories of disease, Miller points out* . . . Miller, "Toxicant-Induced Loss of Tolerance."

CONCLUSION

305 *But only 15 percent of cases are detected at this stage, and once it has spread* . . . Editorial Board, "Ovarian, Fallopian Tube, and Peritoneal Cancer: Statistics," Cancer.net, August 2016, www.cancer.net/cancer-types/ovarian-fallopian-tube -and-peritoneal-cancer/statistics.

306 *In 1942, gynecologist Harry Sturgeon Crossen described the disease* . . . H. S. Crossen, "The Menace of 'Silent' Ovarian Carcinoma," *JAMA* 119, no. 18 (August 1942), doi:10.1001/jama.1942.02830350017004.

306 *But as historian Patricia Jasen has explained* . . . Patricia Jasen, "From the 'Silent Killer' to the 'Whispering Disease': Ovarian Cancer and the Uses of Metaphor," *Medical History* 53, no. 4 (October 2009), www.ncbi.nlm.nih.gov/pmc/articles /PMC2766137/.

306 *but the pattern was common enough that, British gynecologist Stanley Way* . . . Archibald Donald Campbell and Mabel A. Shannon, *Gynecology for Nurses*, (Philadelphia, PA: F. A. Davis, 1946), 144; Stanley Way, *Malignant Disease of the Female Genital Tract* (London: J. and A. Churchill, 1951), 182.

306 *"All too often," gynecologist Hugh Barber lamented* . . . Hugh R. K. Barber, *Ovarian Carcinoma: Etiology, Diagnosis, and Treatment* (New York: Masson, 1978), 97.

307 *"Ovarian cancer, is unfortunately, very insidious . . .* Howard C. Jones III, Anne Colston Wentz, and Lonnie S. Burnett, *Novak's Textbook of Gynecology*, 11th ed. (Baltimore: Williams and Wilkins, 1988), 793.

307 *"We have to rely on the woman and her initiative . . .* C. Wikborn, F. Pettersson, and P. J. Moberg, "Delay in Diagnosis of Epithelial Ovarian Cancer," *International Journal of Gynecology and Obstetrics* 52, no. 3 (March 1996), 266.

307 *Beth, who was diagnosed with ovarian cancer in 1987 . . .* All quotes from author's interview with Beth.

308 *Dr. Barbara Goff, a young gynecologic oncologist, happened to witness this eruption . . .* All quotes from author's interview with Dr. Barbara Goff.

308 *"the majority of women with ovarian carcinoma are symptomatic . . .* B. A. Goff et al., "Ovarian Carcinoma Diagnosis," *Cancer* 89, no. 10 (November 2000), doi:10.1002/1097-0142(20001115)89:10<2068::AID-CNCR6>3.0.CO;2-Z.

309 *In a national consensus statement . . .* Foundation for Women's Cancer, "Ovarian Cancer Symptoms Consensus Statement," www.foundationforwomenscancer.org /about-the-foundation/allied-support-group/ovarian-cancer-symptoms-consensus -statement/.

309 *"For years, women have known that . . .* Ovarian Cancer Research Fund Alliance, "Symptoms and Detection," 2016, https://ocrfa.org/patients/about-ovarian-cancer /symptoms-and-detection/.

310 *The research suggests that the concern about overtesting is unfounded . . .* M. Robyn Anderson, Kimberly A. Lowe, and Barbara A. Goff, "Value of Symptom-Triggered Diagnostic Evaluation for Ovarian Cancer," *Obstetrics and Gynecology* 123, no. 1 (January 2014), doi:10.1097/AOG.0000000000000051.

310 *Back in the sixties, during congressional hearings . . .* Matthew J. Sobnosky, "Experience, Testimony, and the Women's Health Movement," *Women's Studies in Communication* 36, no. 3 (2013), doi:10.1080/07491409.2013.835667.

310 *Other researchers have suggested that improving . . .* Ilana Cass and Beth Y. Karlan, "Ovarian Cancer Symptoms Speak Out—But What Are They Really Saying?" *Journal of the National Cancer Institute* 102, no. 4 (February 2010), doi:10.1093/jnci/djp525.

312 *"I can't even tell you how isolating . . .* All quotes from author's interview with Paula Kamen.

312 *"to confirm or deny the reality of everyone's . . .* Susan Wendell, *The Rejected Body: Feminist Philosophical Reflections on Disability* (New York: Routledge, 1996), 122.

312 *"Whether or not fibromyalgia is a 'real' thing . . .* All quotes from author's interview with Amy Berkowitz.

312 *"What can I know if I can't know what . . .* Wendell, *The Rejected Body*, 125.

315 *In 2006, a study demonstrated that roughly 10 percent . . .* I. Hickie et al., "Post-Infective and Chronic Fatigue Syndromes Precipitated by Viral and Non-Viral Pathogens: Prospective Cohort Study," *BMJ* 333, no. 7568 (September 2006), doi:10.1136/bmj.38933.585764.AE.

315 *"Our patients were telling us that all along . . .* Jose Montoya, "Stanford's Dr. Jose Montoya on Chronic Fatigue Syndrome," Mar 11, 2011, www.youtube.com/watch ?v=Riybtt6SChU.

316 *Julie Rehmeyer "felt betrayed by the institutions . . .* Rehmeyer, *Through the Shadowlands*, 99.

316 *she "felt like a refugee . . .* Rehmeyer, *Through the Shadowlands*, 246.

INDEX